Nursing Home Statistical Yearbook, 1997

C. McKeen Cowles

Cowles Research Group

Distributed by The Johns Hopkins University Press

Acknowledgments

We extend our appreciation to Sheila Carlisle of Selective Communications, Kirkland, Washington, who, in addition to design and layout, acted as the print production manager, bringing everything together on a tight schedule. Any errors or omissions are those of the author.

Nursing Home Statistical Yearbook, 1997

Copyright © 1998 by Cowles Research Group

Published by Cowles Research Group

All rights reserved. No part of this book may be reproduced or transmitted in any form or by any means, electronic, mechanical, photocopying, recording, or otherwise, without the prior written permission of the publisher. For information, contact:

Cowles Research Group	Phone: (360) 299-9027
1004 Commercial Ave., Suite 130	Toll free: (888) 281-0962
Anacortes, WA 98221-4183	Fax: (360) 299-0659
	E-mail: MickCowles@aol.com

Notice of Liability: The information in this book is distributed on an "As Is" basis, without warranty. While every precaution has been taken in the preparation of this book, neither the contributors nor Cowles Research Group shall have any liability to any person or entity with respect to liability, loss, or damage caused or alleged to be caused directly or indirectly by the information contained in this book.

ISBN: 0-8018-5802-X
ISSN: 1085-0309

Printed and bound in the United States of America

Contents

Introduction: Can Data Define Quality? Part II, *Laurence G. Branch*		1
How the Tables Were Constructed, *C. McKeen Cowles*		5

SECTION I RESIDENT ACUITY

Table I-1	Four Measures of Resident Acuity by State, 1997	20
Table I-2	ACUINDEX by Class of Ownership and State, 1997	22
	Fig. I-A ACUINDEX by Class of Ownership, United States, 1997 23	
Table I-3	ACUINDEX by Urban/Rural and State, 1997	24
	Fig. I-B ACUINDEX by Urban/Rural, United States, 1997 25	
Table I-4	ACUINDEX by Bedsize and State, 1997	26
	Fig. I-C ACUINDEX by Bedsize, United States, 1997 27	

SECTION II RESIDENT ADL CHARACTERISTICS

Table II-1	Resident ADL Limitations by ADL and State, 1997	30
	Fig. II-A Resident ADL Limitations by ADL, United States, 1997 31	
Table II-2	Resident Dependence Level by State — Bathing, 1997	32
	Fig. II-B Resident Dependence Level — Bathing, United States, 1997 33	
Table II-3	Resident Dependence Level by State — Dressing, 1997	34
	Fig. II-C Resident Dependence Level — Dressing, United States, 1997 35	
Table II-4	Resident Dependence Level by State — Toileting, 1997	36
	Fig. II-D Resident Dependence Level — Toileting, United States, 1997 37	
Table II-5	Resident Dependence Level by State — Transferring, 1997	38
	Fig. II-E Resident Dependence Level — Transferring, United States, 1997 39	
Table II-6	Resident Dependence Level by State — Eating, 1997	40
	Fig. II-F Resident Dependence Level — Eating, United States, 1997 41	
Table II-7	Residents with Multiple Dependencies by State, 1997	42
	Fig. II-G Residents with Multiple Dependencies, United States, 1997 43	
Table II-8	Resident Continence Characteristics by State, 1997	44
Table II-9	Resident Mobility Characteristics by State, 1997	46
Table II-10	Incidence of Contractures and Use of Restraints by State, 1997	48

SECTION III	**OTHER RESIDENT CHARACTERISTICS**		
	Table III-1	Use of Psychoactive Medication by State, 1997	**52**
	Table III-2	Other Medication Characteristics by State, 1997	**54**
	Table III-3	Resident Skin Care Characteristics by State, 1997	**56**
	Table III-4	Resident Special Treatments by State, 1997	**58**
	Table III-5	Communication and Advance Directives by State, 1997	**60**
	Table III-6	Mental Status by State, 1997	**62**
	Table III-7	Payor Mix and Census by State, 1997	**64**
		Fig. III-A Payor Mix, Percent Medicare, 1994–1997 65	
SECTION IV	**SURVEY DEFICIENCIES**		
	Table IV-1	Total and Nursing Deficiencies by State, 1997	**68**
	Table IV-2	Total Deficiencies by Class of Ownership and State, 1997	**70**
		Fig. IV-A Total Deficiencies by Class of Ownership, United States, 1997 71	
	Table IV-3	Top 40 Deficiencies: United States, 1997	**72**
	Table IV-4	Most Frequently Cited Deficiencies, 1997	**73**

          Alabama, 73   Montana, 99
          Alaska, 74   Nebraska, 100
          Arizona, 75   Nevada, 101
          Arkansas, 76   New Hampshire, 102
          California, 77   New Jersey, 103
          Colorado, 78   New Mexico, 104
          Connecticut, 79   New York, 105
          Delaware, 80   North Carolina, 106
          District of Columbia, 81 North Dakota, 107
          Florida, 82   Ohio, 108
          Georgia, 83   Oklahoma, 109
          Hawaii, 84   Oregon, 110
          Idaho, 85   Pennsylvania, 111
          Illinois, 86   Rhode Island, 112
          Indiana, 87   South Carolina, 113
          Iowa, 88   South Dakota, 114
          Kansas, 89   Tennessee, 115
          Kentucky, 90   Texas, 116
          Louisiana, 91   Utah, 117
          Maine, 92   Vermont, 118
          Maryland, 93   Virginia, 119
          Massachusetts, 94   Washington, 120
          Michigan, 95   West Virginia, 121
          Minnesota, 96   Wisconsin, 122
          Mississippi, 97   Wyoming, 123
          Missouri, 98

	Table IV-5	Scope and Severity Code Utilization by State, 1997	**124**
		Fig. IV-B Scope and Severity Code Utilization, United States, 1997 125	

SECTION V **FACILITY CHARACTERISTICS**

Table V-1	Facilities by Type of Certification and State, 1997		**128**
	Fig. V-A Facilities by Type of Certification, United States, 1997 129		
Table V-2	Facilities by Class of Ownership and State, 1997		**130**
	Fig. V-B Facilities by Class of Ownership, United States, 1997 131		
Table V-3	Facilities by Size Category and State, 1997		**132**
	Fig. V-C Facilities by Size Category, United States, 1997 133		
Table V-4	Beds by Type of Certification and State, 1997		**134**
	Fig. V-D Beds by Type of Certification, United States, 1997 135		
Table V-5	Dedicated Special Care Units and Beds by State, 1997		**136**
Table V-6	Occupancy Rate as a Percent by State, 1994–1997		**138**
	Fig. V-E Occupancy Rate as a Percent, United States, 1994–1997 139		
Table V-7	Facilities by Type of Certification and HSA, 1997		**140**
Table V-8	Beds by Type of Certification and HSA, 1997		**159**
Table V-9	Dedicated Special Care Units and Beds by HSA, 1997		**178**

SECTION VI **STAFFING INFORMATION**

Table VI-1	Physical Therapist Staffing by State, 1997		**208**
	Fig. VI-A Physical Therapist Staffing, United States, 1997 209		
Table VI-2	Occupational Therapist Staffing by State, 1997		**210**
	Fig. VI-B Occupational Therapist Staffing, United States, 1997 211		
Table VI-3	Speech and Language Pathologist Staffing by State, 1997		**212**
	Fig. VI-C Speech and Language Pathologist Staffing, United States, 1997 213		
Table VI-4	Contract Labor Usage for Nursing Services by State, 1997		**214**
	Fig. VI-D Contract Labor Usage for Nursing Services, United States, 1997 215		
Table VI-5	Nurse Staffing Hours Per Patient Day, 1997		**216**
Table VI-6	Nurse Aide Staffing Hours Per Patient Day, 1997		**218**
Table VI-7	Occupational Therapist Hours Per Patient Day, 1997		**220**
Table VI-8	Physical and Speech Therapist Hours Per Patient Day, 1997		**222**

APPENDIX A **HEALTH SERVICE AREA MAPS**

Map A-1	Health Service Areas in Maine, New Hampshire, Vermont, Massachusetts, Rhode Island, and Connecticut	**226**
Map A-2	Health Service Areas in New York, New Jersey, Pennsylvania, Delaware, Maryland, Washington, D.C., Virginia, and West Virginia	**227**
Map A-3	Health Service Areas in Ohio, Indiana, Illinois, Michigan, and Wisconsin	**228**
Map A-4	Health Service Areas in Minnesota, Iowa, Missouri, North Dakota, South Dakota, Nebraska, and Kansas	**229**

Map A-5	Health Service Areas in North Carolina, South Carolina, Georgia, and Florida	**230**
Map A-6	Health Service Areas in Kentucky, Tennessee, Alabama, and Mississippi	**231**
Map A-7	Health Service Areas in Arkansas, Louisiana, Oklahoma, and Texas	**232**
Map A-8	Health Service Areas in Montana, Idaho, Wyoming, Colorado, New Mexico, Arizona, Utah, and Nevada	**233**
Map A-9	Health Service Areas in Washington, Oregon, California, Alaska, and Hawaii	**234**

APPENDIX B *HEALTH SERVICE AREA DEFINITIONS*

Table B-1	Health Service Areas by State and County	**236**
Table B-2	Numeric List of Health Service Areas	**249**

INTRODUCTION:
CAN DATA DEFINE QUALITY? PART II

Laurence G. Branch, Ph.D. Professor, Duke Medical School, and
Associate Director, VA National Center for Health Promotion

Do you remember when you first grasped the real meaning of "this is a necessary but not sufficient condition for that outcome"? The distinction between necessary and sufficient causes ranks right up there with the third law of thermodynamics and the assertion that men are from Mars and women are from Venus. A handful of important insights, when applied correctly, render one's environment much more predictable and therefore comfortable.

So it is with long-term care (LTC) data. They are necessary but not sufficient for defining quality in LTC. Those who think they can understand quality without data are fooling themselves, but they are no bigger fools than those who think the numbers themselves define quality.

A little background

Jody Ann Noon did an excellent job of framing the fundamental issues in the introduction to the *Nursing Home Statistical Yearbook, 1996*.[1] To recapitulate, the 1986 Institute of Medicine report[2] paved the way for the nursing home reform provisions of the Omnibus Budget Reconciliation Act of 1987, which in turn spawned the Resident Assessment Instrument (RAI), the Minimum Data Set (MDS), and the Resident Assessment Protocols (RAPs) that some know and love and other do not. But none can deny that the RAI/MDS/RAP approach produces more systematic data about the LTC system in the United States than we have ever had before. The challenge for LTC researchers and policy makers is to convert the volumes of RAI/MDS/RAP data into useful information, a challenge for which a successful outcome is not automatic. Numbers remain just numbers until someone knows what to do with them.

It may be helpful to recognize that this latest quest to define quality in LTC is not isolated to LTC; defining quality of care is of paramount interest throughout the health care delivery system. Health maintenance organizations are trying to clarify comparative quality by means of uniform data as defined by the

---

1. Noon, J.A. Introduction: Can data define quality? *Nursing Home Statistical Yearbook, 1996.* 1-4, Cowles Research Group, 1997.
2. Institute of Medicine, Committee on Nursing Home Regulation, "Improving the Quality of Care in Nursing Homes," National Academy Press, 1986.

Health Plan Employer Data and Information Set (HEDIS)[3]. The goal of HEDIS is to compare the performance of health plans against defined and measurable outcomes.

Furthermore, the whole of medical care is involved in the revolution of evidence-based medicine. As with HEDIS, the revolution emphasizes the efficacy and efficiency of interventions against agreed-upon outcomes, typically death, disease, disability, discomfort, dissatisfaction, and dollars (the six Ds, adapted from Lohr, 1988)[4]. The bottom line of this approach is "Show me the data" — does the intervention lead to a favorable outcome in any the six Ds? While it may be true that some managed care organizations favor the outcome of dollars over the other outcomes, the evidence-based medicine approach per se does not favor one outcome over another.

The outcomes of importance

What are the outcomes of importance or interest in the context of LTC? Certainly death or mortality is important. We need to know if and when any provider or provider system has an increased mortality rate over the expected rate. We also want to know when rates of disease (i.e., morbidities), disability, discomfort or pain, patient/client/family dissatisfaction, or costs/charges/reimbursements are over the expected rate. But therein are the major challenges. What are the expected rates? What benchmarks should LTC researchers and policy makers use to define these rates? And when are differences from the expected rates meaningful?

The establishment of a benchmark for LTC remains the biggest challenge. Every time the Health Care Financing Administration (HCFA) presents comparative information, the providers raise the issue that the patient population of the providers, be they hospitals or LTC facilities, are not necessarily comparable. Therefore, so the argument goes, unless the comparative data are corrected for these important differences in the patient populations (in the jargon, the case-mix differences of the patients), the differences in the outcome rates cannot be interpreted. That argument is valid, in my opinion.

The question we might ask ourselves is this: Why has the organization that has had sole or shared responsibility for the payment of every Medicare and Medicaid bill since the 1966 implementation of Medicare and Medicaid been unable to convert its data into the useful information policy makers and program evaluators need? Why has HCFA, with its intramural and extramural research office and staff, been unable to provide a case-mix adjustment system for interpreting comparative information? Without a case-mix adjustment system, the data cannot achieve their full potential as information.

Lest we be criticized for characterizing the glass as half empty because the full potential has not been reached, let us return to a glass half full. Including this issue, the Nursing Home Statistical Yearbooks provide state-specific information for three consecutive years (1995, 1996, and 1997) on:

---

3. Committee on Performance Measurement. HEDIS 3.0. National Committee for Quality Assurance, 1996.
4. Lohr, K.N. Outcome measurement: Concepts and questions. Inquiry, 25, 37-50, 1988.

- resident acuity or case-mix as measured by different approaches,
- resident functional characteristics,
- other resident characteristics,
- certification survey deficiencies,
- facility characteristics (also by Health Service Area within states), and
- staffing information.

This state-specific information defines case-mix adjustors and facility-difference adjustors as we have them in 1997 and is an extremely important starting point for understanding quality in LTC. Without this information we have no chance of measuring and monitoring quality in LTC facilities. What will be necessary for the future, however, is systematic clarification of how these differences in resident and facility characteristics (that is, differences in the patient and facility adjustors as we have them) affect differences in the outcomes of interest in LTC — death, disease, disability, discomfort, dissatisfaction, and dollars. Knowing the associations with outcomes admittedly will take a long time. But it likely will take less time than the 30+ years billing data have been collected without providing the salient information. When the outcomes are known, the glass will be full.

Meaningful differences

When are differences salient? Many a late-night debate has pitted academic against academic, practitioner against practitioner, and academic against practitioner in grappling with this topic. Suffice it to say that more heat than light has resulted. My opinion is that a statistically significant difference is a necessary but not sufficient condition for a practical meaningful difference. Without statistical significance, one cannot rely on the probabilities of the scientific conventions to evaluate the differences. Hence, statistical significance is a prerequisite to salience. But the real differences as statistically confirmed may not be practically important or salient, particularly because the reality (statistical significance) of the differences might well be born by the huge sample sizes that national data such as these present. Hence there is a second criterion of salience in addition to statistical significance, and that is professional judgement. In this regard we might be better off to hold out for a consensus professional judgement rather than an individual judgement.

Policy conflicts

Discussions about quality in LTC remind me of an experience I had in the early 1980s as a founding board member (and later president of the board) of a continuing care retirement community (CCRC). The CCRC had just received determination-of-need approval from the state health department to build a 60-bed LTC facility which was intended ultimately to serve the needs of the CCRC residents. However, during the initial years the CCRC intended to accept non-CCRC residents into the LTC facility. It truly made no real difference to the CCRC board whether the initial non-CCRC residents of the LTC facility were private-paying or Medicaid-paying; the financial impact was trivial. However, the CCRC was interested in being helpful to the state, so we offered to take Medicaid-paying residents to fill the LTC beds at the outset if that was what the state wanted. The initial response from the state was that we should take only private-paying residents because the state did not want to incur more Medicaid costs than necessary. Two days later, the state called back to say they wanted the CCRC to accept all Medicaid-paying patients, because those patients would be assured the best-quality LTC (we accepted the implicit compliment, recognizing, however, that it was based on assumptions because there were no data as yet). Two days later, they called back and opted for a return to the private-paying option. Then two days later they called and reversed themselves again. And so it went. The point of this story is that no amount of information would have helped those state administrators in that context. They had two policies (to minimize state Medicaid LTC payments and to maximize quality for Medicaid LTC residents), and the policies can conflict. Information will not solve the problem of policies in conflict.

Another policy conflict has occurred on the supply side. For more than 30 years state and federal policies have constrained the supply of LTC beds in the United States. While these policies have reduced LTC expenditures over the period, they have not improved quality. In many areas, occupancy rates have been too high to provide consumers with easy access to institutional LTC and to allow current residents to act like dissatisfied consumers if their situation warrants and to vote with their feet by changing facilities. High occupancy rates, and the concomitant waiting lists for new residents, simply do not empower the consumer. And a consumer without power or consumer rights — particularly when that consumer by definition is a frail older person dependent on others for basic care needs — seems to be a formula for disaster. Those state and federal policies have, in some markets more than others, created a disaster waiting to happen. We need policy changes to increase the supply of institutional LTC options for the frail and dependent members of our population.

Conclusion The United States health care system is undergoing a revolution of evidence-based medicine. The revolution is outcome-oriented and data-driven, and seeks to define quality in terms of the causal relationships between interventions and outcomes. In the LTC sector there is now more systematic data than ever before. Our challenge is to convert these data into useful information. The cogent characteristics of U.S. nursing homes and nursing home residents presented in this volume define case-mix adjustors and facility-difference adjustors as we have them in 1997.

Dr. Branch is a Research Professor in Duke University's Center for the Study of Aging and Human Development, and Associate Director of the VA National Center for Health Promotion and Disease Prevention located in Durham, North Carolina. He contributes regularly to the health policy field as evidenced by his over 125 peer-reviewed journal articles and 50 book chapters and monographs. He currently is the co-editor of one professional journal, on the editorial boards of two others, and reviews for numerous others annually. He has held elected and appointed leadership positions in the American Public Health Association and the Gerontological Society of America. He has held numerous governmental advisory positions, including membership on the National Committee on Vital and Health Statistics which advises the Secretary of Health and Human Services on the adequacy of the federal statistical system and chairman of its Subcommittee on Long-Term Care Statistics.

How the Tables Were Constructed

C. McKeen Cowles, M.S., Cowles Research Group

The original source of the information presented in the tables and graphs that follow is the Health Care Financing Administration's Online Survey Certification and Reporting (OSCAR) database. OSCAR is extensively used by the Health Care Financing Administration (HCFA), particularly as it relates to the survey and certification process. The OSCAR database contains hundreds of variables on every nursing facility in the United States that is certified by Medicare and/or Medicaid. While OSCAR is an excellent administrative database, some limitations of the file need to be methodologically resolved in order to make the data usable for research. The two major limitations are record duplication and data validity.

The nursing facility portion of OSCAR contains hundreds of duplicate records. These are nursing homes that have been issued multiple "provider numbers" and consequently occur repeatedly in the database. The duplicate records confound research uses of OSCAR in two important ways. First, the total number of facilities is wrong, overstated by the degree of duplication. Second, frequency distributions, which describe the characteristics of the facilities and their residents, are also wrong. Frequency distributions result in double and triple counting the characteristics of the duplicate facilities, reducing the precision by which the population is described.

Before construction any of the tables in this book we "unduplicated" the file, i.e., deleted the duplicates. The duplicates were identified by grouping facilities in various ways, and then evaluating, facility by facility, whether the observations represented duplicates. An example of such grouping would be all nursing homes on the same street in the same town. Where there were multiple nursing homes on the same street, the detailed characteristics of the homes were visually compared and a determination was made.

The validity and accuracy of the OSCAR data varies by data field (variable). Many variables are routinely checked and submitted to various "edits" by HCFA to ensure a high degree of accuracy. Other data fields are entered and forgotten, never to be looked at again. Such variability in the accuracy of the data is characteristic of administrative databases such as OSCAR.

HCFA must necessarily prioritize the resources expended to verify OSCAR data accuracy in proportion to the importance of the specific data element to the organizational function for which OSCAR is maintained, i.e., survey and certification. Unfortunately, the interests of researchers and the administrative needs of HCFA do not always correspond. The fields from which the tables in *Nursing Home Statistical Yearbook, 1997* were constructed were independently subjected to logical edits and, in some instances, the data fields were "backfilled" to improve accuracy. Backfilling describes a situation where data known to be inaccurate are overwritten with the correct information.

All of the tables and graphs presented in *Nursing Home Statistical Yearbook, 1997* were constructed from an unduplicated backfilled OSCAR file representing the database as of December 29, 1997. The data presented are intended to serve as a guide and basis for general comparisons and evaluations, but not as the sole basis upon which any specific material conduct is to be recommended or undertaken.

One of the objectives of this volume was to present data for areas smaller than whole states. After considering county, metropolitan statistical area (MSA), and several other area definitions, we selected health service areas (HSAs) as the most appropriate and potentially useful for defining institutional health care markets in general, and nursing home markets specifically. HSAs were developed by the National Center for Health Statistics (NCHS) to define areas that are "relatively self-contained with respect to the provision of routine hospital care."[5] Using recent data on short-stay hospital utilization, NCHS researchers linked hospital county location to patient county of residence. HSAs were then defined in such a way that patients were less likely to be admitted to a hospital in a different HSA from their residence.[6] Appendix A contains maps showing the HSA boundaries. Appendix B provides the precise definition of each HSA.

SECTION I: RESIDENT ACUITY

The Section I tables report various measures of "resident acuity" (sometimes called "case-mix," "resource need," or "resource intensity") that are based on resident characteristics captured from HCFA Form 672.

The best possible resident acuity measures are going to be computed using the data from the Resident Assessment Instrument (RAI) as captured in the

---

5. Makuc, D.M., et al., 1991. *Health Service Areas for the United States*, National Center for Health Statistics, Vital and Health Statistics (2)112, p.1.
6. NCHS researchers estimated four HSA solutions, two "linked" and two "unlinked." The linking had to do with whether they would allow the computer to freely cross MSA boundaries (unlinked) in defining HSAs. Both the linked and the unlinked solutions were estimated for 800 and 1600 HSAs. The definitions used throughout this book are from the "800 unlinked" solution. By summarizing, we drastically oversimplify the NCHS study, which was a huge and brilliantly executed research project. The reader is encouraged to consult the original research document.

Minimum Data Set (MDS). Unfortunately RAI/MDS data is only available for a few states. HCFA will begin requiring all facilities in all states to submit MDS data beginning in June 1998, and therefore, sometime in 1999 we will be computing RAI-based acuity to compile tables such as those presented in this section. In the meantime, the only case-mix data that is available for all certified facilities in the country will continue to come from Form 672.

Table I-1 Table I-1 combines resident characteristics into four acuity indexes, each representing a different measure of relative resource intensity needed to care for residents. Historically, OSCAR-based measures of resident acuity have been done using a number of slightly different methods, all of which link deficits in activities of daily living (ADLs) to resource need.

The variable "PROPAC," so named because the Prospective Payment Assessment Commission used it in their 1992 Report to Congress entitled *Medicare's Skilled Nursing Facility Payment Reform*, is based on the "Management Minutes" system developed by Thoms in 1975,[7] which assigns weights to nine discrete care-giving activities and characteristics of patients. The weights in Thoms' system were developed using time and motion studies, and theoretically represent the actual minutes of care required on a daily basis for patients requiring specific procedures or with certain levels of functional deficits. PROPAC is calculated as the sum of the products of nine specific patient characteristics and their associated weights. This method of calculating acuity was used by Dor in 1989,[8] Cohen and Dubay in 1990,[9] and the West Virginia Medicaid program. The nine specific patient characteristics and weights that determine the PROPAC acuity score are shown below.

DERIVATION OF PROPAC

#	Weight	Description of Variable
1	46	Proportion of bedfast residents. [bedfast all or most of time / total residents]
2	32	Proportion of residents needing assistance with ambulation. [(chairbound + physically restrained + contractures) / total residents]
3	45	Proportion of residents needing full eating assistance. [eating dependent / total residents]

---

7. Thoms, W., 1975. "Proposed Criteria for Long Term Care Quality and Cost Containment Systems," Unpublished paper. Greenbriar Terrace Nursing Home, Nashua, New Hampshire.
8. Dor, A., 1989. "The Costs of Medicare Patients in Nursing Homes in the United States." *Journal of Health Economics.* 8(3):253-70.
9. Cohen, J., and Dubay, L., 1990. "The Effects of Medicaid Reimbursement Method and Ownership on Nursing Home Costs, Case Mix, and Staffing." *Inquiry.* 27:183-200.

DERIVATION OF PROPAC

#	Weight	Description of Variable
4	20	Proportion of residents requiring the assistance of one or two staff. [eating with assistance of one or two staff / total residents]
5	20	Proportion of residents with indwelling or external catheters. [catheter / total residents]
6	48	Proportion of residents who are incontinent. [(bowel incontinent + bladder incontinent) / total residents]
7	20	Proportion of residents with decubitus ulcers. [with pressure sores / total residents]
8	26	Proportion of residents receiving bowel or bladder training. [(bowel training + bladder training) / total residents]
9	10	Proportion of residents receiving preventative skin care. [preventative skin care / total residents]

However, because the PROPAC weights were developed prior to the enactment of the Omnibus Budget Reconciliation Act of 1987 (OBRA), they may not reflect the relative resource needs of post-OBRA period residents as accurately as possible.

"ADLINDEX" and "ACUINDEX" are newer acuity measures that were developed in conjunction with a research project examining quality of care issues in nursing homes. They are based on work done as part of the minimum data set development for resident assessment. An ADL index (ADLINDEX) is added to a special treatments index (STINDEX) to obtain an acuity index (ACUINDEX). ADLINDEX is derived as the sum of specific resident characteristics and their associated weights as follows.

Derivation of ADLINDEX

ADLINDEX = [proportion of residents totally dependent at eating × 3] + [proportion of residents requiring the assistance one or two staff with eating × 2] + [proportion of residents who are either independent or require supervision eating] + [proportion of residents totally dependent at toileting × 5] + [proportion of residents requiring the assistance of one or two staff with toileting × 3] + [proportion of residents independent or requiring supervision with toileting] + [proportion of residents totally dependent at transferring × 5] + [proportion of residents requiring the assistance of one or two staff with transferring × 3] + [proportion of residents independent or requiring supervision with transferring] + [proportion of residents who are bedfast × 5] + [proportion of residents who are chairbound × 3] + [proportion of residents who are ambulatory]

ACUINDEX is the sum of ADLINDEX and STINDEX, where STINDEX is defined as follows.

Derivation of STINDEX

STINDEX = [proportion of residents receiving respiratory care] + [proportion of residents receiving suctioning] + [proportion of residents receiving intravenous therapy] + [proportion of residents receiving tracheostomy care] + [proportion of residents receiving parenteral feeding]

ADLSCORE is a measure of the average number of ADL dependencies. It is based on ranking the five ADLs (bathing, dressing, toileting, transferring, and eating) with respect to the typical order in which independence is lost. The number of residents dependent at eating are assumed to be dependent at all five ADLs. Similarly, the number of residents requiring no assistance with bathing are assumed to have no ADL limitations. The percentage of residents with one, two, three, and four ADL limitations are calculated as the difference between the intermediate ADLs. The inherent order in which residents are assumed to lose ADLs is bathing, dressing, toileting, transferring, and eating.

All of the averages presented in Table I-1 are weighted, i.e., the resident characteristics are summed by state and then the acuity values were computed from the totals.

Table I-2   Table I-2 breaks out the acuity measure ACUINDEX from Table I-1 by state and class of ownership. As in Table I-1, the averages reported in Table I-2 are weighted (by the number of residents).

Table I-3   Similarly, Table I-3 shows ACUINDEX by state and urban/rural designation. A facility within the boundary of a Metropolitan Statistical Area (MSA) is considered urban, otherwise rural. Averages are weighted.

Table I-4   Table I-4 reports ACUINDEX by state and size category. Averages are weighted.

SECTION II: RESIDENT ADL CHARACTERISTICS

Table II-1   Table II-1 reports the average percentage of residents nationally and by state who are dependent in each of five ADLs. All residents not categorized as "independent" in each ADL are recategorized as "dependent" for the purposes of Table II-1. Averages are weighted.

Table II-2   Table II-2 breaks out the degree to which nursing home residents are dependent at bathing by state. The process of bathing is defined to *exclude* back washing and the shampooing of hair. It includes full-body bath/shower, sponge bath, and transfer into and out of tub or shower. If a facility routinely provides "set up" assistance to all residents, such as drawing water for a tub bath or laying out bathing materials, and a resident requires no other assistance beyond set up, then they are categorized as "independent." Averages are weighted.

Table II-3   Table II-3 breaks out dressing dependencies by state. Dressing is defined as how the resident puts on, fastens, and takes off all items of street clothing, including donning or removing prosthetic devices such as a brace or artificial limb. If a facility routinely sets out clothes for all residents, and this is the only assistance the resident receives, the resident is counted as "independent." However, if a resident receives assistance with donning a brace, elastic stocking, a prosthesis and so on, the resident is counted as needing the assistance of one or two staff. Averages are weighted.

Table II-4 Table II-4 reports ADL dependence information specific to toileting, which is defined as how the resident uses the toilet room (or bedpan, bedside commode, or urinal). It includes transferring on and off toilet, cleansing, adjusting clothing, and so on. If all that is done for the resident is to open a package, the resident is counted as "independent." Averages are weighted.

Table II-5 Table II-5 reports transferring dependence levels by state. Transferring is defined as how the resident moves between surfaces, such as to and from the bed, chair, wheelchair or to and from a standing position. It *excludes* transfers to and from the bath or toilet. If the facility routinely provides "set up" assistance to all residents such as handing the equipment (e.g., sliding board) to the resident, and this is the only assistance required, the resident is counted as "independent." Averages are weighted.

Table II-6 Table II-6 shows eating dependence by state. Eating is defined as how a resident eats and drinks regardless of skill. If the facility routinely provides "set up" activities, such as opening containers, buttering bread, and organizing the tray, and this is the only assistance provided, the resident is categorized as "independent." Averages are weighted.

Table II-7 Table II-7 reports the percentage of residents by state with one, two, three, four, and five ADL dependencies. These are the numbers from which the column "ADLSCORE" in Table I-1 and the column "1996" in Table I-5 were calculated. Averages are weighted.

Table II-8 Table II-8 reports the percent of residents with urinary catheters, the percent of those with catheters who had them on admission, the percent of residents who are bladder or bowel incontinent, and the percentage of residents on bladder or bowel training programs. Catheter use includes both internal and external. "Bladder Incontinence" refers to those occasionally or frequently incontinent of bladder, defined as those who have an incontinent episode two or more times per week. Residents with catheters are not included in this category. "Bowel Incontinence" refers to those residents who are occasionally or frequently incontinent of bowel, defined as residents who have a loss of bowel control one or more times per week. "Bladder Training Program" represents the percentage of residents on individually written bladder training programs, i.e., detailed plan of care to assist the resident to gain and maintain bladder control. The plan of care must be consistently implemented. These include all residents on training programs including those who are incontinent or with catheters. Similarly, "Bowel Training Program" is defined as the percentage of residents on individually written bowel training programs. Averages are weighted.

Table II-9 Resident mobility characteristics by state are reported in Table II-9. "Bedfast" describes residents who were in bed or recliner 22 hours or more per day in a seven-day period and includes bedfast with bathroom privileges. "Chairbound" refers to those who depend on a chair for mobility, and include those residents who can stand with assistance to pivot from bed to wheelchair. Residents categorized as chairbound cannot take steps without extensive or constant weight-bearing support from others. "Ambulatory" residents are independently ambulatory, requiring no help or oversight, or help or oversight was provided only one or two times during a seven-day period. "Ambulation w/Assistance" refers to residents who required oversight, cueing, or physical assistance or who used a cane, walker, crutch, leg splints, braces, or orthotics. "Independent" means no help or oversight, or help was provided only one or two times in a seven-day period. Averages are weighted

Table II-10 The first column of Table II-10 reports the percentage of residents with contractures, which includes residents having a restriction of full range of motion of any joint due to deformity, disuse, pain, etc., and includes loss of range of motion in fingers, wrists, elbows, shoulders, hips, knees and ankles. The next column is the number of residents who had contractures on admission expressed as a percent of the total number of residents with contractures. The next column reports the percent of residents who are physically restrained, defined as residents whose freedom of movement and/or normal access to their own body is restricted by any manual method or physical or mechanical device, material or equipment that is attached or adjacent to his/her body and cannot be easily removed by the resident. The last column reports the number of resident who had orders for restraints upon admission expressed as a percent of the total number of residents physically restrained. Averages are weighted.

SECTION III: OTHER RESIDENT CHARACTERISTICS

Table III-1 Table III-1 reports the use of psychoactive medications by state. The first column represents the percent of residents who receive any psychoactive drug, which includes antipsychotics, antianxiety medications, antidepressants, and hypnotics. The remaining columns break out psychoactive medication use by specific categories. Averages are weighted.

Table III-2 Table III-2 provides information about interstate variation in other medications related variables in nursing homes. The first column is the percentage of residents receiving antibiotics, either for prophylaxis or treatment. "% Pain Management" describes the percent of residents with specific pain control plans, which includes self-medication pumps or regularly scheduled administration of medications. "% IV Therapy/Feed" are the percent of residents receiving fluids, medications, and/or nutritional requirements intravenously. The drug error rates are calculated by the survey team on a facility wide "medications pass" basis, where the denominator is the number of opportunities for medication errors that were evaluated during the medications pass, and the numerator is the number of times that the survey team observing medications pass determined that a drug order was administered differently than written. All of the averages reported in Table III-2 are weighted (by the number of residents) except the medication error rate, which is unweighted, i.e., each facility in the state contributes equally to the average, regardless of the number of residents in the facility.

Table III-3 Table III-3 reports skin care characteristics by state. The first column is the percentage of residents who have pressure sores, defined as ischemic ulcerations and/or necrosis of tissues overlaying a bony prominence, and exclude Stage I sores. The next column, nosocomial pressure sore rate, reports the percentage of residents who developed bedsores after admission, calculated as "total bedsores" less "with bedsores on admission" divided by the total number of residents in the facility. The last two columns are the percent of residents receiving special skin care, defined as non-routine skin care provided according to a physicians order (or in care plan) and the percent with rashes. Averages are weighted.

Table III-4 The percentage of residents receiving special treatments are reported on Table III-4. "Trach Care" refers to tracheostomy care and includes residents receiving care involved in maintenance of the airway, the stoma and surrounding skin, and dressings/coverings for the stoma. "Suctioning" includes those who require use of a mechanical device which provides suction to remove secretions from the respiratory tract via the mouth, nasal passage, or tracheostomy stoma. "Rehab Services" is defined as residents receiving care provided by, or under the direction of, a rehabilitation professional (physical therapist, occupational therapist, speech-language pathologist, or psychiatrist) and designed to improve functional ability. It excludes health rehabilitation for MI/MR. "Ostomy Care" includes residents receiving care for a colostomy, ileostomy, ureterostomy, or other ostomy of the intestinal and/or urinary tract (excludes tracheotomy). "Radiation Therapy" includes any treatment plan involving radiation therapy, and "Hospice Benefit" counts residents who have elected to receive or are receiving the hospice benefit. "Dialysis" represents residents receiving hemodialysis or peritoneal dialysis either within the facility or offsite. "Tube Feeding" is defined as those receiving all or most of their nutritional requirements via a feeding tube that delivers food/nutritional substances directly into the GI system. "Eating Assistive Devices" are the percent of residents who use devices to maintain independence and to provide comfort when eating and include such things as plates with guards, large-handled flatware, large-handled mugs, extended-hand flatware, etc. "Mechanically Altered Diets" include pureed and/or chopped foods, not only meat. "Unplanned Weight Loss/Gain" are the percent of residents who have experienced gain or loss of five percent in one month or ten percent over six months. All averages are weighted.

Table III-5 Table III-5 reports the percent of residents who do not communicate in the dominant language at the facility, the percent who use non-oral communication devices (e.g., picture boards, computers, sign-language), and the percent of residents who have advanced directives, such as a living will or durable power of attorney for health care, recognized under state law and relating to the provisions of care when the individual is incapacitated. All averages are weighted.

Table III-6 The first column of Table III-6 represents the percent of residents in any category of developmental disability regardless of severity, as determined by the State Mental Health or State Mental Retardation authorities. The next column are the percent of residents with documented signs and symptoms of depression as defined by Mood and Behavior Section of the Minimum Data Set. "With Psychiatric Diagnosis" are the percent with primary or secondary psychiatric diagnosis, including but not limited to, schizophrenia, schizo-affective disorder, schizophreniform disorder, delusional disorder, and psychotic mood disorder. "Dementia" refer to residents with a primary or secondary diagnosis of dementia or organic mental syndrome including multi-infarct, senile type, Alzheimer's type, or other than Alzheimer's type. "Behavior Symptoms" refer to residents with one or more of the following symptoms: wandering, verbally abusive, physically abusive, socially inappropriate/disruptive, resistive to care as defined in the Mood and Behavioral Patterns section of the Minimum Data Set. The next column reports the percentage of residents with behavior symptoms who are receiving an individualized care plan/program designed to address those symptoms. The last column in Table III-6 reports the percent of residents for whom the facility is providing health rehabilitative services for MI/MR as defined at 483.45(a). All averages are weighted.

Table III-7 Table III-7 reports the total number of nursing home residents by state (total census) and breaks the number out by payor mix. "Medicare" is defined as residents for whom the primary payor is Medicare and "Medicaid" is defined as residents for whom the primary payor is Medicaid. The residual category "Other" represents residents whose primary payor is neither Medicare nor Medicaid, typically private pays. All averages are weighted.

SECTION IV: SURVEY DEFICIENCIES

Table IV-1 Table IV-1 reports the unweighted average number of health deficiencies cited nationally and by state. The averages reported are the average total number of deficiencies, and the average number of "nursing" deficiencies. The creation of a nursing deficiencies category is an attempt to define a set of deficiency tag numbers that are related to quality of care, modeled after Jean Johnson-Pawlson's doctoral dissertation.[10] Nursing deficiencies are defined as any of the 48 tag numbers listed below.

---

10. Johnson-Pawlson, Jean, 1993. "The Relationship Between Nursing Staff and Quality of Care in Nursing Facilities." The George Washington University.

"Nursing" Deficiencies

TAG	Requirement
F154	Right to be fully informed in advance about care and treatment.
F164	Right to privacy and confidentiality.
F176	Self administration of drugs.
F221	Physical restraints.
F222	Chemical restraints.
F223	Right to be free from abuse.
F224	Staff treatment of residents.
F240	Quality of life.
F241	Dignity.
F242	Right to make choices about life in the facility.
F246	Right to accommodations of individual needs and preferences.
F252	Safe, clean, comfortable and homelike environment.
F272	Comprehensive assessment.
F273	Assessment within 14 days.
F274	Assessment after significant change.
F275	Assessment every 12 months.
F276	Assessment review.
F279	Develop comprehensive care plan.
F280	Care plan developed by interdisciplinary team.
F283	Discharge summary.
F284	Post-discharge plan of care.
F309	Highest practicable care.
F310	ADLs do not diminish unless circumstances of the individual's clinical condition demonstrate that diminution was unavoidable.
F311	Treatments maintain or improve abilities.
F312	ADL dependent residents receive necessary services.
F313	Vision and hearing.
F314	Pressure sores.
F315	Resident's clinical condition demonstrates catheterization necessary.
F316	Urinary incontinence.
F317	No reduction in range of motion.
F318	Range of motion treatment.
F319	Mental treatment.
F320	No development of mental problems.
F321	Naso-gastric tubes.
F322	Naso-gastric treatment.
F323	Environment is free of hazards.
F324	Prevent accidents.
F325	Maintain nutrition.
F326	Therapeutic diet.
F327	Hydration.
F328	Special treatments.

"NURSING" DEFICIENCIES (CONTINUED)

TAG	Requirement
F329	Pharmacy.
F330	Not use antipsychotics.
F331	Antipsychotic dose reductions.
F332	5% medication error.
F333	Residents free of significant medication errors.
F369	Assistive devices while eating.
F444	Hand washing / infection control.

Table IV-2 Table IV-2 breaks out the total number of health deficiencies reported in Table IV-1 by class of ownership and state. Averages are unweighted.

Table IV-3 Table IV-3 reports the forty most frequently cited deficiencies in the United States by tag number in decreasing frequency.

Table IV-4 Table IV-4 reports the top forty deficiencies by decreasing frequency for each state and the District of Columbia. It is just like Table IV-3 except presented on a state-by-state basis.

Table IV-5 This table shows the frequency distribution of the new scope and severity codes. The rows sum to 100 percent.

SECTION V: FACILITY CHARACTERISTICS

Table V-1 Table V-1 shows the number of certified nursing facilities in the United States broken out by state and type of certification.

Table V-2 Table V-2 reports the total number of certified nursing facilities in the United States broken out by state and class of ownership.

Table V-3 Table V-3 reports the total number of certified nursing facilities in the United States broken out by state and facility size category.

Table V-4 Table V-4 reports the total number of beds in certified facilities by state and breaks out the total by type of certification, including uncertified beds in certified facilities.

Table V-5 Table V-5 reports dedicated special care units and beds by special care category and state. These are units with a specific number of beds, identified and dedicated by the facility for residents with specific needs/diagnoses. They need not be certified or recognized by regulatory authorities. For example, a SNF admits a large number of residents with head injuries. They have set aside eight beds, staffed with specially trained personnel. The facility would contribute eight to the total shown in the column "Head Trauma Beds" and one to the column "Head Trauma Units."

Table V-6 Table V-6 reports occupancy rates, which are computed by dividing the total number of nursing home residents (total census as reported on Table III-7) by the total number of beds (as reported on Table V-4).

Table V-7 Table V-7 shows the total number of certified facilities by type of certification by Health Service Area (HSA).

Table V-8 Table V-8 breaks out beds by type of certification and HSA.

Table V-9 Table V-9 reports special care units and beds by HSA.

SECTION VI: STAFFING INFORMATION

Tables VI-1 to VI-3 These tables contain information about staffing patterns for physical therapists, occupational therapists, and speech pathologists respectively. The first column reports the percentage of facilities that report zero staff hours in the referenced labor category. The next column, "On Staff Only" is the percentage of facilities that report all hours as staff hours. The next column reports the percentage of facilities that report all hours as contract hours. The last column is the percentage of facilities that report both staff and contract hours in the referenced labor category.

Table VI-4 This table reports the percentage of facilities that use contract nurses and nurse aides. Facilities reporting non-zero contract hours are counted as using contract labor in the referenced labor category, otherwise not.

Tables VI-5 to VI-8 Tables VI-5 through VI-8 report staffing hours per patient day in fourteen specific staffing categories. The data are compiled from staffing hours reported on page 2 of HCFA Form 671. We used univariate analyses and professional judgement to eliminate unlikely values prior to computing the reported averages. The reported averages are unweighted. Mutually exclusive staffing categories are defined as follows:

RN Director of Nursing. Professional registered nurse(s) administratively responsible for managing and supervising nursing services within the facility.

Nurses with Administrative Duties. Nurses (RN, LPN, LVN) who, as either a facility employee or contractor, perform the Resident Assessment Instrument function in the facility and do not provide direct patient care.

Other Registered Nurses. Licensed in the state of operation to practice as registered nurses, including geriatric nurse practitioners and clinical nurse specialists who primarily perform nursing, not physician-delegated tasks.

Licensed Practical Nurses. Licensed in the state of operation to practice as licensed practical/vocational nurses.

Certified Nurse Aides. Have completed a state approved training and competency evaluation program, or competency evaluation program approved by the state or have been determined competent as provided in 483.150(a) and (3) and who are providing nursing or nursing-related services to residents. Does not include volunteers.

Nurse Aides in Training. In the first four months of employment and who are receiving training in a state approved nurse aide training and competency evaluation program and are providing nursing or nursing-related services for which they have been trained or are under the supervision of a licensed or registered nurse. Excludes volunteers.

Medication Aides/Technicians. Individuals, other than a licensed professional, who fulfill the state requirement for approval to administer medications to residents.

Occupational Therapists. Persons licensed/registered as occupational therapists (OTs) according to state law. Includes OTs who spend less than 50% of their time as activities therapists.

Occupational Therapy Assistants. Have licenses/certification and specialized training to assist a licensed/certified/registered OT to carry out the OT's comprehensive plan of care, without the direct supervision of the therapist. Includes OT Assistants who spend less than 50% of their time as activities therapists.

Occupational Therapy Aides. Have specialized training to assist an OT to carry out the OT's comprehensive plan of care under the direct supervision of the therapist.

Physical Therapists. Licensed/registered as physical therapists (PTs).

Physical Therapy Assistants. Have licenses/certification and specialized training to assist a licensed/certified/registered PT to carry out the PT's comprehensive plan of care, without the direct supervision of a PT.

Physical Therapy Aides. Have specialized training to assist a PT to carry out the PT's comprehensive plan of care under the direct supervision of the therapist.

Speech Language Pathologists. Licensed/registered to provide speech therapy and related services (e.g., teaching a resident to swallow).

APPENDICES A & B: HEALTH SERVICE AREAS

The Appendices provide an improved method to define the health services market area for every county in the United States. Table B-1 lists each county in the United States alphabetically by state and its associated Health Service Area (HSA), while Table B-2 provides the same list sorted by HSA.

The value of these tables can be illustrated using the example of Washington, D.C. From Table B-1, the District of Columbia is in HSA #61. Table B-2 shows that HSA #61 includes Charles, Montgomery, Prince George's, and St. Mary's counties in Maryland. Interestingly, the Metropolitan Statistical Area (MSA) definition of Washington, D.C. includes all counties in the HSA definition plus six counties in northern Virginia and Calvert county, Maryland. From a health care market area perspective, however, Calvert county is more appropriately associated with counties to the north, i.e., Baltimore, as it is in the HSA definition. Similarly, northern Virginia is not strongly a part of Washington, D.C.'s health care market.

SECTION I

RESIDENT ACUITY

TABLE I-1

FOUR MEASURES OF RESIDENT ACUITY BY STATE, 1997

	ADLINDEX	ACUINDEX	PROPAC	ADLSCORE
UNITED STATES	**9.984**	**10.151**	**103.25**	**3.6829**
Alabama	10.553	10.758	109.88	3.7050
Alaska	10.459	10.924	109.71	3.8352
Arizona	10.062	10.254	104.08	3.7089
Arkansas	9.966	10.097	100.66	3.5871
California	10.679	10.909	110.01	3.9063
Colorado	9.058	9.232	91.91	3.4851
Connecticut	9.319	9.450	89.97	3.4528
Delaware	10.294	10.493	110.59	3.5953
District of Columbia	10.939	11.171	116.24	3.7865
Florida	10.222	10.422	103.22	3.7713
Georgia	10.381	10.550	103.89	3.6450
Hawaii	11.563	11.817	124.78	4.1531
Idaho	9.412	9.530	94.82	3.6680
Illinois	8.563	8.690	80.27	3.0662
Indiana	9.608	9.783	96.90	3.5043
Iowa	8.620	8.720	79.38	3.3588
Kansas	8.803	8.909	88.01	3.3453
Kentucky	11.387	11.630	117.13	4.2431
Louisiana	9.554	9.723	93.36	3.2546
Maine	10.485	10.607	116.05	4.1638
Maryland	10.948	11.151	116.21	3.9251
Massachusetts	9.458	9.592	97.43	3.7729
Michigan	9.930	10.079	101.18	3.7289
Minnesota	9.056	9.161	93.20	3.5643
Mississippi	9.924	10.078	104.05	3.5008
Missouri	9.490	9.634	93.45	3.5312
Montana	8.830	8.990	85.34	3.4096
Nebraska	8.878	9.001	79.51	3.4605
Nevada	10.054	10.288	104.97	3.6886
New Hampshire	8.875	8.976	90.69	3.5093
New Jersey	9.968	10.124	97.60	3.6124
New Mexico	9.362	9.526	94.23	3.4796
New York	10.453	10.618	123.60	3.9396
North Carolina	11.049	11.241	116.69	3.8538
North Dakota	9.074	9.181	88.57	3.5113
Ohio	10.109	10.317	110.99	3.8100
Oklahoma	9.608	9.755	92.66	3.4358
Oregon	10.263	10.396	107.08	3.8515
Pennsylvania	10.543	10.733	113.01	3.8698

Table I-1: Four Measures of Resident Acuity by State, 1997 (Continued)

	ADLINDEX	ACUINDEX	PROPAC	ADLSCORE
Rhode Island	8.856	8.963	82.07	3.3950
South Carolina	11.520	11.692	127.69	4.0940
South Dakota	8.845	8.949	97.25	3.4585
Tennessee	10.786	10.963	110.38	3.8785
Texas	10.163	10.329	104.99	3.5660
Utah	9.258	9.397	92.09	3.5141
Vermont	9.419	9.536	97.01	3.9189
Virginia	11.546	11.746	125.47	4.2546
Washington	10.160	10.305	111.77	3.9007
West Virginia	11.363	11.550	100.85	4.1367
Wisconsin	9.157	9.266	94.42	3.4889
Wyoming	8.451	8.616	90.23	3.2655

TABLE I-2

ACUINDEX BY CLASS OF OWNERSHIP AND STATE, 1997

	For Profit	Non-Profit	Government
UNITED STATES	**10.145**	**10.069**	**10.477**
Alabama	10.819	10.845	10.182
Alaska	9.231	11.228	8.431
Arizona	10.257	10.140	11.342
Arkansas	9.980	10.721	10.718
California	10.864	10.884	11.704
Colorado	9.250	9.311	8.754
Connecticut	9.539	9.070	10.387
Delaware	10.341	10.174	11.840
District of Columbia	11.464	11.133	10.429
Florida	10.457	10.215	10.825
Georgia	10.459	10.717	11.229
Hawaii	11.337	11.729	13.234
Idaho	9.567	9.488	9.378
Illinois	8.438	9.122	9.820
Indiana	9.790	9.713	10.340
Iowa	8.607	8.813	9.188
Kansas	8.870	8.924	9.110
Kentucky	11.633	11.786	10.369
Louisiana	9.609	9.924	11.196
Maine	10.501	10.746	11.320
Maryland	11.216	10.943	11.797
Massachusetts	9.589	9.555	10.205
Michigan	9.877	10.151	10.977
Minnesota	9.039	9.126	9.648
Mississippi	10.092	10.361	9.762
Missouri	9.589	9.777	9.585
Montana	8.993	9.168	8.594
Nebraska	8.917	9.027	9.152
Nevada	10.362	10.441	7.790
New Hampshire	8.796	8.759	9.454
New Jersey	10.042	9.969	10.964
New Mexico	9.368	9.868	9.478
New York	10.518	10.600	11.047
North Carolina	11.259	11.215	10.922
North Dakota	9.091	9.207	8.149
Ohio	10.335	10.255	10.346
Oklahoma	9.713	10.047	9.934
Oregon	10.277	10.862	10.219
Pennsylvania	10.775	10.571	11.034

TABLE I-2: ACUINDEX BY CLASS OF OWNERSHIP AND STATE, 1997 (CONTINUED)

	For Profit	Non-Profit	Government
Rhode Island	9.082	8.441	n/a
South Carolina	11.734	11.174	11.793
South Dakota	8.920	8.938	9.381
Tennessee	10.954	10.747	11.313
Texas	10.327	10.369	10.044
Utah	9.277	9.768	10.463
Vermont	9.445	10.108	8.768
Virginia	11.755	11.700	11.854
Washington	10.247	10.206	11.721
West Virginia	11.784	10.967	10.761
Wisconsin	9.364	9.291	8.998
Wyoming	8.510	8.729	8.739

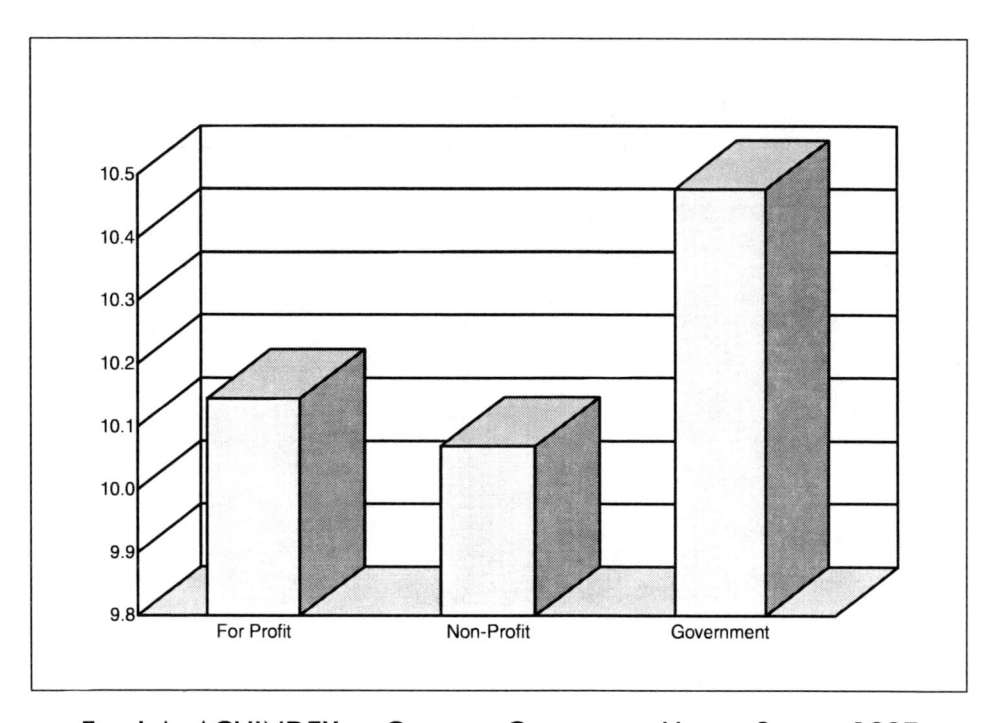

FIG. I-A: ACUINDEX BY CLASS OF OWNERSHIP, UNITED STATES, 1997

SECTION I: RESIDENT ACUITY

TABLE I-3

ACUINDEX BY URBAN/RURAL AND STATE, 1997

	Urban	Rural
UNITED STATES	**10.256**	**9.887**
Alabama	10.876	10.573
Alaska	11.359	10.343
Arizona	10.333	9.751
Arkansas	10.179	10.055
California	10.917	10.684
Colorado	9.387	8.797
Connecticut	9.459	9.174
Delaware	10.336	10.910
District of Columbia	11.171	n/a
Florida	10.441	10.244
Georgia	10.777	10.305
Hawaii	12.138	11.355
Idaho	10.126	9.280
Illinois	8.613	8.909
Indiana	9.851	9.639
Iowa	9.012	8.604
Kansas	9.001	8.851
Kentucky	11.600	11.651
Louisiana	9.741	9.691
Maine	10.396	10.850
Maryland	11.149	11.165
Massachusetts	9.594	9.440
Michigan	10.093	10.036
Minnesota	9.148	9.177
Mississippi	9.813	10.181
Missouri	9.860	9.347
Montana	9.206	8.928
Nebraska	9.678	8.719
Nevada	10.485	9.407
New Hampshire	9.019	8.887
New Jersey	10.124	n/a
New Mexico	9.528	9.524
New York	10.618	10.612
North Carolina	11.226	11.264
North Dakota	9.490	9.049
Ohio	10.444	9.883
Oklahoma	9.969	9.572
Oregon	10.311	10.591
Pennsylvania	10.775	10.536

TABLE I-3: ACUINDEX BY URBAN/RURAL AND STATE, 1997 (CONTINUED)

	Urban	Rural
Rhode Island	8.963	n/a
South Carolina	11.600	11.862
South Dakota	9.063	8.916
Tennessee	11.046	10.857
Texas	10.501	9.985
Utah	9.410	9.360
Vermont	9.214	9.621
Virginia	11.801	11.636
Washington	10.335	10.194
West Virginia	11.774	11.415
Wisconsin	9.404	9.059
Wyoming	8.603	8.622

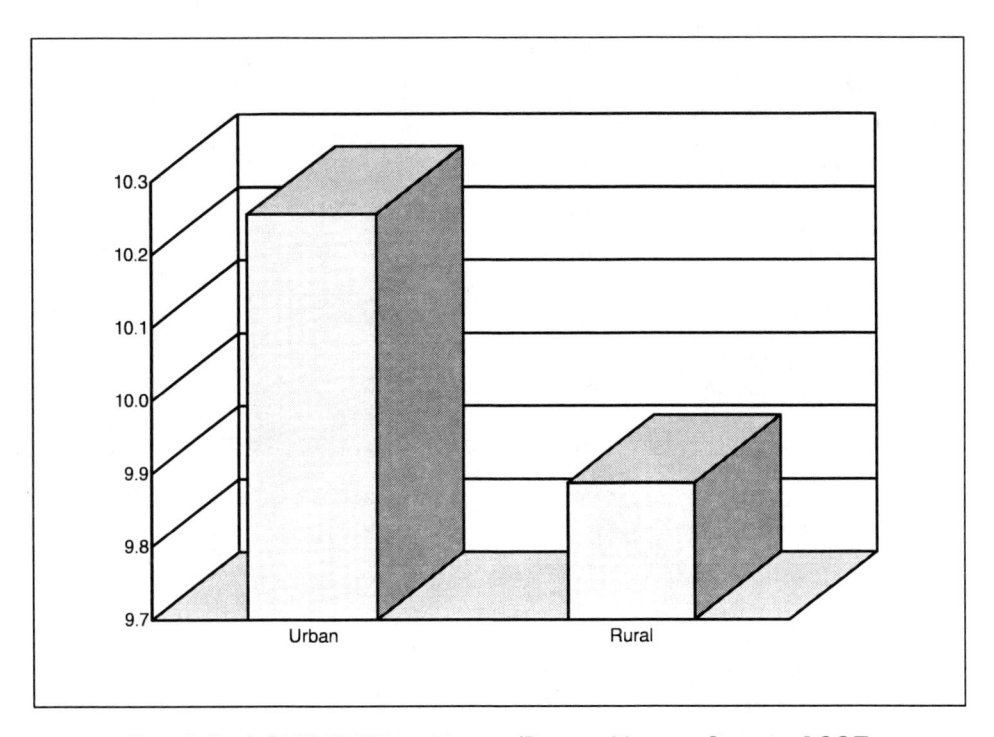

FIG. I-B: ACUINDEX BY URBAN/RURAL, UNITED STATES, 1997

SECTION I: RESIDENT ACUITY

TABLE I-4

ACUINDEX BY BEDSIZE AND STATE, 1997

	< 61 Beds	61–120 Beds	> 120 Beds
UNITED STATES	**9.8871**	**10.0758**	**10.2652**
Alabama	10.8698	10.5483	10.8790
Alaska	9.3365	11.2538	12.2038
Arizona	9.4982	10.1153	10.4266
Arkansas	10.3691	10.0073	10.2208
California	10.9035	10.8932	10.9273
Colorado	9.0759	9.0436	9.5482
Connecticut	9.0352	9.2082	9.6508
Delaware	9.7714	10.0594	11.0370
District of Columbia	10.3665	12.7737	11.1735
Florida	9.9906	10.4435	10.4855
Georgia	11.0353	10.4236	10.6237
Hawaii	11.0936	11.8331	12.0182
Idaho	9.3423	9.4816	9.7737
Illinois	9.2045	8.5994	8.6856
Indiana	9.6477	9.6700	9.8826
Iowa	8.3825	8.6979	9.0489
Kansas	8.7159	9.0372	8.9862
Kentucky	11.6515	11.4965	11.8320
Louisiana	11.6619	9.7317	9.5916
Maine	10.6513	10.5568	10.7364
Maryland	10.1438	11.2597	11.1945
Massachusetts	8.7022	9.6339	9.6852
Michigan	9.5339	9.8844	10.2946
Minnesota	8.9054	9.1408	9.2376
Mississippi	10.1075	10.2182	9.8095
Missouri	9.4804	9.5568	9.8255
Montana	8.6265	9.1518	9.0527
Nebraska	8.9846	8.7608	9.4851
Nevada	8.1065	11.2179	10.2386
New Hampshire	8.5217	8.9079	9.1754
New Jersey	10.0787	10.1776	10.1111
New Mexico	9.5647	9.5568	9.4272
New York	10.8219	10.6666	10.6009
North Carolina	11.1993	11.1524	11.3606
North Dakota	9.0355	9.0533	9.4900
Ohio	9.6522	10.3182	10.4595
Oklahoma	9.7559	9.8027	9.6395
Oregon	10.4015	10.3215	10.5441
Pennsylvania	10.0144	10.7969	10.7978

Table I-4: ACUINDEX by Bedsize and State, 1997 (Continued)

	< 61 Beds	61–120 Beds	> 120 Beds
Rhode Island	8.9244	8.8109	9.0494
South Carolina	10.9366	11.8116	11.6990
South Dakota	8.8698	8.9654	9.0654
Tennessee	10.8180	10.8251	11.0538
Texas	10.3948	10.1508	10.5329
Utah	8.9942	9.4268	9.6240
Vermont	9.5306	9.5392	9.5350
Virginia	11.8073	11.6970	11.7534
Washington	10.1333	10.3393	10.3102
West Virginia	11.1329	11.6629	11.5636
Wisconsin	9.1191	9.1442	9.3723
Wyoming	9.0278	8.1100	8.9281

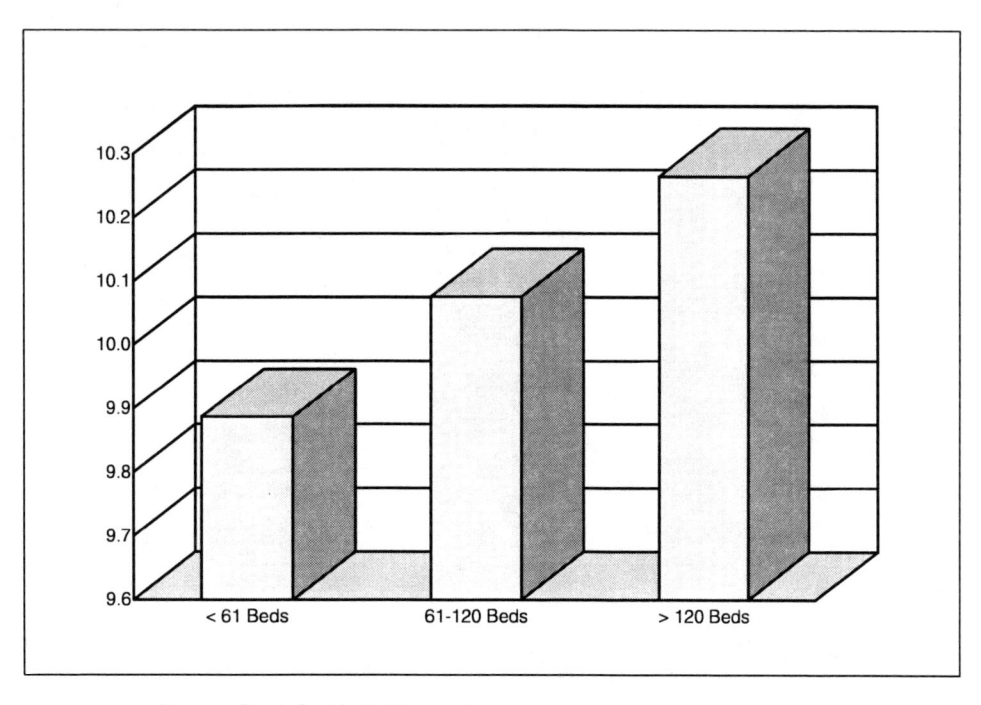

Fig. I-C: ACUINDEX by Bedsize, United States, 1997

Section I: Resident Acuity

Section II

Resident ADL Characteristics

TABLE II-1

RESIDENT ADL LIMITATIONS BY ADL AND STATE, 1997

	% Bathing	% Dressing	% Toileting	% Transferring	% Eating
UNITED STATES	**92.44**	**84.46**	**75.20**	**70.28**	**45.91**
Alabama	91.89	84.85	74.37	70.30	49.08
Alaska	94.02	86.43	81.10	73.99	47.98
Arizona	93.17	84.94	77.05	71.35	44.38
Arkansas	92.98	82.19	69.53	65.46	48.55
California	93.62	88.50	81.23	77.82	49.47
Colorado	93.34	79.49	71.27	63.31	41.10
Connecticut	88.28	81.91	69.22	65.46	40.41
Delaware	89.63	83.80	75.47	68.56	42.07
District of Columbia	92.58	87.61	77.32	72.97	48.18
Florida	91.84	85.69	78.25	73.60	47.75
Georgia	91.35	83.52	73.66	69.89	46.09
Hawaii	96.35	92.25	87.26	84.49	54.96
Idaho	94.48	83.75	77.03	70.02	41.53
Illinois	80.57	71.50	62.54	57.63	34.39
Indiana	90.85	81.13	70.66	65.60	42.18
Iowa	94.46	79.74	67.18	60.79	33.70
Kansas	92.18	76.45	67.94	61.42	36.54
Kentucky	97.68	94.74	85.21	81.07	65.62
Louisiana	87.28	75.49	63.73	59.73	39.23
Maine	97.11	94.85	89.98	85.93	48.51
Maryland	94.09	88.65	80.12	76.04	53.61
Massachusetts	92.36	89.48	75.84	72.99	46.62
Michigan	92.49	85.99	77.75	71.41	45.24
Minnesota	95.96	82.12	72.26	63.64	42.46
Mississippi	91.75	79.52	70.77	65.41	42.64
Missouri	92.35	80.75	71.99	66.10	41.93
Montana	96.93	78.84	69.31	62.41	33.48
Nebraska	94.53	78.90	69.99	64.50	38.14
Nevada	93.53	85.77	77.50	71.46	40.60
New Hampshire	92.30	84.50	71.30	64.33	38.51
New Jersey	91.21	84.82	73.63	68.27	43.32
New Mexico	93.05	81.21	72.02	64.15	37.53
New York	94.98	88.08	80.50	75.38	55.02
North Carolina	92.26	87.70	79.99	75.69	49.74
North Dakota	94.71	81.18	72.04	65.15	38.05
Ohio	94.24	86.88	78.61	73.03	48.23
Oklahoma	91.71	79.04	67.43	62.81	42.59
Oregon	94.95	88.20	81.10	75.34	45.56
Pennsylvania	92.96	88.53	80.84	76.90	47.75

TABLE II-1: RESIDENT ADL LIMITATIONS BY ADL AND STATE, 1997 (CONTINUED)

	% Bathing	% Dressing	% Toileting	% Transferring	% Eating
Rhode Island	88.51	81.69	67.38	62.18	39.75
South Carolina	96.10	93.03	85.49	80.39	54.39
South Dakota	96.35	79.02	70.57	63.88	36.03
Tennessee	94.49	88.81	77.42	73.50	53.63
Texas	92.73	81.96	71.05	67.58	43.29
Utah	92.18	81.78	72.46	64.53	40.46
Vermont	97.15	90.98	82.11	75.82	45.82
Virginia	97.15	94.02	85.44	80.94	67.91
Washington	95.93	88.39	82.57	74.49	48.69
West Virginia	97.39	92.66	84.20	79.40	60.03
Wisconsin	92.22	81.93	71.56	65.90	37.27
Wyoming	93.18	75.49	66.14	58.60	33.14

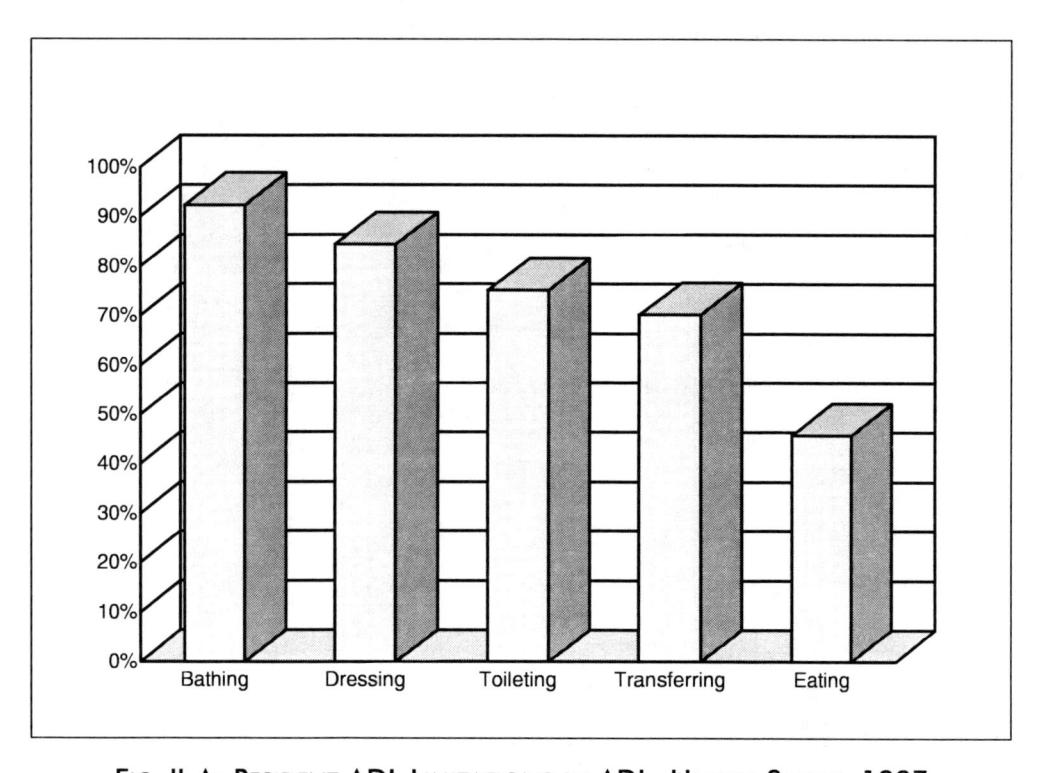

FIG. II-A: RESIDENT ADL LIMITATIONS BY ADL, UNITED STATES, 1997

SECTION II: RESIDENT ADL CHARACTERISTICS

TABLE II-2

RESIDENT DEPENDENCE LEVEL BY STATE — BATHING, 1997

	% Independent	% Assistance of 1–2 Staff	% Dependent
UNITED STATES	**7.56**	**48.89**	**43.56**
Alabama	8.11	45.37	46.52
Alaska	5.98	54.60	39.42
Arizona	6.83	52.99	40.19
Arkansas	7.02	46.13	46.85
California	6.38	46.23	47.40
Colorado	6.66	62.51	30.83
Connecticut	11.73	43.53	44.75
Delaware	10.38	40.70	48.93
District of Columbia	7.42	34.73	57.85
Florida	8.16	52.13	39.71
Georgia	8.65	44.76	46.59
Hawaii	3.65	47.29	49.06
Idaho	5.52	62.09	32.39
Illinois	19.44	54.79	25.78
Indiana	9.15	51.64	39.21
Iowa	5.54	62.36	32.11
Kansas	7.82	55.82	36.36
Kentucky	2.32	36.76	60.91
Louisiana	12.73	43.33	43.95
Maine	2.89	49.27	47.84
Maryland	5.91	34.51	59.58
Massachusetts	7.65	44.77	47.58
Michigan	7.51	54.83	37.66
Minnesota	4.04	57.01	38.95
Mississippi	8.25	55.29	36.46
Missouri	7.65	55.24	37.11
Montana	3.08	55.68	41.25
Nebraska	5.47	58.36	36.17
Nevada	6.47	50.46	43.07
New Hampshire	7.70	56.07	36.23
New Jersey	8.79	44.30	46.91
New Mexico	6.95	54.10	38.95
New York	5.02	46.34	48.64
North Carolina	7.74	40.32	51.95
North Dakota	5.29	57.69	37.03
Ohio	5.76	48.88	45.37
Oklahoma	8.29	51.77	39.93
Oregon	5.05	55.48	39.47
Pennsylvania	7.04	45.00	47.96

TABLE II-2: RESIDENT DEPENDENCE LEVEL BY STATE — BATHING, 1997 (CONTINUED)

	% Independent	% Assistance of 1–2 Staff	% Dependent
Rhode Island	11.49	44.02	44.49
South Carolina	3.90	40.34	55.76
South Dakota	3.65	63.32	33.03
Tennessee	5.51	42.92	51.57
Texas	7.27	47.59	45.14
Utah	7.83	59.98	32.20
Vermont	2.85	57.88	39.28
Virginia	2.85	34.48	62.67
Washington	4.07	57.36	38.56
West Virginia	2.61	36.92	60.47
Wisconsin	7.78	56.53	35.70
Wyoming	6.82	62.24	30.95

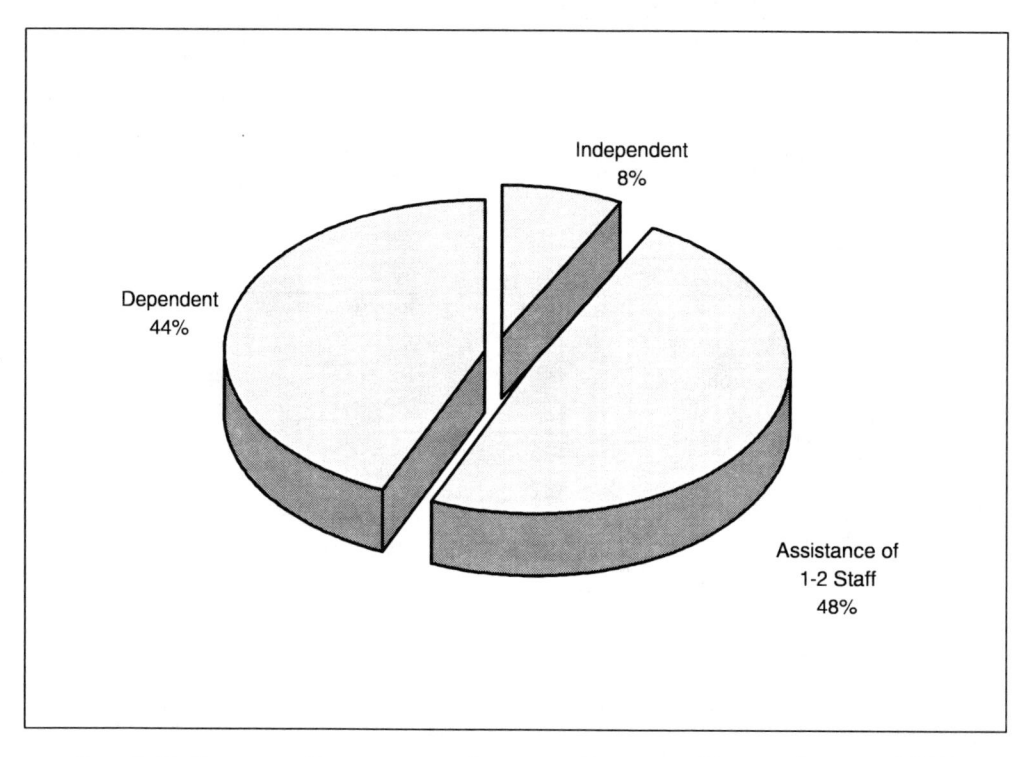

FIG. II-B: RESIDENT DEPENDENCE LEVEL — BATHING, UNITED STATES, 1997

TABLE II-3

RESIDENT DEPENDENCE LEVEL BY STATE — DRESSING, 1997

	% Independent	% Assistance of 1–2 Staff	% Dependent
UNITED STATES	**15.54**	**45.89**	**38.57**
Alabama	15.15	42.88	41.97
Alaska	13.57	56.70	29.73
Arizona	15.06	49.71	35.24
Arkansas	17.82	41.31	40.87
California	11.50	49.12	39.37
Colorado	20.51	52.80	26.69
Connecticut	18.09	39.31	42.60
Delaware	16.20	38.09	45.72
District of Columbia	12.39	31.77	55.84
Florida	14.31	48.54	37.15
Georgia	16.48	42.06	41.46
Hawaii	7.75	49.52	42.73
Idaho	16.26	57.89	25.86
Illinois	28.50	48.16	23.34
Indiana	18.87	46.72	34.41
Iowa	20.26	50.47	29.27
Kansas	23.55	47.13	29.32
Kentucky	5.26	37.13	57.61
Louisiana	24.51	38.33	37.16
Maine	5.16	54.23	40.61
Maryland	11.35	35.11	53.54
Massachusetts	10.52	43.47	46.01
Michigan	14.01	52.69	33.30
Minnesota	17.88	46.78	35.34
Mississippi	20.49	53.07	26.45
Missouri	19.25	47.76	32.99
Montana	21.16	46.85	31.99
Nebraska	21.11	48.68	30.22
Nevada	14.23	50.52	35.25
New Hampshire	15.50	54.12	30.38
New Jersey	15.18	40.94	43.88
New Mexico	18.79	49.30	31.91
New York	11.92	46.17	41.92
North Carolina	12.30	40.22	47.48
North Dakota	18.82	50.42	30.76
Ohio	13.12	48.72	38.16
Oklahoma	20.96	42.79	36.25
Oregon	11.80	55.25	32.95
Pennsylvania	11.47	43.52	45.01

Table II-3: Resident Dependence Level by State — Dressing, 1997 (Continued)

	% Independent	% Assistance of 1–2 Staff	% Dependent
Rhode Island	18.31	40.43	41.26
South Carolina	6.97	42.08	50.95
South Dakota	20.98	55.42	23.60
Tennessee	11.20	42.46	46.35
Texas	18.05	42.06	39.90
Utah	18.23	53.74	28.03
Vermont	9.02	60.89	30.09
Virginia	5.98	35.96	58.05
Washington	11.61	58.63	29.75
West Virginia	7.34	37.92	54.74
Wisconsin	18.07	51.68	30.25
Wyoming	24.51	48.52	26.97

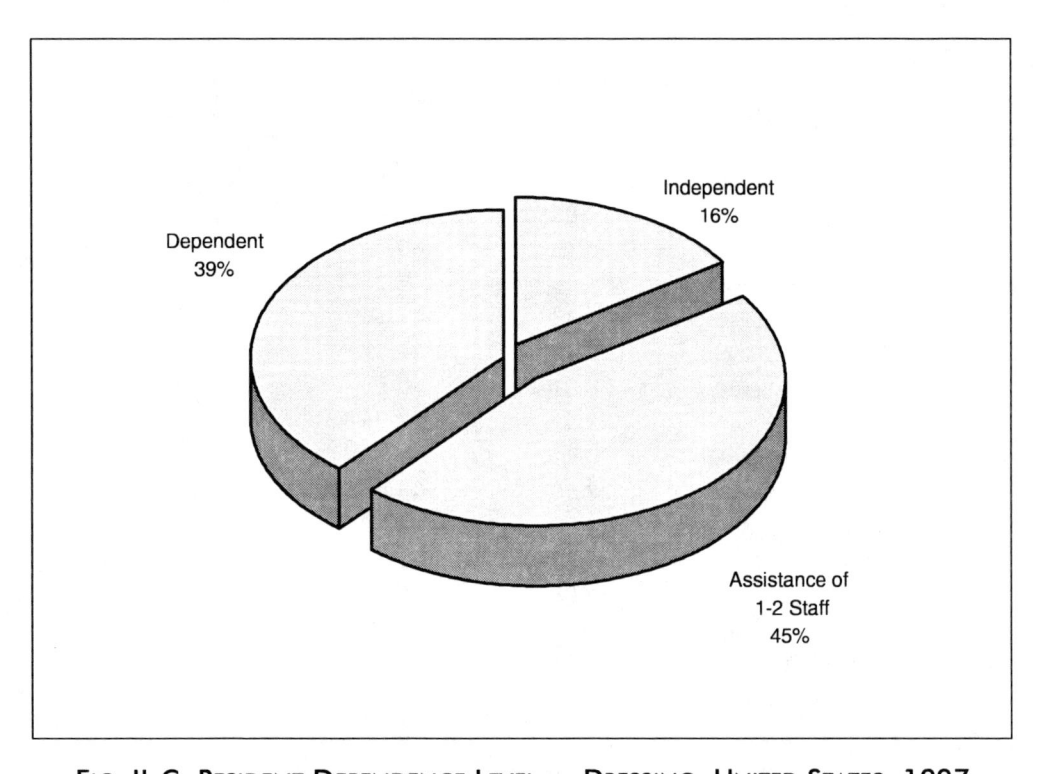

Fig. II-C: Resident Dependence Level — Dressing, United States, 1997

- Independent 16%
- Assistance of 1-2 Staff 45%
- Dependent 39%

Section II: Resident ADL Characteristics

TABLE II-4

RESIDENT DEPENDENCE LEVEL BY STATE — TOILETING, 1997

	% Independent	% Assistance of 1–2 Staff	% Dependent
UNITED STATES	**24.80**	**37.91**	**37.28**
Alabama	25.63	31.92	42.45
Alaska	18.90	42.49	38.61
Arizona	22.95	40.02	37.03
Arkansas	30.47	30.99	38.54
California	18.77	38.90	42.33
Colorado	28.73	44.14	27.13
Connecticut	30.78	34.57	34.65
Delaware	24.53	32.99	42.48
District of Columbia	22.68	27.07	50.26
Florida	21.75	41.44	36.81
Georgia	26.34	31.87	41.79
Hawaii	12.74	38.34	48.92
Idaho	22.97	49.87	27.16
Illinois	37.46	38.36	24.18
Indiana	29.34	37.60	33.06
Iowa	32.82	40.90	26.29
Kansas	32.06	39.71	28.23
Kentucky	14.79	34.71	50.51
Louisiana	36.27	27.84	35.89
Maine	10.02	50.81	39.17
Maryland	19.88	29.98	50.14
Massachusetts	24.16	40.20	35.64
Michigan	22.25	42.76	34.99
Minnesota	27.74	41.13	31.13
Mississippi	29.23	37.57	33.20
Missouri	28.01	40.56	31.43
Montana	30.69	40.96	28.35
Nebraska	30.01	41.12	28.87
Nevada	22.50	38.22	39.28
New Hampshire	28.70	42.80	28.50
New Jersey	26.37	33.75	39.88
New Mexico	27.98	40.30	31.72
New York	19.50	40.96	39.53
North Carolina	20.01	32.66	47.34
North Dakota	27.96	42.64	29.41
Ohio	21.39	40.67	37.94
Oklahoma	32.57	33.66	33.77
Oregon	18.90	44.72	36.39
Pennsylvania	19.16	38.19	42.66

TABLE II-4: RESIDENT DEPENDENCE LEVEL BY STATE — TOILETING, 1997 (CONTINUED)

	% Independent	% Assistance of 1–2 Staff	% Dependent
Rhode Island	32.62	32.12	35.26
South Carolina	14.51	33.88	51.61
South Dakota	29.43	46.58	23.99
Tennessee	22.58	32.69	44.74
Texas	28.95	30.39	40.65
Utah	27.54	44.04	28.42
Vermont	17.89	50.47	31.64
Virginia	14.56	34.98	50.45
Washington	17.43	49.37	33.20
West Virginia	15.80	32.54	51.66
Wisconsin	28.44	43.23	28.33
Wyoming	33.86	44.55	21.59

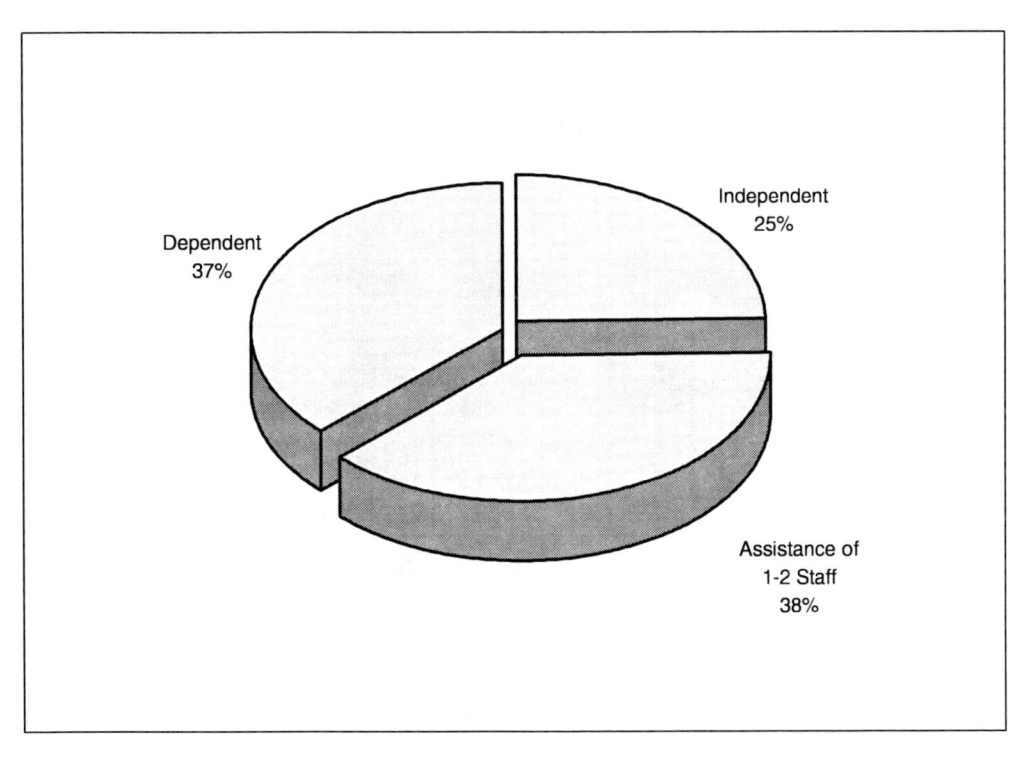

FIG. II-D: RESIDENT DEPENDENCE LEVEL — TOILETING, UNITED STATES, 1997

- Independent 25%
- Assistance of 1-2 Staff 38%
- Dependent 37%

SECTION II: RESIDENT ADL CHARACTERISTICS

TABLE II-5

RESIDENT DEPENDENCE LEVEL BY STATE — TRANSFERRING, 1997

	% Independent	% Assistance of 1–2 Staff	% Dependent
UNITED STATES	**29.72**	**40.55**	**29.74**
Alabama	29.70	34.34	35.95
Alaska	26.01	45.40	28.60
Arizona	28.65	43.97	27.38
Arkansas	34.54	32.73	32.73
California	22.18	43.67	34.15
Colorado	36.69	42.48	20.83
Connecticut	34.54	37.91	27.54
Delaware	31.44	34.93	33.64
District of Columbia	27.03	29.69	43.28
Florida	26.40	43.10	30.51
Georgia	30.11	35.46	34.43
Hawaii	15.51	44.58	39.91
Idaho	29.98	47.74	22.28
Illinois	42.38	37.72	19.90
Indiana	34.40	38.86	26.74
Iowa	39.21	39.38	21.41
Kansas	38.58	38.77	22.65
Kentucky	18.93	40.98	40.08
Louisiana	40.27	29.79	29.94
Maine	14.07	56.57	29.36
Maryland	23.96	35.20	40.84
Massachusetts	27.01	47.71	25.28
Michigan	28.59	44.50	26.91
Minnesota	36.36	40.39	23.25
Mississippi	34.59	37.30	28.11
Missouri	33.90	39.97	26.13
Montana	37.59	42.37	20.04
Nebraska	35.50	41.12	23.39
Nevada	28.55	42.67	28.78
New Hampshire	35.67	43.20	21.13
New Jersey	31.73	36.59	31.68
New Mexico	35.85	39.31	24.85
New York	24.62	45.33	30.05
North Carolina	24.31	37.15	38.54
North Dakota	34.86	42.86	22.29
Ohio	26.97	43.53	29.50
Oklahoma	37.19	33.31	29.50
Oregon	24.66	47.35	27.99
Pennsylvania	23.10	42.60	34.30

TABLE II-5: RESIDENT DEPENDENCE LEVEL BY STATE — TRANSFERRING, 1997 (CONTINUED)

	% Independent	% Assistance of 1–2 Staff	% Dependent
Rhode Island	37.82	34.48	27.69
South Carolina	19.61	39.68	40.70
South Dakota	36.12	44.82	19.06
Tennessee	26.50	36.12	37.39
Texas	32.42	35.52	32.06
Utah	35.47	42.77	21.77
Vermont	24.18	52.61	23.22
Virginia	19.06	39.17	41.77
Washington	25.51	50.55	23.94
West Virginia	20.61	35.78	43.62
Wisconsin	34.10	42.94	22.97
Wyoming	41.40	41.33	17.27

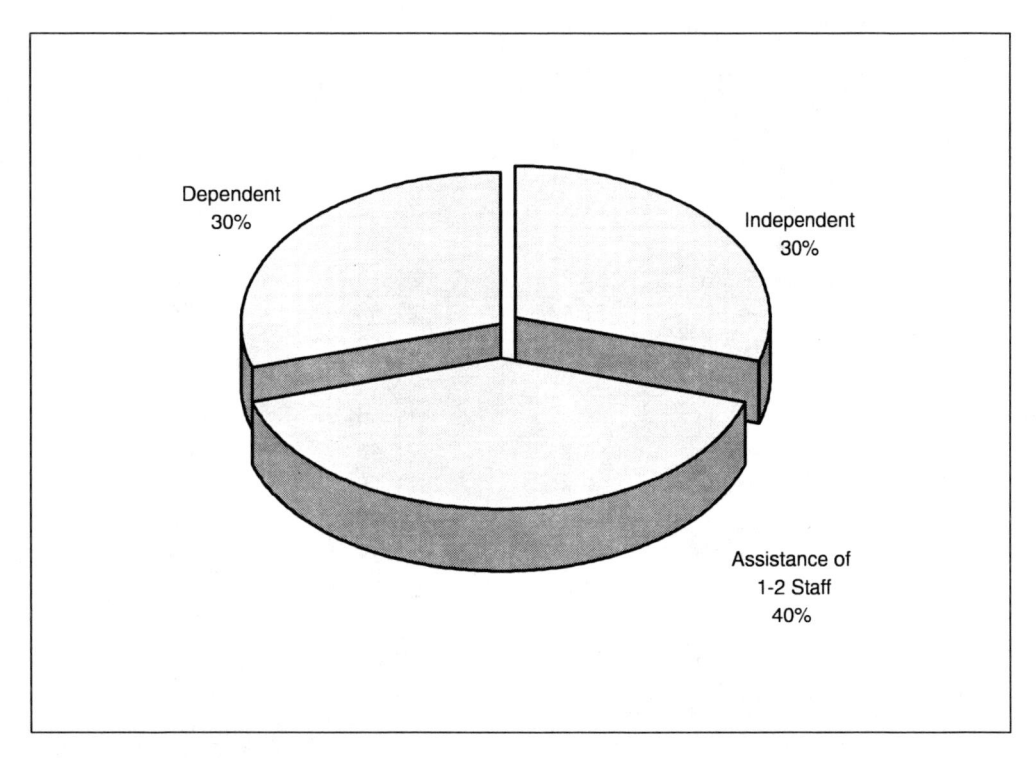

FIG. II-E: RESIDENT DEPENDENCE LEVEL — TRANSFERRING, UNITED STATES, 1997

SECTION II: RESIDENT ADL CHARACTERISTICS

TABLE II-6

RESIDENT DEPENDENCE LEVEL BY STATE — EATING, 1997

	% Independent	% Assistance of 1–2 Staff	% Dependent
UNITED STATES	**54.09**	**24.95**	**20.96**
Alabama	50.92	20.59	28.49
Alaska	52.02	25.69	22.29
Arizona	55.62	27.06	17.32
Arkansas	51.45	23.68	24.87
California	50.54	24.88	24.58
Colorado	58.90	27.76	13.34
Connecticut	59.59	20.86	19.55
Delaware	57.93	18.84	23.23
District of Columbia	51.82	20.29	27.89
Florida	52.25	25.81	21.94
Georgia	53.91	21.70	24.39
Hawaii	45.04	23.63	31.33
Idaho	58.47	27.09	14.44
Illinois	65.61	20.03	14.36
Indiana	57.82	23.56	18.61
Iowa	66.30	21.44	12.27
Kansas	63.46	23.17	13.37
Kentucky	34.39	33.61	32.01
Louisiana	60.77	18.68	20.55
Maine	51.49	28.64	19.87
Maryland	46.39	24.21	29.41
Massachusetts	53.38	27.90	18.72
Michigan	54.76	26.88	18.36
Minnesota	57.54	27.60	14.86
Mississippi	57.36	20.69	21.95
Missouri	58.07	24.64	17.29
Montana	66.52	19.85	13.63
Nebraska	61.86	24.43	13.71
Nevada	59.40	21.15	19.45
New Hampshire	61.49	24.19	14.32
New Jersey	56.68	21.39	21.93
New Mexico	62.47	22.36	15.17
New York	44.98	31.22	23.80
North Carolina	50.26	22.43	27.32
North Dakota	61.96	21.74	16.31
Ohio	51.77	27.74	20.49
Oklahoma	57.41	21.86	20.73
Oregon	54.44	25.19	20.37
Pennsylvania	52.25	24.96	22.79

TABLE II-6: RESIDENT DEPENDENCE LEVEL BY STATE — EATING, 1997 (CONTINUED)

	% Independent	% Assistance of 1–2 Staff	% Dependent
Rhode Island	60.25	20.89	18.86
South Carolina	45.61	26.78	27.61
South Dakota	63.97	23.82	12.21
Tennessee	46.37	26.59	27.04
Texas	56.71	21.28	22.01
Utah	59.54	26.73	13.74
Vermont	54.18	29.73	16.09
Virginia	32.09	39.37	28.54
Washington	51.31	30.05	18.65
West Virginia	39.97	25.70	34.33
Wisconsin	62.73	23.09	14.19
Wyoming	66.86	21.25	11.89

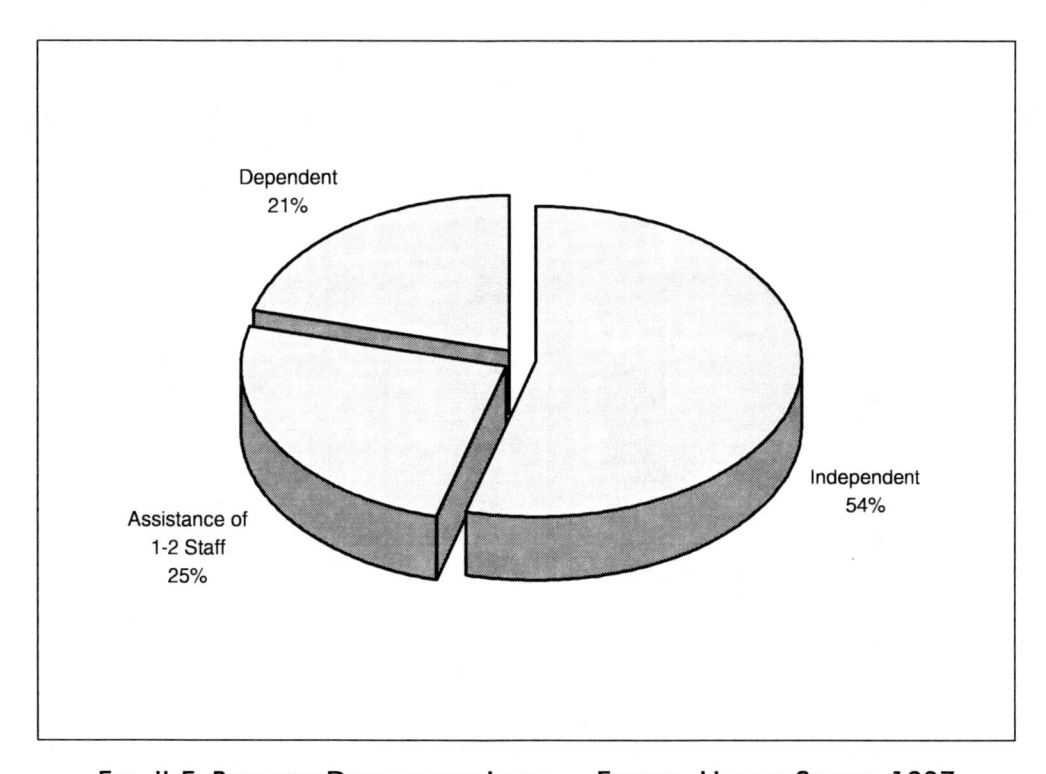

FIG. II-F: RESIDENT DEPENDENCE LEVEL — EATING, UNITED STATES, 1997

SECTION II: RESIDENT ADL CHARACTERISTICS

TABLE II-7

RESIDENTS WITH MULTIPLE DEPENDENCIES BY STATE, 1997

	% 0 ADLs	% 1 ADL	% 2 ADLs	% 3 ADLs	% 4 ADLs	% 5 ADLs
UNITED STATES	**7.56**	**7.99**	**9.26**	**4.91**	**24.38**	**45.91**
Alabama	8.11	7.04	10.48	4.07	21.22	49.08
Alaska	5.98	7.59	5.33	7.11	26.01	47.98
Arizona	6.83	8.23	7.90	5.70	26.97	44.38
Arkansas	7.02	10.80	12.66	4.06	16.91	48.55
California	6.38	5.13	7.27	3.41	28.35	49.47
Colorado	6.66	13.86	8.22	7.96	22.21	41.10
Connecticut	11.73	6.36	12.69	3.76	25.05	40.41
Delaware	10.38	5.82	8.33	6.91	26.49	42.07
District of Columbia	7.42	4.97	10.28	4.36	24.79	48.18
Florida	8.16	6.15	7.44	4.65	25.85	47.75
Georgia	8.65	7.83	9.86	3.77	23.79	46.09
Hawaii	3.65	4.11	4.99	2.77	29.53	54.96
Idaho	5.52	10.73	6.72	7.01	28.49	41.53
Illinois	19.44	9.07	8.96	4.92	23.24	34.39
Indiana	9.15	9.72	10.47	5.06	23.42	42.18
Iowa	5.54	14.73	12.56	6.39	27.09	33.70
Kansas	7.82	15.73	8.51	6.52	24.88	36.54
Kentucky	2.32	2.93	9.53	4.15	15.45	65.62
Louisiana	12.73	11.78	11.76	4.00	20.50	39.23
Maine	2.89	2.27	4.86	4.05	37.42	48.51
Maryland	5.91	5.44	8.53	4.08	22.43	53.61
Massachusetts	7.65	2.87	13.64	2.85	26.37	46.62
Michigan	7.51	6.50	8.24	6.34	26.17	45.24
Minnesota	4.04	13.85	9.86	8.62	21.18	42.46
Mississippi	8.25	12.23	8.75	5.36	22.77	42.64
Missouri	7.65	11.60	8.76	5.89	24.17	41.93
Montana	3.08	18.08	9.53	6.90	28.93	33.48
Nebraska	5.47	15.63	8.91	5.49	26.37	38.14
Nevada	6.47	7.77	8.27	6.04	30.85	40.60
New Hampshire	7.70	7.80	13.20	6.97	25.83	38.51
New Jersey	8.79	6.40	11.19	5.36	24.95	43.32
New Mexico	6.95	11.84	9.19	7.87	26.62	37.53
New York	5.02	6.89	7.59	5.12	20.36	55.02
North Carolina	7.74	4.57	7.70	4.30	25.95	49.74
North Dakota	5.29	13.53	9.14	6.90	27.10	38.05
Ohio	5.76	7.36	8.27	5.58	24.80	48.23
Oklahoma	8.29	12.67	11.61	4.62	20.22	42.59
Oregon	5.05	6.75	7.10	5.77	29.78	45.56
Pennsylvania	7.04	4.43	7.68	3.95	29.15	47.75

TABLE II-7: RESIDENTS WITH MULTIPLE DEPENDENCIES BY STATE, 1997 (CONTINUED)

	% 0 ADLs	% 1 ADL	% 2 ADLs	% 3 ADLs	% 4 ADLs	% 5 ADLs
Rhode Island	11.49	6.82	14.31	5.20	22.43	39.75
South Carolina	3.90	3.07	7.54	5.11	26.00	54.39
South Dakota	3.65	17.33	8.45	6.69	27.85	36.03
Tennessee	5.51	5.69	11.38	3.92	19.87	53.63
Texas	7.27	10.77	10.91	3.46	24.30	43.29
Utah	7.83	10.40	9.32	7.93	24.07	40.46
Vermont	2.85	6.17	8.88	6.28	30.01	45.82
Virginia	2.85	3.13	8.58	4.50	13.03	67.91
Washington	4.07	7.54	5.82	8.08	25.80	48.69
West Virginia	2.61	4.73	8.46	4.81	19.37	60.03
Wisconsin	7.78	10.29	10.37	5.65	28.63	37.27
Wyoming	6.82	17.69	9.36	7.54	25.46	33.14

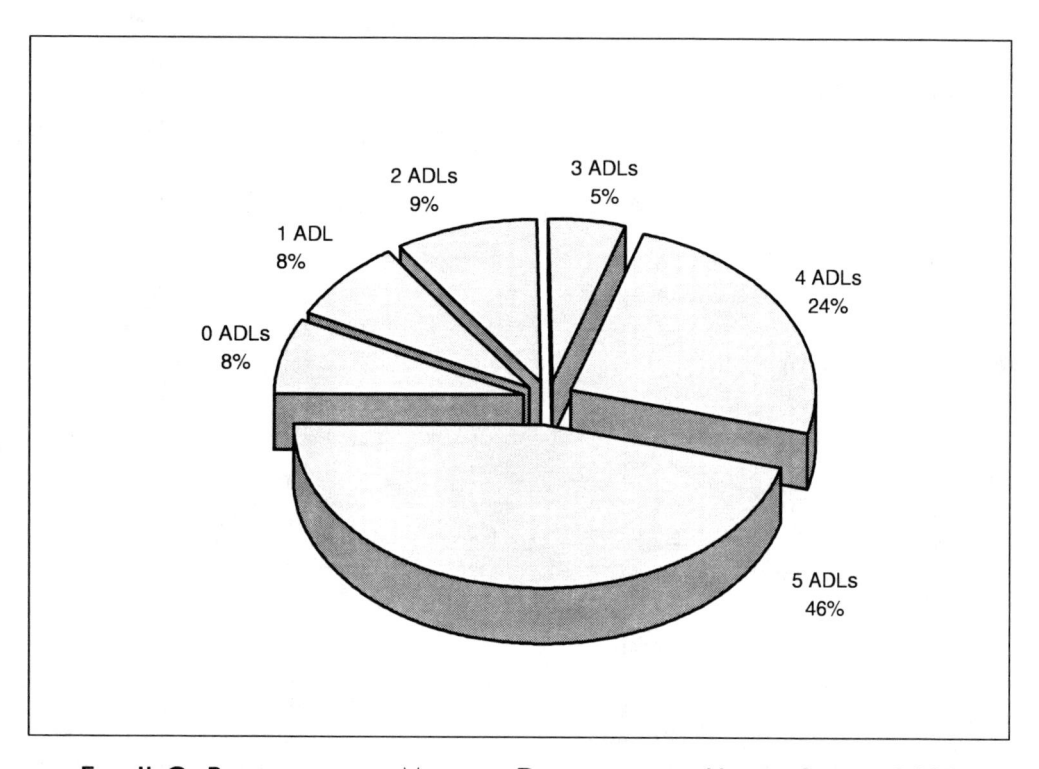

FIG. II-G: RESIDENTS WITH MULTIPLE DEPENDENCIES, UNITED STATES, 1997

SECTION II: RESIDENT ADL CHARACTERISTICS

TABLE II-8

RESIDENT CONTINENCE CHARACTERISTICS BY STATE, 1997

	% With Catheter	% Catheters with Catheters on Admission	% Bladder Incontinence	% Bladder Training Program	% Bowel Incontinence	% Bowel Training Program
UNITED STATES	**6.65**	**71.02**	**52.27**	**5.85**	**43.73**	**4.23**
Alabama	5.50	77.02	53.50	10.70	49.61	7.59
Alaska	8.40	55.77	47.98	7.92	38.61	7.11
Arizona	8.59	88.54	52.78	2.45	46.61	2.11
Arkansas	7.53	61.61	47.24	3.83	42.49	3.61
California	7.84	87.04	51.92	3.04	46.33	2.37
Colorado	6.73	68.40	50.55	3.28	37.88	2.41
Connecticut	4.22	58.85	51.00	4.02	40.87	2.81
Delaware	5.12	61.62	57.90	10.30	50.40	6.13
District of Columbia	6.37	69.52	62.21	10.15	50.94	4.26
Florida	7.56	80.49	50.93	8.10	46.30	5.83
Georgia	6.19	62.61	50.87	5.21	46.24	4.34
Hawaii	4.82	70.41	56.36	5.53	50.77	4.05
Idaho	6.07	74.83	51.11	5.90	37.32	4.87
Illinois	6.56	74.02	41.96	5.01	31.78	2.60
Indiana	8.31	62.15	48.25	5.74	39.67	3.84
Iowa	4.89	68.54	49.44	3.83	30.15	3.34
Kansas	5.23	68.77	49.26	7.58	34.65	5.01
Kentucky	8.95	70.83	58.01	3.79	53.84	2.98
Louisiana	9.32	59.52	41.12	3.59	38.96	2.47
Maine	5.71	67.09	63.16	15.88	45.15	11.72
Maryland	5.37	76.11	58.03	8.61	51.97	8.26
Massachusetts	4.85	65.37	55.68	3.53	44.72	1.47
Michigan	5.79	75.95	52.49	7.40	40.93	4.88
Minnesota	4.50	62.18	54.99	6.32	36.94	10.15
Mississippi	6.45	59.34	45.48	3.95	40.16	3.44
Missouri	6.18	70.29	50.16	4.97	42.15	4.44
Montana	4.89	64.26	47.49	9.47	31.91	7.51
Nebraska	5.70	64.76	45.18	7.37	28.52	4.58
Nevada	9.36	75.35	51.66	4.24	48.08	0.90
New Hampshire	4.73	68.88	51.19	8.44	33.42	8.85
New Jersey	5.49	77.71	52.78	4.25	46.33	3.14
New Mexico	6.17	77.51	48.17	4.21	41.97	3.13
New York	4.81	68.79	60.77	5.21	51.48	2.86
North Carolina	6.38	69.33	55.53	10.27	51.71	6.31
North Dakota	4.64	56.37	50.61	3.66	30.60	2.91

TABLE II-8: RESIDENT CONTINENCE CHARACTERISTICS BY STATE, 1997 (CONTINUED)

	% With Catheter	% Catheters with Catheters on Admission	% Bladder Incontinence	% Bladder Training Program	% Bowel Incontinence	% Bowel Training Program
Ohio	7.22	72.10	50.72	11.80	40.55	6.14
Oklahoma	8.24	57.65	46.06	3.38	40.60	2.50
Oregon	7.51	70.91	57.10	4.11	45.90	3.94
Pennsylvania	7.30	69.16	59.16	7.82	51.12	5.79
Rhode Island	4.38	70.63	47.53	5.46	36.55	2.94
South Carolina	5.39	76.06	64.75	3.43	61.99	2.14
South Dakota	5.76	63.80	44.78	12.90	25.77	6.57
Tennessee	7.78	65.55	53.06	5.64	49.19	3.75
Texas	8.66	72.16	51.75	0.96	48.22	0.71
Utah	7.03	99.28	49.49	7.11	37.52	5.81
Vermont	5.35	67.37	53.68	5.33	38.74	7.69
Virginia	6.84	70.01	62.85	7.52	57.75	7.19
Washington	8.45	70.37	57.17	3.87	42.19	5.15
West Virginia	7.56	55.63	35.62	3.16	28.74	2.47
Wisconsin	6.37	63.78	49.22	9.17	35.37	7.18
Wyoming	6.63	46.86	45.08	20.64	29.21	14.02

TABLE II-9

RESIDENT MOBILITY CHARACTERISTICS BY STATE, 1997

	% Ambulatory	% Ambulation w/ Assistance	% Bedfast	% Chairbound
UNITED STATES	**21.01**	**30.46**	**7.14**	**49.96**
Alabama	19.87	26.50	13.42	48.21
Alaska	18.74	35.22	7.27	58.64
Arizona	18.70	28.75	8.06	53.31
Arkansas	25.27	21.77	8.94	46.87
California	16.59	28.49	7.93	55.52
Colorado	24.98	33.62	3.23	48.37
Connecticut	25.72	35.67	3.29	45.36
Delaware	22.10	25.23	10.17	50.30
District of Columbia	21.49	16.55	8.10	56.08
Florida	17.46	28.48	6.89	54.08
Georgia	20.87	21.94	10.03	52.35
Hawaii	7.55	28.02	12.60	59.44
Idaho	20.00	39.73	4.02	50.71
Illinois	32.38	28.00	3.91	42.37
Indiana	24.29	33.02	6.62	50.18
Iowa	23.58	41.88	3.17	41.75
Kansas	23.82	31.51	3.85	42.29
Kentucky	15.35	30.72	11.53	51.45
Louisiana	29.60	26.51	11.67	43.02
Maine	13.68	39.94	7.33	46.99
Maryland	20.21	25.10	8.54	51.51
Massachusetts	18.51	42.37	3.26	42.05
Michigan	19.70	31.80	6.00	52.53
Minnesota	23.33	39.64	2.50	43.97
Mississippi	21.00	29.67	12.29	50.14
Missouri	22.59	28.97	6.38	48.01
Montana	22.97	36.43	4.57	43.30
Nebraska	22.75	40.01	3.55	40.67
Nevada	15.82	27.06	10.42	47.79
New Hampshire	25.48	40.28	3.98	39.60
New Jersey	24.52	25.56	5.79	50.41
New Mexico	19.96	37.48	6.48	48.55
New York	17.33	28.33	4.97	57.81
North Carolina	16.57	25.76	12.80	54.72
North Dakota	22.69	36.92	2.57	46.60
Ohio	22.62	40.47	6.90	48.97
Oklahoma	27.56	25.16	9.85	44.54
Oregon	18.19	31.24	8.24	53.11
Pennsylvania	15.57	29.31	7.98	52.97

Table II-9: Resident Mobility Characteristics by State, 1997 (Continued)

	% Ambulatory	% Ambulation w/ Assistance	% Bedfast	% Chairbound
Rhode Island	28.42	39.11	4.00	31.20
South Carolina	13.09	24.94	11.55	60.93
South Dakota	24.53	39.24	3.27	46.77
Tennessee	19.59	26.02	12.68	49.62
Texas	21.95	19.31	11.11	50.28
Utah	25.69	31.67	6.27	46.75
Vermont	23.05	47.25	4.11	36.94
Virginia	12.23	27.77	9.64	60.16
Washington	17.37	38.38	6.20	57.30
West Virginia	14.63	25.49	13.04	48.12
Wisconsin	23.20	36.29	3.30	49.00
Wyoming	29.39	41.93	3.33	42.27

TABLE II-10

INCIDENCE OF CONTRACTURES AND USE OF RESTRAINTS BY STATE, 1997

	% With Contractures	% Contractures With Contractures on Admission	% Physically Restrained	% Restrained with Orders on Admission
UNITED STATES	**24.67**	**66.07**	**15.93**	**38.52**
Alabama	23.72	65.94	7.26	23.58
Alaska	18.58	75.65	33.76	26.32
Arizona	19.16	63.32	19.69	39.85
Arkansas	17.44	57.03	24.16	36.27
California	24.11	68.28	26.08	43.66
Colorado	17.45	56.52	18.64	30.61
Connecticut	13.54	55.29	14.97	33.72
Delaware	23.86	54.23	15.52	23.00
District of Columbia	19.68	76.47	15.70	36.23
Florida	18.23	71.03	9.39	30.78
Georgia	21.67	63.11	11.97	31.97
Hawaii	38.91	67.62	20.84	53.22
Idaho	23.43	55.00	16.36	35.29
Illinois	18.50	62.28	11.08	37.12
Indiana	19.78	55.24	16.50	34.45
Iowa	22.87	57.53	3.52	29.14
Kansas	27.78	61.56	5.80	22.99
Kentucky	22.47	67.08	11.52	35.79
Louisiana	15.62	55.62	27.34	38.64
Maine	34.22	67.60	10.59	31.73
Maryland	18.99	63.71	18.41	44.49
Massachusetts	16.87	61.93	17.26	37.36
Michigan	22.99	68.00	14.90	36.49
Minnesota	18.91	52.74	16.47	42.20
Mississippi	35.25	56.62	18.72	22.05
Missouri	18.59	56.97	8.35	30.62
Montana	21.64	53.89	12.19	34.43
Nebraska	21.25	57.15	3.43	27.00
Nevada	19.40	70.63	22.90	53.59
New Hampshire	25.74	70.13	12.82	18.72
New Jersey	18.30	71.62	8.68	22.77
New Mexico	15.80	60.64	20.29	42.08
New York	58.22	79.92	11.92	40.13
North Carolina	29.27	71.09	9.10	29.67
North Dakota	29.26	49.42	15.74	29.74

TABLE II-10 INCIDENCE OF CONTRACTURES AND USE OF RESTRAINTS BY STATE, 1997 (CONTINUED)

	% With Contractures	% Contractures With Contractures on Admission	% Physically Restrained	% Restrained with Orders on Admission
Ohio	41.51	67.46	16.82	44.70
Oklahoma	14.61	63.50	16.23	33.89
Oregon	24.51	62.56	14.93	38.27
Pennsylvania	19.70	62.65	19.11	41.30
Rhode Island	15.65	50.65	11.84	28.48
South Carolina	34.63	72.46	9.86	33.74
South Dakota	39.24	66.37	26.97	35.54
Tennessee	20.03	59.42	16.52	34.93
Texas	17.52	66.40	23.98	47.67
Utah	12.42	64.94	18.24	33.98
Vermont	27.05	49.48	15.98	18.17
Virginia	21.88	68.28	13.85	47.99
Washington	33.42	56.29	18.99	29.48
West Virginia	29.10	46.53	20.26	24.87
Wisconsin	18.03	55.68	26.39	41.35
Wyoming	23.22	41.76	15.91	26.19

Section III

Other Resident Characteristics

TABLE III-1

USE OF PSYCHOACTIVE MEDICATION BY STATE, 1997

	% Psychoactive Medications	% Antipsychotic Medications	% Antianxiety Medications	% Antidepressants	% Hypnotic Medications
UNITED STATES	**45.47**	**17.45**	**15.09**	**24.51**	**5.17**
Alabama	42.53	15.45	13.67	22.98	5.05
Alaska	52.50	16.32	15.02	36.19	6.95
Arizona	44.83	14.41	14.43	26.03	4.79
Arkansas	50.93	23.37	15.13	22.26	4.75
California	39.39	17.59	11.33	18.96	6.20
Colorado	45.80	14.95	13.14	26.50	3.24
Connecticut	49.37	21.62	19.11	25.69	6.08
Delaware	38.19	16.92	17.65	21.35	6.13
District of Columbia	37.25	15.94	9.43	11.95	2.52
Florida	43.02	13.79	15.00	23.32	6.80
Georgia	45.43	20.31	15.25	22.89	6.77
Hawaii	18.02	5.59	4.53	10.38	1.85
Idaho	49.04	14.16	14.16	32.62	3.77
Illinois	43.79	21.60	14.01	20.66	4.29
Indiana	48.65	17.89	17.81	24.85	6.36
Iowa	42.49	12.13	13.94	26.52	3.02
Kansas	48.51	17.61	14.44	28.20	4.52
Kentucky	46.99	17.56	18.13	22.49	7.64
Louisiana	51.54	23.26	16.72	25.52	9.08
Maine	50.85	17.43	18.01	29.50	8.30
Maryland	44.72	17.63	14.47	24.26	3.84
Massachusetts	52.29	20.88	18.45	30.70	4.08
Michigan	39.85	12.65	11.67	22.22	3.61
Minnesota	47.23	16.49	15.58	29.10	3.27
Mississippi	47.15	18.61	15.82	24.11	6.98
Missouri	48.09	17.07	16.34	29.41	5.47
Montana	46.55	13.70	15.75	26.27	4.32
Nebraska	44.93	14.83	15.48	26.83	4.46
Nevada	39.41	13.84	10.42	20.33	6.10
New Hampshire	52.25	16.50	20.37	31.67	3.75
New Jersey	37.06	14.74	10.34	19.54	3.30
New Mexico	37.46	12.15	10.69	23.16	4.03
New York	37.42	16.67	8.58	18.57	2.45
North Carolina	46.63	14.17	17.83	24.06	6.08
North Dakota	47.48	15.37	13.66	29.23	3.50
Ohio	51.09	18.60	17.85	28.99	5.66
Oklahoma	43.11	18.77	15.07	21.90	6.99
Oregon	47.71	15.59	12.90	30.19	3.19
Pennsylvania	47.87	16.89	16.94	27.93	5.68

TABLE III-1: USE OF PSYCHOACTIVE MEDICATION BY STATE, 1997 (CONTINUED)

	% Psychoactive Medications	% Antipsychotic Medications	% Antianxiety Medications	% Antidepressants	% Hypnotic Medications
Rhode Island	51.15	19.87	12.87	30.94	4.56
South Carolina	44.56	14.75	18.18	22.60	5.49
South Dakota	44.74	14.92	14.97	24.75	3.42
Tennessee	51.48	19.24	20.80	26.07	5.07
Texas	48.89	20.42	18.23	23.53	8.25
Utah	53.74	19.70	17.16	31.86	5.79
Vermont	51.37	16.65	14.40	31.87	3.97
Virginia	47.52	17.16	18.20	24.11	5.97
Washington	46.34	13.83	14.34	30.45	3.28
West Virginia	44.40	16.26	15.83	23.71	4.93
Wisconsin	48.16	16.28	16.17	29.16	3.10
Wyoming	45.76	14.89	12.01	26.89	3.83

TABLE III-2

OTHER MEDICATION CHARACTERISTICS BY STATE, 1997

	% Antibiotic Medication	% Pain Management	% Chemotherapy	% IV Therapy / Feed	Drug Error Rate (%)
UNITED STATES	**7.87**	**7.84**	**0.28**	**0.99**	**0.84**
Alabama	7.06	5.14	0.15	0.66	1.89
Alaska	10.34	8.40	0.65	2.75	0.00
Arizona	9.95	8.59	0.18	2.56	1.37
Arkansas	7.49	4.67	0.08	0.99	2.01
California	8.36	5.63	0.14	1.78	0.93
Colorado	7.79	11.34	0.16	0.90	0.68
Connecticut	6.35	4.33	0.29	0.43	0.23
Delaware	8.41	7.22	0.03	0.98	0.70
District of Columbia	4.97	7.63	0.24	0.65	1.67
Florida	8.53	5.07	0.10	1.26	1.04
Georgia	7.00	5.04	0.15	0.55	1.77
Hawaii	7.01	5.73	0.20	1.00	0.07
Idaho	9.06	15.59	0.15	0.94	0.06
Illinois	6.78	5.19	0.16	0.94	0.66
Indiana	8.22	7.02	0.21	1.41	0.62
Iowa	8.36	15.71	0.27	0.46	0.65
Kansas	9.29	12.36	0.27	0.74	0.25
Kentucky	9.43	3.81	0.16	1.33	1.05
Louisiana	7.01	5.07	0.17	1.16	2.55
Maine	8.33	10.93	0.63	0.78	0.28
Maryland	7.57	6.52	0.16	0.88	0.37
Massachusetts	7.46	5.22	0.18	0.74	0.67
Michigan	7.49	14.59	0.19	0.60	0.19
Minnesota	7.09	16.06	0.19	0.34	0.29
Mississippi	9.33	5.21	0.69	1.31	0.59
Missouri	7.76	6.02	0.23	1.32	1.31
Montana	7.69	13.47	0.21	0.48	1.32
Nebraska	8.23	17.04	0.42	0.81	0.20
Nevada	7.95	6.12	0.27	2.23	1.20
New Hampshire	6.60	15.05	0.30	0.37	0.43
New Jersey	5.68	6.56	0.15	0.43	1.15
New Mexico	6.37	8.60	0.10	0.91	0.79
New York	6.93	8.10	1.21	0.47	0.17
North Carolina	8.42	7.42	0.19	0.81	0.82
North Dakota	8.55	16.72	0.27	0.44	0.34
Ohio	9.05	6.51	0.36	1.27	0.39
Oklahoma	7.67	6.71	0.14	0.98	1.52
Oregon	8.86	20.73	0.20	1.18	0.36
Pennsylvania	8.10	7.07	0.35	1.22	0.54

TABLE III-2: OTHER MEDICATION CHARACTERISTICS BY STATE, 1997 (CONTINUED)

	% Antibiotic Medication	% Pain Management	% Chemotherapy	% IV Therapy / Feed	Drug Error Rate (%)
Rhode Island	6.84	5.21	0.20	0.61	0.24
South Carolina	7.10	6.45	0.21	0.65	1.03
South Dakota	10.09	14.87	0.63	0.98	0.85
Tennessee	7.76	5.68	0.13	0.92	0.45
Texas	8.33	3.64	0.18	1.12	1.73
Utah	10.54	13.79	0.08	1.51	0.33
Vermont	7.64	8.12	1.07	0.82	0.86
Virginia	8.38	5.68	0.17	1.02	0.44
Washington	8.81	15.56	0.19	1.52	0.63
West Virginia	10.43	7.78	0.46	1.63	0.88
Wisconsin	7.81	18.44	0.26	0.62	0.54
Wyoming	9.28	11.59	0.00	0.64	0.11

TABLE III-3

RESIDENT SKIN CARE CHARACTERISTICS BY STATE, 1997

	% With Pressure Sores	Nosocomial pressure sore rate (%)	% Receiving Preventative Skin Care	% With Rashes
UNITED STATES	**6.62**	**3.38**	**52.08**	**4.23**
Alabama	6.26	3.26	48.24	3.45
Alaska	6.46	4.36	72.38	9.05
Arizona	7.75	3.89	55.17	3.55
Arkansas	7.18	4.35	43.60	3.31
California	8.28	3.36	47.07	4.97
Colorado	5.45	3.25	54.79	2.91
Connecticut	4.60	2.61	42.15	3.01
Delaware	6.73	4.17	43.62	3.67
District of Columbia	10.73	4.46	51.65	2.79
Florida	7.66	2.77	55.37	4.13
Georgia	7.44	4.21	46.17	3.31
Hawaii	4.79	2.48	61.86	6.50
Idaho	4.73	2.53	46.95	4.79
Illinois	6.73	3.53	49.49	3.89
Indiana	6.30	3.96	54.87	3.50
Iowa	3.79	2.28	45.03	3.03
Kansas	5.44	3.32	56.25	4.99
Kentucky	6.74	3.83	47.74	3.23
Louisiana	7.12	3.80	41.87	4.28
Maine	4.88	2.62	73.56	6.90
Maryland	8.39	3.84	58.11	2.57
Massachusetts	5.67	3.42	59.49	3.44
Michigan	6.74	3.32	52.98	3.84
Minnesota	3.74	2.29	43.96	5.17
Mississippi	6.72	3.76	54.11	5.16
Missouri	5.86	3.16	46.54	3.58
Montana	3.76	2.56	41.98	4.18
Nebraska	3.59	2.15	55.78	5.40
Nevada	8.40	0.58	56.00	3.95
New Hampshire	4.61	3.18	55.97	4.62
New Jersey	7.85	3.56	38.68	3.11
New Mexico	5.75	2.20	53.10	3.38
New York	6.87	3.16	51.03	5.58
North Carolina	7.54	4.08	56.67	3.45
North Dakota	2.79	1.77	42.14	5.57

TABLE III-3: RESIDENT SKIN CARE CHARACTERISTICS BY STATE, 1997 (CONTINUED)

	% With Pressure Sores	Nosocomial pressure sore rate (%)	% Receiving Preventative Skin Care	% With Rashes
Ohio	6.01	2.85	75.96	5.76
Oklahoma	6.81	4.03	41.74	3.32
Oregon	6.48	3.47	51.41	4.81
Pennsylvania	7.35	3.89	53.18	3.86
Rhode Island	5.10	2.14	43.48	3.66
South Carolina	6.87	3.05	61.27	3.51
South Dakota	4.50	2.53	83.61	6.68
Tennessee	6.82	3.49	50.35	3.29
Texas	7.80	4.36	46.46	3.77
Utah	5.51	2.49	52.78	4.76
Vermont	4.79	3.01	65.68	7.75
Virginia	8.15	3.79	49.22	3.41
Washington	6.25	3.41	64.29	7.51
West Virginia	6.79	4.02	78.44	8.28
Wisconsin	4.93	3.01	48.91	4.32
Wyoming	4.17	2.88	62.16	4.70

Table III-4
Resident Special Treatments by State, 1997

	% Trach Care	% Suctioning	% Rehab. Services	% Ostomy Care	% Radiation Therapy	% Hospice Benefit	% Dialysis	% Tube Feeding	% Eating Assistive Devices	% Mechanically Altered Diets	% Unplanned Weight Loss/Gain
UNITED STATES	0.76	1.67	15.16	2.66	0.12	0.91	0.72	6.86	9.24	37.25	7.69
Alabama	0.37	2.28	11.66	4.70	0.07	0.42	0.54	12.15	6.43	40.60	6.64
Alaska	3.55	5.98	40.07	4.36	0.48	0.00	0.81	14.22	14.70	36.51	10.99
Arizona	1.27	2.12	16.95	1.77	0.13	1.78	1.01	5.02	9.05	38.36	8.72
Arkansas	0.39	1.27	10.83	2.35	0.09	0.55	0.56	5.82	4.20	35.56	9.61
California	1.83	3.21	13.53	2.91	0.18	1.26	0.92	10.37	7.13	41.81	7.36
Colorado	0.62	0.87	17.71	2.03	0.09	1.33	0.53	3.41	11.61	35.43	8.23
Connecticut	0.49	1.10	16.60	1.90	0.15	0.36	0.78	4.51	10.59	36.75	5.69
Delaware	1.37	2.30	20.18	2.43	0.10	0.78	0.91	8.77	6.75	33.74	8.41
District of Columbia	0.85	2.55	10.25	2.15	0.10	0.27	5.89	13.96	2.38	35.99	5.24
Florida	0.76	1.71	20.72	2.57	0.14	2.18	0.81	8.80	9.95	39.71	6.15
Georgia	0.47	2.09	13.60	1.94	0.05	1.13	0.97	8.64	6.97	38.31	7.14
Hawaii	1.43	4.48	17.42	4.53	0.26	0.14	0.88	15.11	7.84	55.87	7.13
Idaho	0.17	0.90	19.50	1.44	0.08	0.36	0.67	1.93	13.39	38.79	7.91
Illinois	0.69	1.29	14.80	3.37	0.12	1.08	0.64	5.17	5.97	30.28	8.64
Indiana	0.72	1.71	13.85	2.44	0.12	0.78	0.63	6.19	9.08	34.64	8.63
Iowa	0.33	0.73	11.74	2.05	0.07	0.67	0.35	2.07	17.64	31.12	7.25
Kansas	0.19	0.70	12.31	1.75	0.07	0.92	0.32	2.25	11.37	34.68	8.10
Kentucky	0.93	2.87	12.27	2.83	0.09	0.93	0.49	10.94	8.17	40.48	6.89
Louisiana	0.74	1.86	10.83	3.13	0.17	0.41	0.98	8.48	3.10	24.17	7.96
Maine	0.45	1.06	13.38	2.68	0.19	0.30	0.30	2.69	13.80	45.04	8.96
Maryland	0.68	2.72	13.63	2.45	0.13	0.72	0.99	10.25	5.14	37.65	6.66
Massachusetts	0.70	1.26	16.58	2.16	0.14	0.49	0.57	4.18	12.56	39.79	6.68
Michigan	0.70	1.38	16.05	2.31	0.07	0.94	0.74	5.60	11.52	36.71	7.80

TABLE III-4: RESIDENT SPECIAL TREATMENTS BY STATE, 1997 (CONTINUED)

	% Trach Care	% Suctioning	% Rehab. Services	% Ostomy Care	% Radiation Therapy	% Hospice Benefit	% Dialysis	% Tube Feeding	% Eating Assistive Devices	% Mechanically Altered Diets	% Unplanned Weight Loss/Gain
Minnesota	0.35	0.60	16.08	2.15	0.06	0.55	0.61	2.30	13.33	27.84	7.34
Mississippi	0.28	0.95	13.18	4.86	0.11	0.08	0.50	8.71	4.87	42.82	8.25
Missouri	0.54	1.25	16.15	2.13	0.36	1.69	0.70	4.96	8.36	36.18	8.84
Montana	0.30	0.82	15.25	1.73	0.13	0.35	0.26	2.34	12.53	30.71	8.92
Nebraska	0.70	1.04	11.43	2.53	0.15	0.79	0.47	2.86	14.89	29.00	7.86
Nevada	0.93	2.12	18.42	2.25	0.16	1.06	0.56	8.88	4.27	38.56	7.53
New Hampshire	0.23	0.50	22.73	1.94	0.07	0.97	0.19	1.80	13.89	38.57	8.92
New Jersey	1.14	2.03	13.94	2.30	0.10	0.59	0.70	8.14	5.38	36.51	6.62
New Mexico	0.34	1.03	17.71	1.73	0.13	1.00	0.90	3.53	10.56	40.99	10.09
New York	1.08	1.80	19.12	4.22	0.11	0.43	0.76	8.31	12.14	36.62	6.03
North Carolina	0.58	1.87	14.13	2.65	0.10	0.67	0.91	9.93	7.88	43.49	7.91
North Dakota	0.46	0.86	22.30	2.42	0.19	0.64	0.41	2.76	17.52	28.21	9.85
Ohio	0.99	1.88	13.47	3.63	0.11	1.05	0.80	8.26	10.99	37.68	8.33
Oklahoma	0.47	1.47	14.54	1.90	0.11	2.44	0.52	6.19	3.83	33.41	9.57
Oregon	0.62	1.55	13.25	2.19	0.08	0.75	0.58	4.44	13.88	42.38	9.17
Pennsylvania	0.73	1.63	17.93	2.32	0.15	0.86	0.71	7.14	11.02	41.55	8.19
Rhode Island	0.30	0.88	10.32	1.96	0.07	0.85	0.55	3.28	8.44	38.60	6.11
South Carolina	0.43	1.64	15.27	3.30	0.05	0.53	0.67	9.80	7.14	46.77	5.78
South Dakota	0.22	0.50	13.33	2.26	0.13	0.39	0.35	2.03	16.82	33.25	8.27
Tennessee	0.54	2.01	16.22	1.79	0.09	0.28	0.68	8.20	6.21	39.82	9.17
Texas	0.56	1.52	11.87	2.15	0.12	1.66	0.80	7.70	4.33	37.73	8.01
Utah	0.54	1.08	21.34	1.95	0.03	0.53	0.53	2.68	8.28	34.32	8.96
Vermont	0.37	0.48	14.77	2.56	0.03	0.39	0.37	3.33	12.17	36.29	11.05
Virginia	0.97	2.68	13.35	2.53	0.08	0.25	0.95	8.03	8.43	39.35	6.85
Washington	0.51	1.23	18.47	2.29	0.18	0.82	0.55	4.92	16.03	42.77	9.63
West Virginia	0.46	1.37	13.45	3.60	0.34	0.07	1.14	7.18	7.13	48.29	9.68
Wisconsin	0.42	0.81	16.45	1.91	0.08	0.40	0.54	2.85	13.95	34.11	7.43
Wyoming	0.27	0.61	12.01	1.52	0.08	0.19	0.42	1.52	14.09	32.73	10.68

SECTION III: OTHER RESIDENT CHARACTERISTICS

TABLE III-5

COMMUNICATION AND ADVANCE DIRECTIVES BY STATE, 1997

	% Not Dominant Language	% Non-Oral Communication Devices	% With Advance Directives
UNITED STATES	**2.39**	**2.38**	**54.84**
Alabama	0.49	2.17	33.71
Alaska	6.79	9.21	56.87
Arizona	5.13	2.66	74.87
Arkansas	0.64	1.38	53.49
California	7.58	2.91	45.90
Colorado	2.13	2.71	77.65
Connecticut	3.06	0.86	64.46
Delaware	1.32	1.19	61.27
District of Columbia	1.12	0.92	27.07
Florida	3.16	1.48	58.57
Georgia	0.46	0.92	41.72
Hawaii	15.56	6.84	61.09
Idaho	1.17	4.46	58.18
Illinois	1.84	1.99	56.40
Indiana	1.02	2.56	60.86
Iowa	0.37	2.11	64.63
Kansas	0.55	3.72	68.53
Kentucky	0.55	0.97	49.57
Louisiana	1.69	2.69	46.89
Maine	4.54	3.01	75.01
Maryland	1.45	1.56	49.15
Massachusetts	3.26	1.49	54.62
Michigan	1.27	1.94	69.18
Minnesota	0.79	2.36	47.20
Mississippi	1.00	4.11	32.05
Missouri	0.63	2.41	51.83
Montana	0.69	2.95	76.17
Nebraska	0.63	4.14	69.93
Nevada	2.17	4.51	50.52
New Hampshire	1.66	3.46	78.35
New Jersey	3.37	2.16	38.79
New Mexico	7.79	6.61	65.88
New York	5.02	1.33	58.38
North Carolina	0.44	1.44	42.33
North Dakota	0.28	1.98	56.62
Ohio	1.19	5.10	58.11
Oklahoma	0.98	1.78	33.44
Oregon	1.65	4.46	46.42
Pennsylvania	1.22	1.08	57.97

TABLE III-5: COMMUNICATION AND ADVANCE DIRECTIVES BY STATE, 1997 (CONTINUED)

	% Not Dominant Language	% Non-Oral Communication Devices	% With Advance Directives
Rhode Island	3.13	2.18	58.80
South Carolina	0.40	1.44	47.84
South Dakota	1.10	9.85	60.57
Tennessee	0.54	1.85	44.14
Texas	4.21	1.94	49.09
Utah	2.58	3.71	70.22
Vermont	1.24	4.79	65.37
Virginia	0.77	1.57	52.99
Washington	2.14	5.21	69.37
West Virginia	1.06	11.11	70.72
Wisconsin	0.77	2.17	74.48
Wyoming	1.55	7.31	80.72

TABLE III-6

MENTAL STATUS BY STATE, 1997

	% Retarded	% Depressed	% With Psychiatric Diagnosis	% With Dementia	% With Behavior Symptoms	% of Behavior Symptoms Receiving Behavior Management Program	% Receiving Health Rehab for MI/MR
UNITED STATES	**2.79**	**24.04**	**13.09**	**43.97**	**29.10**	**53.90**	**4.14**
Alabama	5.15	21.14	11.73	49.58	24.48	66.82	3.20
Alaska	6.14	27.14	12.12	33.44	32.47	24.88	5.33
Arizona	0.99	25.20	8.61	42.07	28.29	35.11	0.99
Arkansas	4.86	20.73	15.30	36.61	26.66	39.28	1.94
California	2.88	22.26	14.02	38.36	29.22	53.52	5.77
Colorado	1.97	27.27	11.98	48.40	33.88	52.50	8.98
Connecticut	1.86	18.76	12.47	42.79	23.26	44.98	2.90
Delaware	2.46	22.43	9.26	42.61	38.55	63.02	1.89
District of Columbia	1.67	11.00	14.51	45.66	18.73	79.27	6.10
Florida	1.32	21.87	10.27	43.05	22.80	55.99	2.78
Georgia	4.43	17.72	13.21	45.51	23.52	36.91	5.27
Hawaii	2.54	12.43	3.45	50.57	22.15	63.58	0.09
Idaho	2.62	36.93	9.18	46.90	35.11	76.52	1.63
Illinois	2.23	23.91	19.47	33.12	33.69	65.82	9.10
Indiana	4.29	25.59	12.27	40.66	28.97	48.83	4.03
Iowa	3.60	27.89	10.26	47.18	27.98	41.82	2.70
Kansas	2.82	32.22	14.75	44.90	30.50	59.75	3.40
Kentucky	4.51	18.39	11.27	47.01	29.57	60.08	1.31
Louisiana	3.50	21.75	18.62	35.26	21.52	21.74	1.45
Maine	3.13	31.08	8.05	53.49	33.07	62.91	3.14
Maryland	2.50	21.35	13.74	44.26	21.96	49.49	4.45
Massachusetts	3.17	25.30	17.10	44.35	35.81	53.37	12.31
Michigan	2.08	22.93	10.61	53.42	29.43	64.02	7.97
Minnesota	1.98	27.69	14.59	42.33	48.57	73.16	3.56
Mississippi	2.69	25.19	17.19	51.40	26.90	42.78	2.26
Missouri	3.42	28.32	14.38	41.11	29.02	47.11	2.58
Montana	2.63	26.81	11.28	46.76	29.46	55.57	1.68
Nebraska	3.53	32.29	12.33	39.03	34.24	46.44	2.17
Nevada	1.83	31.30	12.19	41.56	29.71	34.52	1.48
New Hampshire	1.87	33.30	12.44	45.28	36.94	34.81	8.52
New Jersey	2.66	20.43	12.90	39.83	22.87	55.63	1.77
New Mexico	2.12	23.13	7.57	48.86	28.68	39.67	1.63
New York	2.38	15.57	11.29	47.90	26.95	55.87	1.33
North Carolina	2.30	20.96	9.87	46.73	25.41	38.58	1.54
North Dakota	3.10	26.98	13.17	42.87	35.65	83.89	6.00

TABLE III-6: MENTAL STATUS BY STATE, 1997 (CONTINUED)

	% Retarded	% Depressed	% With Psychiatric Diagnosis	% With Dementia	% With Behavior Symptoms	% of Behavior Symptoms Receiving Behavior Management Program	% Receiving Health Rehab for MI/MR
Ohio	2.75	38.17	18.04	49.44	37.80	66.99	4.81
Oklahoma	4.03	22.23	10.91	39.94	25.42	52.35	3.52
Oregon	3.04	31.86	10.87	48.67	29.90	71.78	3.25
Pennsylvania	2.15	23.38	10.21	45.78	28.42	57.63	2.00
Rhode Island	1.67	18.97	10.03	49.21	23.62	36.94	7.54
South Carolina	2.14	17.78	8.71	55.97	27.15	40.17	1.02
South Dakota	2.93	28.79	10.33	43.17	33.06	69.98	5.61
Tennessee	2.83	25.14	12.25	47.78	28.20	57.59	9.97
Texas	2.80	19.12	13.00	42.14	23.02	34.34	1.86
Utah	3.37	28.93	11.48	46.66	28.96	23.10	3.66
Vermont	1.92	38.60	11.86	43.51	38.88	35.65	3.49
Virginia	3.92	20.52	10.98	45.26	27.64	39.22	2.40
Washington	4.40	36.70	10.62	53.13	33.22	70.02	9.05
West Virginia	4.45	36.14	12.47	47.33	33.75	20.26	1.90
Wisconsin	1.54	26.60	12.72	42.66	30.58	51.14	2.38
Wyoming	2.65	28.07	9.55	46.06	25.49	41.01	1.29

TABLE III-7

PAYOR MIX AND CENSUS BY STATE, 1997

	Medicare Census	Medicare %	Medicaid Census	Medicaid %	Other Census	Other %	Total Census
UNITED STATES	**138,211**	**9.20**	**1,015,742**	**67.58**	**349,149**	**23.23**	**1,503,102**
Alabama	2,149	9.46	16,454	72.39	4,126	18.15	22,729
Alaska	60	9.69	496	80.13	63	10.18	619
Arizona	1,675	12.13	7,811	56.54	4,329	31.34	13,815
Arkansas	1,556	7.60	15,358	74.98	3,569	17.42	20,483
California	10,018	9.27	70,191	64.92	27,911	25.82	108,120
Colorado	1,379	8.17	10,437	61.82	5,066	30.01	16,882
Connecticut	3,545	11.77	20,231	67.18	6,340	21.05	30,116
Delaware	520	13.45	2,019	52.24	1,326	34.31	3,865
District of Columbia	232	7.90	2,466	83.96	239	8.14	2,937
Florida	9,433	14.48	41,632	63.92	14,066	21.60	65,131
Georgia	2,674	7.46	28,168	78.60	4,996	13.94	35,838
Hawaii	262	7.47	2,589	73.80	657	18.73	3,508
Idaho	572	11.97	3,013	63.03	1,195	25.00	4,780
Illinois	6,043	7.10	54,361	63.91	24,655	28.99	85,059
Indiana	4,347	9.72	29,024	64.90	11,349	25.38	44,720
Iowa	1,184	3.88	15,214	49.84	14,129	46.28	30,527
Kansas	1,379	5.74	12,526	52.18	10,102	42.08	24,007
Kentucky	2,202	9.88	16,691	74.88	3,396	15.24	22,289
Louisiana	1,768	5.72	24,907	80.55	4,248	13.74	30,923
Maine	846	10.26	6,031	73.16	1,367	16.58	8,244
Maryland	2,369	9.10	17,118	65.75	6,548	25.15	26,035
Massachusetts	5,625	10.92	36,321	70.49	9,578	18.59	51,524
Michigan	5,619	12.75	29,223	66.33	9,215	20.92	44,057
Minnesota	3,231	7.73	26,236	62.79	12,318	29.48	41,785
Mississippi	1,346	8.48	12,352	77.86	2,167	13.66	15,865
Missouri	3,787	9.29	26,076	63.96	10,907	26.75	40,770
Montana	486	7.79	3,683	58.99	2,074	33.22	6,243
Nebraska	872	5.58	8,368	53.50	6,401	40.92	15,641
Nevada	436	11.56	2,353	62.36	984	26.08	3,773
New Hampshire	462	6.30	5,091	69.42	1,781	24.28	7,334
New Jersey	3,328	7.39	32,235	71.55	9,489	21.06	45,052
New Mexico	423	6.91	4,280	69.87	1,423	23.23	6,126
New York	11,431	11.00	78,860	75.87	13,657	13.14	103,948
North Carolina	4,268	11.51	27,159	73.25	5,651	15.24	37,078
North Dakota	281	4.15	3,742	55.27	2,748	40.59	6,771
Ohio	7,318	8.77	55,616	66.68	20,474	24.55	83,408
Oklahoma	1,233	4.86	16,898	66.55	7,262	28.60	25,393
Oregon	912	8.07	6,814	60.28	3,578	31.65	11,304
Pennsylvania	8,525	9.80	55,043	63.24	23,469	26.96	87,037

TABLE III-7: PAYOR MIX AND CENSUS BY STATE, 1997 (CONTINUED)

	Medicare Census	Medicare %	Medicaid Census	Medicaid %	Other Census	Other %	Total Census
Rhode Island	832	8.85	6,900	73.41	1,667	17.74	9,399
South Carolina	1,632	10.91	10,670	71.30	2,662	17.79	14,964
South Dakota	509	6.64	4,473	58.33	2,687	35.04	7,669
Tennessee	3,574	10.23	25,383	72.62	5,995	17.15	34,952
Texas	7,794	8.90	65,160	74.41	14,614	16.69	87,568
Utah	685	11.60	3,583	60.69	1,636	27.71	5,904
Vermont	327	9.21	2,283	64.33	939	26.46	3,549
Virginia	2,289	8.45	18,274	67.46	6,524	24.09	27,087
Washington	2,383	10.39	14,621	63.77	5,925	25.84	22,929
West Virginia	886	8.57	7,670	74.16	1,786	17.27	10,342
Wisconsin	3,333	7.87	27,944	65.96	11,086	26.17	42,363
Wyoming	171	6.48	1,694	64.17	775	29.36	2,640

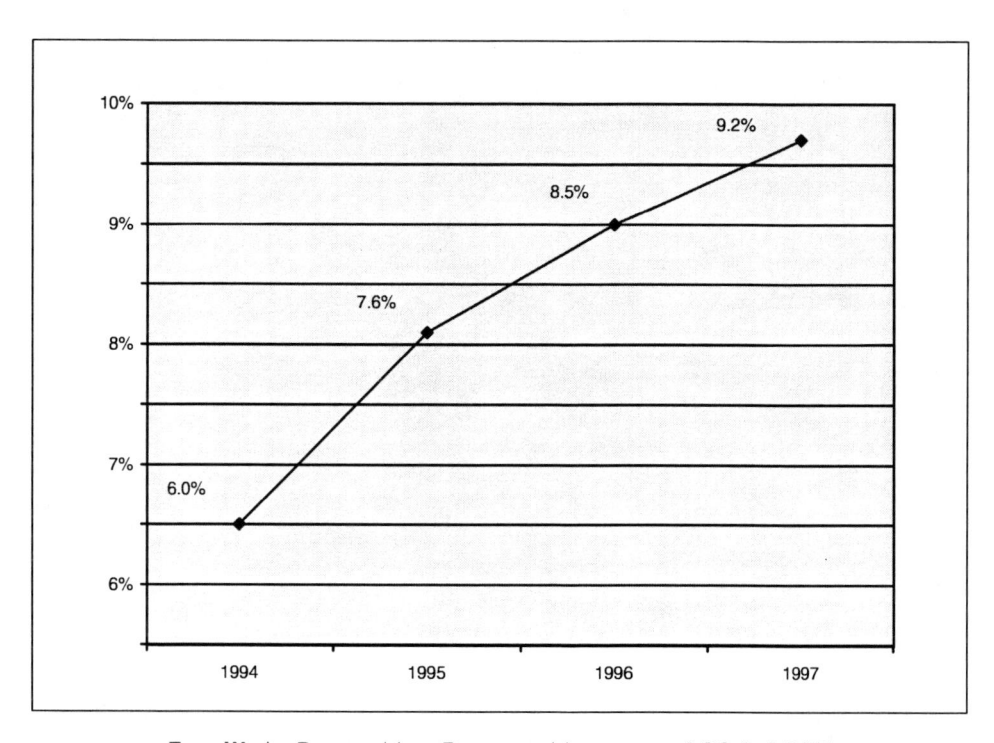

FIG. III-A: PAYOR MIX, PERCENT MEDICARE, 1994–1997

SECTION IV

SURVEY DEFICIENCIES

TABLE IV-1

TOTAL AND NURSING DEFICIENCIES BY STATE, 1997

	Total Deficiencies	Nursing Deficiencies
UNITED STATES	**5.49**	**3.06**
Alabama	6.25	3.53
Alaska	4.06	3.13
Arizona	5.15	2.22
Arkansas	7.29	4.20
California	10.48	5.66
Colorado	3.24	2.36
Connecticut	2.75	1.98
Delaware	7.86	4.02
District of Columbia	5.57	1.52
Florida	6.59	3.38
Georgia	4.20	2.39
Hawaii	5.16	2.81
Idaho	6.94	3.76
Illinois	6.19	3.55
Indiana	6.99	3.25
Iowa	5.09	2.77
Kansas	6.42	3.86
Kentucky	4.23	2.65
Louisiana	4.84	2.05
Maine	3.41	2.06
Maryland	3.45	1.96
Massachusetts	4.10	2.43
Michigan	8.93	5.10
Minnesota	3.79	2.44
Mississippi	4.53	2.61
Missouri	4.60	2.76
Montana	4.83	3.23
Nebraska	4.09	2.27
Nevada	13.80	7.40
New Hampshire	4.20	2.75
New Jersey	3.57	1.73
New Mexico	2.92	1.60
New York	3.15	2.07
North Carolina	4.64	2.89
North Dakota	6.84	3.60
Ohio	4.75	2.80
Oklahoma	4.98	2.69
Oregon	5.67	4.06
Pennsylvania	3.98	2.32

TABLE IV-1: TOTAL AND NURSING DEFICIENCIES BY STATE, 1997 (CONTINUED)

	Total Deficiencies	Nursing Deficiencies
Rhode Island	3.59	1.96
South Carolina	7.59	4.74
South Dakota	4.31	3.05
Tennessee	3.96	2.27
Texas	4.68	2.12
Utah	4.29	2.41
Vermont	3.64	2.34
Virginia	4.46	2.36
Washington	8.65	5.13
West Virginia	6.00	2.43
Wisconsin	3.90	2.37
Wyoming	6.42	4.05

TABLE IV-2

TOTAL DEFICIENCIES BY CLASS OF OWNERSHIP AND STATE, 1997

	For Profit	Non-Profit	Government
UNITED STATES	**5.99**	**4.49**	**4.80**
Alabama	6.50	4.40	6.77
Alaska	4.00	4.78	3.00
Arizona	5.43	4.50	7.25
Arkansas	7.46	6.85	5.92
California	11.03	8.54	10.63
Colorado	3.63	2.46	2.86
Connecticut	2.84	2.36	4.50
Delaware	7.63	8.10	7.75
District of Columbia	7.43	5.08	2.00
Florida	7.20	4.58	4.75
Georgia	4.24	4.47	3.00
Hawaii	5.67	4.93	4.64
Idaho	6.94	4.93	8.35
Illinois	6.76	5.09	5.59
Indiana	7.36	5.84	6.20
Iowa	5.35	4.91	3.78
Kansas	7.43	5.61	4.54
Kentucky	4.47	3.60	5.70
Louisiana	5.17	4.43	2.65
Maine	3.30	3.81	3.20
Maryland	3.85	2.84	3.75
Massachusetts	4.43	3.23	3.33
Michigan	9.41	8.41	7.30
Minnesota	4.07	3.46	4.37
Mississippi	4.67	3.54	5.00
Missouri	5.01	3.86	3.63
Montana	5.38	5.02	3.35
Nebraska	4.36	3.51	4.37
Nevada	14.40	12.80	10.60
New Hampshire	4.63	3.76	3.62
New Jersey	3.99	2.85	2.75
New Mexico	3.22	2.54	2.38
New York	3.05	3.19	3.57
North Carolina	5.20	3.04	3.39
North Dakota	9.00	6.61	5.00
Ohio	4.96	4.20	4.06
Oklahoma	5.31	3.61	3.56
Oregon	5.70	5.00	8.83
Pennsylvania	4.84	3.34	3.72

Table IV-2: Total Deficiencies by Class of Ownership and State, 1997 (Continued)

	For Profit	Non-Profit	Government
Rhode Island	3.91	2.58	n/a
South Carolina	8.14	5.77	6.00
South Dakota	4.15	4.41	4.20
Tennessee	3.97	3.73	4.43
Texas	4.99	3.55	2.21
Utah	4.22	4.67	4.25
Vermont	3.61	3.90	2.00
Virginia	5.09	3.13	4.92
Washington	9.38	7.06	6.82
West Virginia	6.40	5.34	4.93
Wisconsin	4.07	3.88	3.39
Wyoming	6.22	6.83	6.50

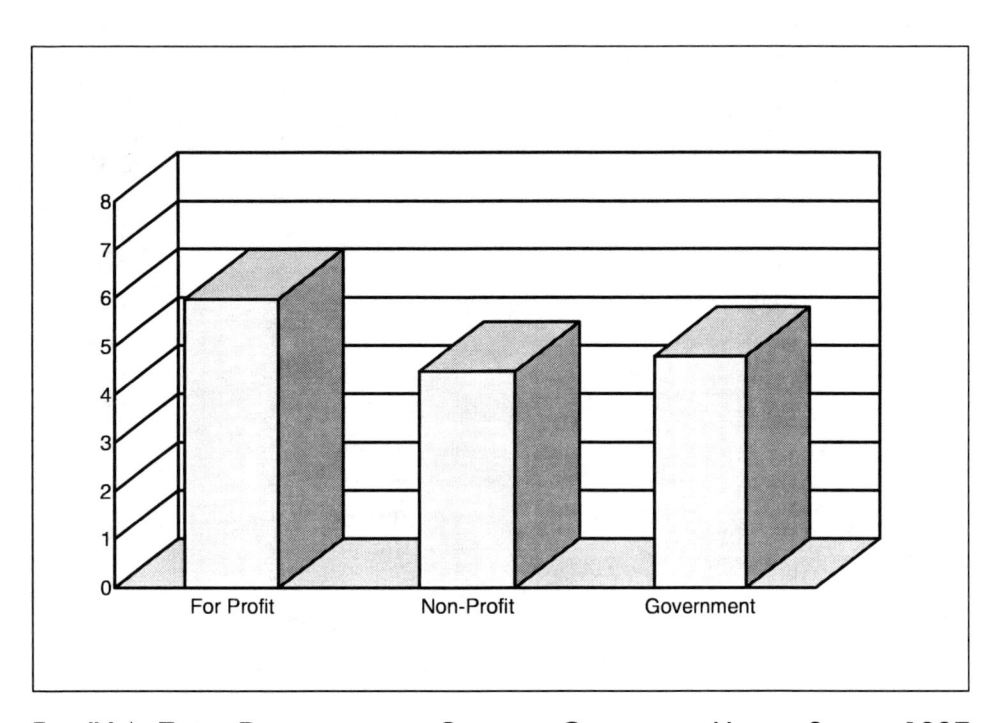

Fig. IV-A: Total Deficiencies by Class of Ownership, United States, 1997

Section IV: Survey Deficiencies

TABLE IV-3

TOP 40 DEFICIENCIES: UNITED STATES, 1997

Rank	Tag	Requirement	% of Facilities Cited
1	F371	Food sanitation	24.85
2	F272	Comprehensive assessments	21.93
3	F279	Comprehensive care plan	20.65
4	F323	Hazard-free environment	18.46
5	F314	Pressure sores	17.00
6	F221	Physical restraints	15.85
7	F309	Highest practicable care	15.51
8	F253	Housekeeping	15.10
9	F241	Dignity	14.84
10	F324	Accident prevention	11.87
11	F329	Drugs	11.74
12	F316	Bladder treatment	11.30
13	F312	ADL services	11.05
14	F441	Infection control	10.79
15	F514	Records complete	10.11
16	F246	Accommodate needs	9.87
17	F248	Activities program	9.61
18	F318	Range of motion treatment	9.23
19	F325	Nutrition	9.13
20	F281	Professional standards	8.84
21	F250	Social services	8.73
22	F364	Food quality	8.45
23	F465	Other environment	8.12
24	F252	Environment-safe, clean	8.01
25	F164	Privacy/confidentiality	7.59
26	F332	Medication errors >5%	5.93
27	F280	Plan requirements	5.85
28	F157	Notice of changes	5.83
29	F311	Appropriate ADL treatment	5.67
30	F225	Criminal staff/abuse	5.65
31	F274	Assessment-condition change	5.60
32	F444	Hand washing	5.29
33	F276	Assessment review	5.22
34	F282	Assessment by qualified staff	5.13
35	F278	Accuracy of assessments	4.95
36	F363	Menus/nutritional adequacy	4.88
37	F322	NG treatment	4.55
38	F458	Square footage	4.35
39	F353	Sufficient staff	4.26
40	F156	Notice of rights/services	4.22

Table IV-4

Most Frequently Cited Deficiencies, 1997: Alabama

Rank	Tag	Requirement	% of Facilities Cited
1	F279	Comprehensive care plan	43.30
2	F314	Pressure sores	42.86
3	F371	Food sanitation	30.36
4	F250	Social services	27.23
5	F316	Bladder treatment	26.79
6	F272	Comprehensive assessments	23.66
7	F221	Physical restraints	19.64
8	F353	Sufficient staff	16.52
9	F241	Dignity	14.73
10	F274	Assessment-condition change	14.73
11	F323	Hazard-free environment	14.29
12	F329	Drugs	14.29
13	F332	Medication errors >5%	13.84
14	F325	Nutrition	12.95
15	F281	Professional standards	12.50
16	F312	ADL services	12.50
17	F166	Resolve grievances	10.27
18	F282	Assessment by qualified staff	10.27
19	F322	NG treatment	9.38
20	F363	Menus/nutritional adequacy	8.93
21	F432	Act on drug reports	8.93
22	F246	Accommodate needs	8.48
23	F324	Accident prevention	8.48
24	F225	Criminal staff/abuse	8.04
25	F248	Activities program	7.14
26	F318	Range of motion treatment	6.70
27	F364	Food quality	6.70
28	F465	Other environment	6.70
29	F254	Clean linens	6.25
30	F156	Notice of rights/services	5.80
31	F252	Environment-safe, clean	5.80
32	F327	Hydration	5.80
33	F309	Highest practicable care	5.36
34	F311	Appropriate ADL treatment	5.36
35	F458	Square footage	4.91
36	F498	N.A. proficiency	4.91
37	F331	Antipsychotic dose reductions	4.46
38	F333	Significant medication errors	4.46
39	F366	Food substitutions	4.46
40	F469	Pest control	4.46

Table IV-4 (continued)

Most Frequently Cited Deficiencies, 1997: Alaska

Rank	Tag	Requirement	% of Facilities Cited
1	F272	Comprehensive assessments	50.00
2	F279	Comprehensive care plan	31.25
3	F309	Highest practicable care	31.25
4	F274	Assessment-condition change	25.00
5	F221	Physical restraints	18.75
6	F324	Accident prevention	18.75
7	F246	Accommodate needs	12.50
8	F248	Activities program	12.50
9	F273	Assessment 14 days after adm.	12.50
10	F275	Annual assessments	12.50
11	F276	Assessment review	12.50
12	F318	Range of motion treatment	12.50
13	F322	NG treatment	12.50
14	F323	Hazard-free environment	12.50
15	F371	Food sanitation	12.50
16	F157	Notice of changes	6.25
17	F159	Manage funds-facility	6.25
18	F241	Dignity	6.25
19	F242	Self determination	6.25
20	F250	Social services	6.25
21	F252	Environment-safe, clean	6.25
22	F253	Housekeeping	6.25
23	F258	Comfortable sound	6.25
24	F278	Accuracy of assessments	6.25
25	F312	ADL services	6.25
26	F319	Mental/psychosocial services	6.25
27	F325	Nutrition	6.25
28	F327	Hydration	6.25
29	F353	Sufficient staff	6.25
30	F372	Garbage	6.25
31	F428	Drug regimen review monthly	6.25
32	F429	Drug records	6.25
33	F441	Infection control	6.25
34	F496	N.A. verification	6.25

TABLE IV-4 (CONTINUED)

MOST FREQUENTLY CITED DEFICIENCIES, 1997: ARIZONA

Rank	Tag	Requirement	% of Facilities Cited
1	F371	Food sanitation	53.94
2	F323	Hazard-free environment	45.45
3	F253	Housekeeping	31.52
4	F441	Infection control	27.88
5	F221	Physical restraints	18.79
6	F272	Comprehensive assessments	17.58
7	F279	Comprehensive care plan	14.55
8	F241	Dignity	13.33
9	F281	Professional standards	11.52
10	F164	Privacy/confidentiality	10.30
11	F431	Report drug irregularities	10.30
12	F278	Accuracy of assessments	9.70
13	F496	N.A. verification	9.70
14	F176	Self-administration of drugs	9.09
15	F518	Staff training	8.48
16	F246	Accommodate needs	7.88
17	F363	Menus/nutritional adequacy	7.88
18	F250	Social services	6.06
19	F329	Drugs	6.06
20	F332	Medication errors >5%	6.06
21	F463	Call system in rooms	6.06
22	F502	Provide or obtain lab services	6.06
23	F157	Notice of changes	5.45
24	F282	Assessment by qualified staff	5.45
25	F364	Food quality	5.45
26	F372	Garbage	5.45
27	F465	Other environment	5.45
28	F274	Assessment-condition change	4.85
29	F309	Highest practicable care	4.85
30	F426	Pharmacy procedures	4.85
31	F248	Activities program	4.24
32	F284	Post-discharge plan of care	4.24
33	F316	Bladder treatment	4.24
34	F494	N.A.s are trained	4.24
35	F514	Records complete	4.24
36	F156	Notice of rights/services	3.64
37	F252	Environment-safe, clean	3.64
38	F283	Assessment recap	3.64
39	F314	Pressure sores	3.64
40	F225	Criminal staff/abuse	3.03

Table IV-4 (continued)

Most Frequently Cited Deficiencies, 1997: Arkansas

Rank	Tag	Requirement	% of Facilities Cited
1	F371	Food sanitation	42.15
2	F253	Housekeeping	36.40
3	F279	Comprehensive care plan	29.12
4	F314	Pressure sores	28.74
5	F309	Highest practicable care	25.67
6	F323	Hazard-free environment	24.90
7	F312	ADL services	24.14
8	F316	Bladder treatment	21.07
9	F318	Range of motion treatment	20.31
10	F272	Comprehensive assessments	19.92
11	F325	Nutrition	17.62
12	F329	Drugs	17.24
13	F328	Special treatments	16.48
14	F326	Therapeutic diet	14.56
15	F164	Privacy/confidentiality	14.18
16	F221	Physical restraints	13.79
17	F332	Medication errors >5%	13.03
18	F469	Pest control	13.03
19	F248	Activities program	12.64
20	F333	Significant medication errors	12.64
21	F363	Menus/nutritional adequacy	12.64
22	F514	Records complete	12.64
23	F241	Dignity	11.88
24	F364	Food quality	11.11
25	F274	Assessment-condition change	9.58
26	F441	Infection control	9.58
27	F458	Square footage	9.58
28	F246	Accommodate needs	8.05
29	F254	Clean linens	8.05
30	F250	Social services	7.28
31	F174	Telephone access	6.51
32	F176	Self-administration of drugs	6.51
33	F431	Report drug irregularities	6.51
34	F463	Call system in rooms	6.51
35	F280	Plan requirements	6.13
36	F432	Act on drug reports	6.13
37	F278	Accuracy of assessments	5.75
38	F322	NG treatment	5.75
39	F330	Antipsychotic drug use	5.75
40	F502	Provide or obtain lab services	5.75

TABLE IV-4 (CONTINUED)

MOST FREQUENTLY CITED DEFICIENCIES, 1997: CALIFORNIA

Rank	Tag	Requirement	% of Facilities Cited
1	F279	Comprehensive care plan	43.83
2	F514	Records complete	42.71
3	F371	Food sanitation	41.93
4	F241	Dignity	39.25
5	F272	Comprehensive assessments	29.18
6	F246	Accommodate needs	28.26
7	F323	Hazard-free environment	27.91
8	F221	Physical restraints	25.93
9	F329	Drugs	25.65
10	F253	Housekeeping	25.51
11	F250	Social services	25.02
12	F309	Highest practicable care	23.26
13	F276	Assessment review	20.72
14	F441	Infection control	20.58
15	F280	Plan requirements	19.94
16	F314	Pressure sores	19.31
17	F248	Activities program	18.18
18	F324	Accident prevention	17.69
19	F312	ADL services	15.86
20	F316	Bladder treatment	15.86
21	F252	Environment-safe, clean	15.36
22	F157	Notice of changes	15.01
23	F164	Privacy/confidentiality	14.45
24	F318	Range of motion treatment	14.45
25	F426	Pharmacy procedures	14.31
26	F465	Other environment	13.11
27	F282	Assessment by qualified staff	13.04
28	F281	Professional standards	12.54
29	F325	Nutrition	11.77
30	F444	Hand washing	11.63
31	F364	Food quality	11.13
32	F156	Notice of rights/services	10.64
33	F328	Special treatments	10.36
34	F166	Resolve grievances	10.29
35	F278	Accuracy of assessments	9.80
36	F322	NG treatment	9.44
37	F225	Criminal staff/abuse	9.09
38	F432	Act on drug reports	8.32
39	F167	Examine survey results	8.10
40	F368	Food schedule	7.96

Table IV-4 (continued)

Most Frequently Cited Deficiencies, 1997: Colorado

Rank	Tag	Requirement	% of Facilities Cited
1	F323	Hazard-free environment	26.67
2	F371	Food sanitation	21.78
3	F272	Comprehensive assessments	20.44
4	F314	Pressure sores	18.22
5	F309	Highest practicable care	14.67
6	F252	Environment-safe, clean	13.78
7	F253	Housekeeping	12.44
8	F221	Physical restraints	11.11
9	F329	Drugs	10.67
10	F312	ADL services	10.22
11	F279	Comprehensive care plan	9.33
12	F318	Range of motion treatment	9.33
13	F246	Accommodate needs	8.89
14	F316	Bladder treatment	8.00
15	F241	Dignity	7.56
16	F325	Nutrition	7.56
17	F164	Privacy/confidentiality	6.67
18	F467	Outside ventilation	6.67
19	F248	Activities program	6.22
20	F441	Infection control	5.78
21	F250	Social services	4.89
22	F332	Medication errors >5%	4.44
23	F319	Mental/psychosocial services	3.56
24	F324	Accident prevention	3.56
25	F157	Notice of changes	3.11
26	F274	Assessment-condition change	3.11
27	F176	Self-administration of drugs	2.67
28	F257	Comfortable/safe temperatures	2.67
29	F273	Assessment 14 days after adm.	2.67
30	F364	Food quality	2.67
31	F432	Act on drug reports	2.67
32	F460	Privacy	2.67
33	F170	Mail service	2.22
34	F310	ADLs don't diminish	2.22
35	F311	Appropriate ADL treatment	2.22
36	F333	Significant medication errors	2.22
37	F225	Criminal staff/abuse	1.78
38	F328	Special treatments	1.78
39	F469	Pest control	1.78
40	F159	Manage funds-facility	1.33

Table IV-4 (continued)

Most Frequently Cited Deficiencies, 1997: Connecticut

Rank	Tag	Requirement	% of Facilities Cited
1	F309	Highest practicable care	26.92
2	F324	Accident prevention	24.23
3	F314	Pressure sores	22.69
4	F272	Comprehensive assessments	17.69
5	F279	Comprehensive care plan	17.31
6	F312	ADL services	13.08
7	F281	Professional standards	11.54
8	F221	Physical restraints	7.31
9	F241	Dignity	6.92
10	F371	Food sanitation	6.92
11	F157	Notice of changes	5.77
12	F318	Range of motion treatment	5.00
13	F225	Criminal staff/abuse	4.62
14	F441	Infection control	4.62
15	F159	Manage funds-facility	3.85
16	F223	Abuse	3.85
17	F248	Activities program	3.85
18	F280	Plan requirements	3.85
19	F322	NG treatment	3.46
20	F329	Drugs	3.46
21	F333	Significant medication errors	3.46
22	F364	Food quality	3.46
23	F246	Accommodate needs	3.08
24	F311	Appropriate ADL treatment	2.69
25	F316	Bladder treatment	2.69
26	F325	Nutrition	2.69
27	F164	Privacy/confidentiality	2.31
28	F274	Assessment-condition change	2.31
29	F310	ADLs don't diminish	2.31
30	F156	Notice of rights/services	1.92
31	F242	Self determination	1.92
32	F323	Hazard-free environment	1.92
33	F332	Medication errors >5%	1.92
34	F162	Double-charging program and resident	1.54
35	F167	Examine survey results	1.54
36	F170	Mail service	1.54
37	F176	Self-administration of drugs	1.54
38	F250	Social services	1.54
39	F253	Housekeeping	1.54
40	F454	Facility is designed/maintained safely	1.54

TABLE IV-4 (CONTINUED)

MOST FREQUENTLY CITED DEFICIENCIES, 1997: DELAWARE

Rank	Tag	Requirement	% of Facilities Cited
1	F225	Criminal staff/abuse	48.84
2	F371	Food sanitation	37.21
3	F279	Comprehensive care plan	34.88
4	F314	Pressure sores	34.88
5	F323	Hazard-free environment	34.88
6	F309	Highest practicable care	30.23
7	F316	Bladder treatment	27.91
8	F514	Records complete	25.58
9	F280	Plan requirements	23.26
10	F324	Accident prevention	23.26
11	F276	Assessment review	20.93
12	F426	Pharmacy procedures	20.93
13	F456	Equipment maintenance	18.60
14	F157	Notice of changes	16.28
15	F311	Appropriate ADL treatment	16.28
16	F425	Provide drugs	16.28
17	F221	Physical restraints	13.95
18	F281	Professional standards	13.95
19	F497	N.A. in-service	13.95
20	F156	Notice of rights/services	11.63
21	F205	Bedhold notice	11.63
22	F248	Activities program	11.63
23	F327	Hydration	11.63
24	F444	Hand washing	11.63
25	F241	Dignity	9.30
26	F325	Nutrition	9.30
27	F441	Infection control	9.30
28	F161	Surety bond	6.98
29	F310	ADLs don't diminish	6.98
30	F322	NG treatment	6.98
31	F329	Drugs	6.98
32	F333	Significant medication errors	6.98
33	F353	Sufficient staff	6.98
34	F368	Food schedule	6.98
35	F372	Garbage	6.98
36	F429	Drug records	6.98
37	F442	Isolate residents	6.98
38	F494	NAs are trained and competent	6.98
39	F151	Rights	4.65
40	F159	Manage funds-facility	4.65

TABLE IV-4 (CONTINUED)

MOST FREQUENTLY CITED DEFICIENCIES, 1997: DISTRICT OF COLUMBIA

Rank	Tag	Requirement	% of Facilities Cited
1	F371	Food sanitation	66.67
2	F253	Housekeeping	57.14
3	F514	Records complete	52.38
4	F441	Infection control	42.86
5	F333	Significant medication errors	33.33
6	F386	Physician documentation	28.57
7	F456	Equipment maintenance	23.81
8	F279	Comprehensive care plan	19.05
9	F314	Pressure sores	19.05
10	F385	Physician services	19.05
11	F278	Accuracy of assessments	14.29
12	F309	Highest practicable care	14.29
13	F176	Self-administration of drugs	9.52
14	F241	Dignity	9.52
15	F254	Clean linens	9.52
16	F272	Comprehensive assessments	9.52
17	F276	Assessment review	9.52
18	F323	Hazard-free environment	9.52
19	F372	Garbage	9.52
20	F406	Rehab	9.52
21	F426	Pharmacy procedures	9.52
22	F428	Drug regimen review – monthly	9.52
23	F430	Act on pharmacist's report	9.52
24	F499	Employ licensed professionals	9.52
25	F161	Surety bond	4.76
26	F252	Environment-safe, clean	4.76
27	F275	Annual assessments	4.76
28	F285	Pasarr MI/MR	4.76
29	F332	Medication errors >5%	4.76
30	F353	Sufficient staff	4.76
31	F387	Physician visits	4.76
32	F445	Handle linens	4.76
33	F469	Pest control	4.76
34	F490	Administration	4.76
35	F502	Provide or obtain lab services	4.76

Table IV-4 (continued)

Most Frequently Cited Deficiencies, 1997: Florida

Rank	Tag	Requirement	% of Facilities Cited
1	F371	Food sanitation	30.13
2	F279	Comprehensive care plan	28.55
3	F272	Comprehensive assessments	25.97
4	F241	Dignity	22.38
5	F441	Infection control	15.64
6	F316	Bladder treatment	15.35
7	F314	Pressure sores	14.92
8	F325	Nutrition	14.92
9	F221	Physical restraints	14.20
10	F329	Drugs	13.63
11	F253	Housekeeping	13.06
12	F248	Activities program	12.20
13	F250	Social services	11.33
14	F156	Notice of rights/services	10.90
15	F514	Records complete	10.47
16	F246	Accommodate needs	10.33
17	F324	Accident prevention	10.33
18	F364	Food quality	10.04
19	F252	Environment-safe, clean	9.76
20	F353	Sufficient staff	9.47
21	F309	Highest practicable care	9.33
22	F368	Food schedule	9.18
23	F323	Hazard-free environment	9.04
24	F274	Assessment-condition change	8.75
25	F164	Privacy/confidentiality	8.32
26	F432	Act on drug reports	8.32
27	F311	Appropriate ADL treatment	8.03
28	F332	Medication errors >5%	8.03
29	F327	Hydration	7.89
30	F225	Criminal staff/abuse	7.75
31	F203	Transfer notice	7.60
32	F166	Resolve grievances	7.17
33	F205	Bedhold notice	7.03
34	F278	Accuracy of assessments	6.89
35	F282	Assessment by qualified staff	6.74
36	F280	Plan requirements	6.46
37	F167	Examine survey results	6.03
38	F426	Pharmacy procedures	6.03
39	F224	Staff treatment of residents	5.74
40	F465	Other environment	5.45

TABLE IV-4 (CONTINUED)

MOST FREQUENTLY CITED DEFICIENCIES, 1997: GEORGIA

Rank	Tag	Requirement	% of Facilities Cited
1	F371	Food sanitation	30.79
2	F252	Environment-safe, clean	21.47
3	F309	Highest practicable care	20.90
4	F253	Housekeeping	20.34
5	F323	Hazard-free environment	17.51
6	F312	ADL services	15.82
7	F241	Dignity	14.12
8	F314	Pressure sores	12.43
9	F332	Medication errors >5%	11.86
10	F465	Other environment	11.30
11	F272	Comprehensive assessments	10.17
12	F324	Accident prevention	10.17
13	F318	Range of motion treatment	9.04
14	F364	Food quality	8.76
15	F164	Privacy/confidentiality	7.63
16	F469	Pest control	7.34
17	F166	Resolve grievances	6.78
18	F242	Self determination	6.78
19	F333	Significant medication errors	6.50
20	F363	Menus/nutritional adequacy	6.21
21	F368	Food schedule	5.93
22	F159	Manage funds-facility	5.65
23	F254	Clean linens	5.37
24	F514	Records complete	5.37
25	F221	Physical restraints	5.08
26	F353	Sufficient staff	5.08
27	F316	Bladder treatment	4.24
28	F248	Activities program	3.95
29	F274	Assessment-condition change	3.95
30	F365	Food form	3.95
31	F372	Garbage	3.95
32	F441	Infection control	3.67
33	F310	ADLs don't diminish	3.39
34	F325	Nutrition	3.39
35	F246	Accommodate needs	3.11
36	F258	Comfortable sound	3.11
37	F322	NG treatment	3.11
38	F456	Equipment maintenance	3.11
39	F162	Double-charging program and resident	2.82
40	F225	Criminal staff/abuse	2.82

Table IV-4 (continued)

Most Frequently Cited Deficiencies, 1997: Hawaii

Rank	Tag	Requirement	% of Facilities Cited
1	F272	Comprehensive assessments	60.47
2	F279	Comprehensive care plan	48.84
3	F454	Facil.is designed/maintained safely	44.19
4	F371	Food sanitation	32.56
5	F441	Infection control	23.26
6	F241	Dignity	20.93
7	F325	Nutrition	20.93
8	F248	Activities program	16.28
9	F274	Assessment-condition change	16.28
10	F329	Drugs	16.28
11	F362	Sufficient dietary staff	13.95
12	F314	Pressure sores	11.63
13	F319	Mental/psychosocial services	11.63
14	F465	Other environment	11.63
15	F221	Physical restraints	9.30
16	F225	Criminal staff/abuse	6.98
17	F246	Accommodate needs	6.98
18	F250	Social services	6.98
19	F276	Assessment review	6.98
20	F364	Food quality	6.98
21	F426	Pharmacy procedures	6.98
22	F444	Hand washing	6.98
23	F456	Equipment maintenance	6.98
24	F514	Records complete	6.98
25	F154	Informed of medical condition	4.65
26	F164	Privacy/confidentiality	4.65
27	F242	Self determination	4.65
28	F323	Hazard-free environment	4.65
29	F328	Special treatments	4.65
30	F353	Sufficient staff	4.65
31	F367	Therapeutic diets	4.65
32	F432	Act on drug reports	4.65
33	F156	Notice of rights/services	2.33
34	F157	Notice of changes	2.33
35	F159	Manage funds-facility	2.33
36	F162	Double-charging program and resident	2.33
37	F176	Self-administration of drugs	2.33
38	F252	Environment-safe, clean	2.33
39	F253	Housekeeping	2.33
40	F281	Professional standards	2.33

Table IV-4 (continued)

Most Frequently Cited Deficiencies, 1997: Idaho

Rank	Tag	Requirement	% of Facilities Cited
1	F371	Food sanitation	34.88
2	F309	Highest practicable care	33.72
3	F272	Comprehensive assessments	32.56
4	F324	Accident prevention	27.91
5	F279	Comprehensive care plan	25.58
6	F248	Activities program	24.42
7	F514	Records complete	24.42
8	F329	Drugs	23.26
9	F250	Social services	22.09
10	F312	ADL services	22.09
11	F441	Infection control	22.09
12	F221	Physical restraints	20.93
13	F253	Housekeeping	20.93
14	F323	Hazard-free environment	18.60
15	F314	Pressure sores	17.44
16	F363	Menus/nutritional adequacy	16.28
17	F246	Accommodate needs	15.12
18	F316	Bladder treatment	15.12
19	F354	RN staff	12.79
20	F318	Range of motion treatment	11.63
21	F325	Nutrition	11.63
22	F225	Criminal staff/abuse	10.47
23	F280	Plan requirements	10.47
24	F241	Dignity	9.30
25	F311	Appropriate ADL treatment	9.30
26	F330	Antipsychotic drug use	9.30
27	F387	Physician visits	9.30
28	F157	Notice of changes	8.14
29	F364	Food quality	8.14
30	F208	Admissions policy	6.98
31	F252	Environment-safe, clean	6.98
32	F331	Antipsychotic dose reductions	6.98
33	F368	Food schedule	5.81
34	F458	Square footage	5.81
35	F460	Privacy	5.81
36	F166	Resolve grievances	4.65
37	F223	Abuse	4.65
38	F258	Comfortable sound	4.65
39	F445	Handle linens	4.65
40	F520	Quality assessment committee	4.65

Table IV-4 (continued)

Most Frequently Cited Deficiencies, 1997: Illinois

Rank	Tag	Requirement	% of Facilities Cited
1	F323	Hazard-free environment	36.26
2	F272	Comprehensive assessments	35.80
3	F371	Food sanitation	32.91
4	F279	Comprehensive care plan	27.60
5	F253	Housekeeping	27.02
6	F281	Professional standards	20.55
7	F314	Pressure sores	19.86
8	F221	Physical restraints	18.24
9	F316	Bladder treatment	17.21
10	F441	Infection control	15.82
11	F241	Dignity	15.36
12	F282	Assessment by qualified staff	15.13
13	F324	Accident prevention	13.63
14	F309	Highest practicable care	13.05
15	F318	Range of motion treatment	12.01
16	F248	Activities program	10.97
17	F458	Square footage	10.97
18	F246	Accommodate needs	10.85
19	F363	Menus/nutritional adequacy	10.62
20	F252	Environment-safe, clean	10.39
21	F312	ADL services	9.24
22	F164	Privacy/confidentiality	9.01
23	F364	Food quality	9.01
24	F322	NG treatment	8.78
25	F444	Hand washing	8.08
26	F311	Appropriate ADL treatment	7.97
27	F325	Nutrition	7.85
28	F329	Drugs	7.16
29	F157	Notice of changes	7.04
30	F445	Handle linens	6.70
31	F167	Examine survey results	6.58
32	F276	Assessment review	6.00
33	F274	Assessment-condition change	5.54
34	F469	Pest control	5.08
35	F174	Telephone access	4.85
36	F326	Therapeutic diet	4.73
37	F319	Mental/psychosocial services	4.62
38	F250	Social services	4.39
39	F368	Food schedule	4.39
40	F465	Other environment	4.39

TABLE IV-4 (CONTINUED)

MOST FREQUENTLY CITED DEFICIENCIES, 1997: INDIANA

Rank	Tag	Requirement	% of Facilities Cited
1	F323	Hazard-free environment	36.74
2	F371	Food sanitation	30.85
3	F272	Comprehensive assessments	30.50
4	F281	Professional standards	29.12
5	F282	Assessment by qualified staff	25.48
6	F465	Other environment	24.96
7	F250	Social services	23.57
8	F221	Physical restraints	22.53
9	F279	Comprehensive care plan	22.53
10	F458	Square footage	18.37
11	F241	Dignity	16.81
12	F253	Housekeeping	15.60
13	F314	Pressure sores	14.90
14	F329	Drugs	14.04
15	F514	Records complete	13.69
16	F248	Activities program	13.34
17	F225	Criminal staff/abuse	13.17
18	F318	Range of motion treatment	13.17
19	F324	Accident prevention	11.61
20	F441	Infection control	11.44
21	F364	Food quality	11.09
22	F312	ADL services	10.92
23	F157	Notice of changes	10.40
24	F325	Nutrition	10.23
25	F280	Plan requirements	9.88
26	F363	Menus/nutritional adequacy	9.71
27	F274	Assessment-condition change	9.36
28	F316	Bladder treatment	8.84
29	F309	Highest practicable care	8.32
30	F353	Sufficient staff	7.97
31	F164	Privacy/confidentiality	7.28
32	F224	Staff treatment of residents	6.07
33	F444	Hand washing	6.07
34	F278	Accuracy of assessments	5.55
35	F156	Notice of rights/services	5.37
36	F159	Manage funds-facility	5.03
37	F319	Mental/psychosocial services	5.03
38	F463	Call system in rooms	4.85
39	F516	Safeguard records	4.85
40	F246	Accommodate needs	4.68

TABLE IV-4 (CONTINUED)

MOST FREQUENTLY CITED DEFICIENCIES, 1997: IOWA

Rank	Tag	Requirement	% of Facilities Cited
1	F281	Professional standards	24.73
2	F371	Food sanitation	24.52
3	F272	Comprehensive assessments	22.60
4	F498	N.A. proficiency	22.60
5	F314	Pressure sores	20.47
6	F316	Bladder treatment	18.76
7	F309	Highest practicable care	17.48
8	F324	Accident prevention	17.27
9	F323	Hazard-free environment	16.84
10	F279	Comprehensive care plan	16.20
11	F329	Drugs	15.57
12	F318	Range of motion treatment	15.35
13	F444	Hand washing	12.79
14	F465	Other environment	11.73
15	F441	Infection control	11.09
16	F363	Menus/nutritional adequacy	10.23
17	F221	Physical restraints	10.02
18	F364	Food quality	9.59
19	F253	Housekeeping	8.74
20	F312	ADL services	8.74
21	F164	Privacy/confidentiality	8.32
22	F274	Assessment-condition change	8.32
23	F157	Notice of changes	7.89
24	F429	Drug records	7.46
25	F241	Dignity	6.61
26	F282	Assessment by qualified staff	6.61
27	F310	ADLs don't diminish	6.61
28	F353	Sufficient staff	6.18
29	F368	Food schedule	5.76
30	F250	Social services	5.54
31	F311	Appropriate ADL treatment	5.54
32	F246	Accommodate needs	5.33
33	F252	Environment-safe, clean	5.33
34	F325	Nutrition	5.12
35	F248	Activities program	4.48
36	F170	Mail service	4.26
37	F445	Handle linens	4.26
38	F332	Medication errors >5%	3.84
39	F278	Accuracy of assessments	3.62
40	F362	Sufficient dietary staff	3.62

TABLE IV-4 (CONTINUED)

MOST FREQUENTLY CITED DEFICIENCIES, 1997: KANSAS

Rank	Tag	Requirement	% of Facilities Cited
1	F279	Comprehensive care plan	31.21
2	F309	Highest practicable care	30.73
3	F323	Hazard-free environment	28.13
4	F314	Pressure sores	27.90
5	F371	Food sanitation	27.90
6	F272	Comprehensive assessments	24.82
7	F253	Housekeeping	23.17
8	F496	N.A. verification	22.46
9	F324	Accident prevention	21.99
10	F316	Bladder treatment	21.51
11	F312	ADL services	20.09
12	F221	Physical restraints	16.55
13	F325	Nutrition	15.37
14	F465	Other environment	15.13
15	F248	Activities program	13.48
16	F159	Manage funds-facility	11.82
17	F318	Range of motion treatment	11.82
18	F281	Professional standards	11.35
19	F274	Assessment-condition change	11.11
20	F444	Hand washing	11.11
21	F164	Privacy/confidentiality	10.64
22	F329	Drugs	10.40
23	F241	Dignity	9.46
24	F250	Social services	8.75
25	F225	Criminal staff/abuse	8.27
26	F246	Accommodate needs	7.80
27	F353	Sufficient staff	7.09
28	F441	Infection control	6.86
29	F252	Environment-safe, clean	6.62
30	F322	NG treatment	6.15
31	F498	N.A. proficiency	5.91
32	F157	Notice of changes	5.67
33	F328	Special treatments	5.20
34	F364	Food quality	5.20
35	F156	Notice of rights/services	4.96
36	F280	Plan requirements	4.73
37	F311	Appropriate ADL treatment	4.49
38	F319	Mental/psychosocial services	4.26
39	F310	ADLs don't diminish	4.02
40	F160	Funds conveyed upon death	3.78

Table IV-4 (continued)

Most Frequently Cited Deficiencies, 1997: Kentucky

Rank	Tag	Requirement	% of Facilities Cited
1	F272	Comprehensive assessments	27.62
2	F279	Comprehensive care plan	27.30
3	F221	Physical restraints	18.73
4	F371	Food sanitation	15.87
5	F329	Drugs	11.75
6	F364	Food quality	11.11
7	F316	Bladder treatment	10.16
8	F252	Environment-safe, clean	9.84
9	F332	Medication errors >5%	8.89
10	F241	Dignity	8.57
11	F248	Activities program	8.57
12	F250	Social services	8.57
13	F325	Nutrition	7.94
14	F253	Housekeeping	7.62
15	F309	Highest practicable care	7.62
16	F314	Pressure sores	7.62
17	F157	Notice of changes	7.30
18	F327	Hydration	6.67
19	F311	Appropriate ADL treatment	6.35
20	F353	Sufficient staff	6.03
21	F318	Range of motion treatment	5.71
22	F274	Assessment-condition change	5.40
23	F280	Plan requirements	5.40
24	F441	Infection control	5.40
25	F310	ADLs don't diminish	5.08
26	F312	ADL services	5.08
27	F363	Menus/nutritional adequacy	5.08
28	F514	Records complete	5.08
29	F222	Chemical restraints	4.76
30	F278	Accuracy of assessments	4.76
31	F323	Hazard-free environment	4.76
32	F333	Significant medication errors	4.76
33	F444	Hand washing	4.76
34	F319	Mental/psychosocial services	4.44
35	F324	Accident prevention	4.44
36	F225	Criminal staff/abuse	3.81
37	F246	Accommodate needs	3.81
38	F322	NG treatment	3.81
39	F164	Privacy/confidentiality	3.49
40	F276	Assessment review	3.49

TABLE IV-4 (CONTINUED)

MOST FREQUENTLY CITED DEFICIENCIES, 1997: LOUISIANA

Rank	Tag	Requirement	% of Facilities Cited
1	F281	Professional standards	37.76
2	F371	Food sanitation	25.96
3	F279	Comprehensive care plan	22.12
4	F332	Medication errors >5%	16.81
5	F252	Environment-safe, clean	12.39
6	F514	Records complete	12.09
7	F363	Menus/nutritional adequacy	11.21
8	F241	Dignity	10.91
9	F465	Other environment	10.62
10	F314	Pressure sores	10.03
11	F164	Privacy/confidentiality	9.44
12	F329	Drugs	9.44
13	F272	Comprehensive assessments	8.85
14	F309	Highest practicable care	8.85
15	F498	N.A. proficiency	8.85
16	F248	Activities program	8.55
17	F253	Housekeeping	8.26
18	F323	Hazard-free environment	7.96
19	F333	Significant medication errors	7.96
20	F368	Food schedule	7.37
21	F429	Drug records	7.08
22	F278	Accuracy of assessments	6.78
23	F497	N.A. in-service	6.78
24	F246	Accommodate needs	6.49
25	F364	Food quality	5.90
26	F496	N.A. verification	5.60
27	F254	Clean linens	5.31
28	F325	Nutrition	5.31
29	F162	Double-charging program and resident	5.01
30	F318	Range of motion treatment	5.01
31	F157	Notice of changes	4.72
32	F274	Assessment-condition change	4.72
33	F426	Pharmacy procedures	4.72
34	F432	Act on drug reports	4.72
35	F221	Physical restraints	4.13
36	F354	RN staff	4.13
37	F280	Plan requirements	3.83
38	F316	Bladder treatment	3.83
39	F431	Report drug irregularities	3.83
40	F441	Infection control	3.83

Table IV-4 (continued)

Most Frequently Cited Deficiencies, 1997: Maine

Rank	Tag	Requirement	% of Facilities Cited
1	F272	Comprehensive assessments	40.00
2	F279	Comprehensive care plan	37.78
3	F371	Food sanitation	24.44
4	F323	Hazard-free environment	17.78
5	F221	Physical restraints	11.85
6	F274	Assessment-condition change	10.37
7	F329	Drugs	10.37
8	F246	Accommodate needs	9.63
9	F253	Housekeeping	9.63
10	F309	Highest practicable care	9.63
11	F156	Notice of rights/services	6.67
12	F225	Criminal staff/abuse	6.67
13	F281	Professional standards	6.67
14	F167	Examine survey results	5.93
15	F314	Pressure sores	5.93
16	F465	Other environment	5.93
17	F164	Privacy/confidentiality	5.19
18	F241	Dignity	5.19
19	F441	Infection control	5.19
20	F469	Pest control	5.19
21	F248	Activities program	4.44
22	F252	Environment-safe, clean	4.44
23	F311	Appropriate ADL treatment	4.44
24	F460	Privacy	4.44
25	F324	Accident prevention	3.70
26	F331	Antipsychotic dose reductions	3.70
27	F445	Handle linens	3.70
28	F174	Telephone access	2.96
29	F203	Transfer notice	2.96
30	F353	Sufficient staff	2.96
31	F364	Food quality	2.96
32	F432	Act on drug reports	2.96
33	F458	Square footage	2.96
34	F159	Manage funds-facility	2.22
35	F242	Self determination	2.22
36	F258	Comfortable sound	2.22
37	F319	Mental/psychosocial services	2.22
38	F464	Dining/activity rooms	2.22
39	F151	Rights	1.48
40	F222	Chemical restraints	1.48

TABLE IV-4 (CONTINUED)

MOST FREQUENTLY CITED DEFICIENCIES, 1997: MARYLAND

Rank	Tag	Requirement	% of Facilities Cited
1	F309	Highest practicable care	39.11
2	F314	Pressure sores	16.53
3	F371	Food sanitation	16.13
4	F325	Nutrition	15.32
5	F324	Accident prevention	12.90
6	F364	Food quality	12.50
7	F241	Dignity	10.89
8	F279	Comprehensive care plan	9.27
9	F157	Notice of changes	8.47
10	F323	Hazard-free environment	8.47
11	F469	Pest control	8.47
12	F253	Housekeeping	7.66
13	F514	Records complete	7.66
14	F326	Therapeutic diet	7.26
15	F463	Call system in rooms	7.26
16	F221	Physical restraints	6.85
17	F316	Bladder treatment	6.85
18	F327	Hydration	6.85
19	F332	Medication errors >5%	5.65
20	F272	Comprehensive assessments	5.24
21	F159	Manage funds-facility	4.84
22	F333	Significant medication errors	4.84
23	F365	Food form	4.84
24	F458	Square footage	4.84
25	F322	NG treatment	4.44
26	F363	Menus/nutritional adequacy	4.44
27	F315	Catheter use	4.03
28	F248	Activities program	3.23
29	F318	Range of motion treatment	3.23
30	F467	Outside ventilation	3.23
31	F164	Privacy/confidentiality	2.82
32	F246	Accommodate needs	2.82
33	F278	Accuracy of assessments	2.82
34	F368	Food schedule	2.82
35	F386	Physician documentation	2.82
36	F167	Examine survey results	2.42
37	F283	Assessment recap	2.42
38	F312	ADL services	2.42
39	F329	Drugs	2.42
40	F367	Therapeutic diets	2.42

Table IV-4 (continued)

Most Frequently Cited Deficiencies, 1997: Massachusetts

Rank	Tag	Requirement	% of Facilities Cited
1	F272	Comprehensive assessments	38.72
2	F221	Physical restraints	26.11
3	F324	Accident prevention	18.29
4	F316	Bladder treatment	15.28
5	F282	Assessment by qualified staff	14.92
6	F278	Accuracy of assessments	12.61
7	F279	Comprehensive care plan	11.37
8	F281	Professional standards	10.48
9	F314	Pressure sores	9.59
10	F250	Social services	7.99
11	F252	Environment-safe, clean	7.28
12	F276	Assessment review	7.28
13	F325	Nutrition	7.10
14	F225	Criminal staff/abuse	6.75
15	F332	Medication errors >5%	6.57
16	F371	Food sanitation	6.39
17	F246	Accommodate needs	6.22
18	F329	Drugs	6.22
19	F203	Transfer notice	5.86
20	F157	Notice of changes	5.68
21	F156	Notice of rights/services	5.51
22	F364	Food quality	5.33
23	F497	N.A. in-service	4.80
24	F241	Dignity	4.62
25	F274	Assessment-condition change	4.62
26	F311	Appropriate ADL treatment	4.62
27	F323	Hazard-free environment	4.62
28	F318	Range of motion treatment	4.44
29	F248	Activities program	4.26
30	F328	Special treatments	4.26
31	F368	Food schedule	4.26
32	F280	Plan requirements	4.09
33	F312	ADL services	3.37
34	F319	Mental/psychosocial services	3.37
35	F441	Infection control	3.37
36	F253	Housekeeping	3.20
37	F521	Q.A. committee meets/plans	3.20
38	F310	ADLs don't diminish	3.02
39	F167	Examine survey results	2.84
40	F496	N.A. verification	2.84

Table IV-4 (continued)

Most Frequently Cited Deficiencies, 1997: Michigan

Rank	Tag	Requirement	% of Facilities Cited
1	F371	Food sanitation	41.89
2	F314	Pressure sores	35.36
3	F323	Hazard-free environment	33.56
4	F329	Drugs	32.21
5	F253	Housekeeping	29.95
6	F246	Accommodate needs	27.25
7	F312	ADL services	27.03
8	F318	Range of motion treatment	25.45
9	F309	Highest practicable care	23.65
10	F316	Bladder treatment	23.20
11	F324	Accident prevention	22.75
12	F325	Nutrition	22.52
13	F252	Environment-safe, clean	21.40
14	F221	Physical restraints	19.82
15	F465	Other environment	17.79
16	F241	Dignity	17.12
17	F328	Special treatments	17.12
18	F248	Activities program	16.22
19	F456	Equipment maintenance	14.64
20	F322	NG treatment	14.19
21	F458	Square footage	14.19
22	F319	Mental/psychosocial services	12.39
23	F164	Privacy/confidentiality	12.16
24	F311	Appropriate ADL treatment	11.94
25	F364	Food quality	11.26
26	F353	Sufficient staff	11.04
27	F497	N.A. in-service	10.81
28	F426	Pharmacy procedures	10.36
29	F441	Infection control	9.91
30	F326	Therapeutic diet	9.68
31	F327	Hydration	9.46
32	F432	Act on drug reports	8.78
33	F250	Social services	8.33
34	F460	Privacy	8.33
35	F368	Food schedule	8.11
36	F463	Call system in rooms	8.11
37	F225	Criminal staff/abuse	7.66
38	F445	Handle linens	7.66
39	F429	Drug records	7.21
40	F310	ADLs don't diminish	6.76

Table IV-4 (continued)

Most Frequently Cited Deficiencies, 1997: Minnesota

Rank	Tag	Requirement	% of Facilities Cited
1	F272	Comprehensive assessments	39.42
2	F221	Physical restraints	24.94
3	F241	Dignity	17.37
4	F316	Bladder treatment	15.37
5	F465	Other environment	11.14
6	F318	Range of motion treatment	10.69
7	F309	Highest practicable care	10.47
8	F314	Pressure sores	10.47
9	F164	Privacy/confidentiality	10.24
10	F312	ADL services	10.24
11	F276	Assessment review	9.35
12	F311	Appropriate ADL treatment	8.91
13	F371	Food sanitation	7.80
14	F441	Infection control	7.35
15	F444	Hand washing	7.35
16	F323	Hazard-free environment	6.46
17	F458	Square footage	6.01
18	F176	Self-administration of drugs	5.79
19	F329	Drugs	5.57
20	F364	Food quality	5.35
21	F246	Accommodate needs	5.12
22	F319	Mental/psychosocial services	5.12
23	F460	Privacy	4.90
24	F274	Assessment-condition change	4.45
25	F242	Self determination	4.23
26	F426	Pharmacy procedures	4.23
27	F157	Notice of changes	3.79
28	F170	Mail service	3.79
29	F248	Activities program	3.79
30	F253	Housekeeping	3.56
31	F156	Notice of rights/services	3.34
32	F310	ADLs don't diminish	3.34
33	F167	Examine survey results	3.12
34	F250	Social services	3.12
35	F279	Comprehensive care plan	3.12
36	F324	Accident prevention	3.12
37	F353	Sufficient staff	3.12
38	F159	Manage funds-facility	2.90
39	F354	RN staff	2.90
40	F205	Bedhold notice	2.67

TABLE IV-4 (CONTINUED)

MOST FREQUENTLY CITED DEFICIENCIES, 1997: MISSISSIPPI

Rank	Tag	Requirement	% of Facilities Cited
1	F272	Comprehensive assessments	34.98
2	F323	Hazard-free environment	30.05
3	F371	Food sanitation	22.17
4	F253	Housekeeping	19.21
5	F314	Pressure sores	19.21
6	F441	Infection control	16.75
7	F279	Comprehensive care plan	15.76
8	F329	Drugs	14.29
9	F514	Records complete	12.81
10	F164	Privacy/confidentiality	11.82
11	F325	Nutrition	10.84
12	F252	Environment-safe, clean	9.36
13	F309	Highest practicable care	8.37
14	F326	Therapeutic diet	7.88
15	F157	Notice of changes	7.39
16	F432	Act on drug reports	7.39
17	F316	Bladder treatment	6.90
18	F174	Telephone access	6.40
19	F221	Physical restraints	6.40
20	F224	Staff treatment of residents	6.40
21	F225	Criminal staff/abuse	6.40
22	F241	Dignity	6.40
23	F497	N.A. in-service	6.40
24	F248	Activities program	5.42
25	F167	Examine survey results	4.93
26	F246	Accommodate needs	4.93
27	F280	Plan requirements	4.93
28	F463	Call system in rooms	4.93
29	F258	Comfortable sound	4.43
30	F318	Range of motion treatment	4.43
31	F324	Accident prevention	4.43
32	F332	Medication errors >5%	4.43
33	F364	Food quality	4.43
34	F429	Drug records	4.43
35	F430	Act on pharmacist's report	3.94
36	F444	Hand washing	3.94
37	F468	Handrails	3.94
38	F322	NG treatment	3.45
39	F353	Sufficient staff	3.45
40	F274	Assessment-condition change	2.96

Table IV-4 (continued)

Most Frequently Cited Deficiencies, 1997: Missouri

Rank	Tag	Requirement	% of Facilities Cited
1	F454	Facil.is designed/maintained safely	28.60
2	F371	Food sanitation	22.63
3	F279	Comprehensive care plan	20.88
4	F312	ADL services	20.70
5	F272	Comprehensive assessments	20.00
6	F465	Other environment	15.61
7	F364	Food quality	14.39
8	F314	Pressure sores	14.04
9	F253	Housekeeping	12.63
10	F311	Appropriate ADL treatment	12.28
11	F221	Physical restraints	12.11
12	F241	Dignity	12.11
13	F325	Nutrition	10.70
14	F252	Environment-safe, clean	10.53
15	F323	Hazard-free environment	10.53
16	F324	Accident prevention	9.65
17	F332	Medication errors >5%	9.65
18	F309	Highest practicable care	9.47
19	F318	Range of motion treatment	9.47
20	F329	Drugs	9.47
21	F274	Assessment-condition change	8.95
22	F248	Activities program	8.42
23	F164	Privacy/confidentiality	8.25
24	F319	Mental/psychosocial services	6.49
25	F316	Bladder treatment	6.32
26	F246	Accommodate needs	5.79
27	F250	Social services	5.79
28	F363	Menus/nutritional adequacy	5.79
29	F281	Professional standards	5.26
30	F444	Hand washing	5.26
31	F469	Pest control	4.39
32	F167	Examine survey results	3.68
33	F353	Sufficient staff	3.51
34	F278	Accuracy of assessments	3.33
35	F310	ADLs don't diminish	3.16
36	F242	Self determination	2.98
37	F276	Assessment review	2.81
38	F456	Equipment maintenance	2.81
39	F282	Assessment by qualified staff	2.63
40	F322	NG treatment	2.63

TABLE IV-4 (CONTINUED)

MOST FREQUENTLY CITED DEFICIENCIES, 1997: MONTANA

Rank	Tag	Requirement	% of Facilities Cited
1	F309	Highest practicable care	22.33
2	F312	ADL services	20.39
3	F316	Bladder treatment	17.48
4	F272	Comprehensive assessments	15.53
5	F327	Hydration	15.53
6	F314	Pressure sores	14.56
7	F324	Accident prevention	14.56
8	F329	Drugs	14.56
9	F310	ADLs don't diminish	13.59
10	F318	Range of motion treatment	13.59
11	F248	Activities program	12.62
12	F325	Nutrition	10.68
13	F274	Assessment-condition change	9.71
14	F353	Sufficient staff	9.71
15	F460	Privacy	9.71
16	F311	Appropriate ADL treatment	8.74
17	F332	Medication errors >5%	8.74
18	F371	Food sanitation	8.74
19	F387	Physician visits	8.74
20	F221	Physical restraints	7.77
21	F225	Criminal staff/abuse	7.77
22	F241	Dignity	7.77
23	F246	Accommodate needs	7.77
24	F319	Mental/psychosocial services	7.77
25	F444	Hand washing	7.77
26	F452	Tag does not exist	7.77
27	F514	Records complete	7.77
28	F323	Hazard-free environment	6.80
29	F164	Privacy/confidentiality	5.83
30	F166	Resolve grievances	5.83
31	F280	Plan requirements	5.83
32	F223	Abuse	4.85
33	F252	Environment-safe, clean	4.85
34	F279	Comprehensive care plan	4.85
35	F333	Significant medication errors	4.85
36	F368	Food schedule	4.85
37	F429	Drug records	4.85
38	F431	Report drug irregularities	4.85
39	F465	Other environment	4.85
40	F176	Self-administration of drugs	3.88

Table IV-4 (continued)

Most Frequently Cited Deficiencies, 1997: Nebraska

Rank	Tag	Requirement	% of Facilities Cited
1	F314	Pressure sores	22.78
2	F309	Highest practicable care	18.99
3	F248	Activities program	14.35
4	F279	Comprehensive care plan	14.35
5	F221	Physical restraints	13.92
6	F465	Other environment	13.50
7	F498	N.A. proficiency	11.39
8	F371	Food sanitation	10.97
9	F318	Range of motion treatment	10.55
10	F246	Accommodate needs	9.70
11	F323	Hazard-free environment	9.28
12	F441	Infection control	9.28
13	F325	Nutrition	8.86
14	F329	Drugs	8.86
15	F364	Food quality	8.86
16	F312	ADL services	8.44
17	F241	Dignity	8.02
18	F166	Resolve grievances	7.59
19	F316	Bladder treatment	7.59
20	F324	Accident prevention	7.17
21	F272	Comprehensive assessments	6.75
22	F280	Plan requirements	6.75
23	F250	Social services	6.33
24	F274	Assessment-condition change	5.91
25	F444	Hand washing	5.49
26	F497	N.A. in-service	5.49
27	F157	Notice of changes	5.06
28	F311	Appropriate ADL treatment	5.06
29	F319	Mental/psychosocial services	5.06
30	F310	ADLs don't diminish	4.64
31	F253	Housekeeping	4.22
32	F284	Post-discharge plan of care	4.22
33	F518	Staff training	4.22
34	F164	Privacy/confidentiality	3.80
35	F429	Drug records	3.80
36	F520	Quality assessment committee	3.80
37	F225	Criminal staff/abuse	3.38
38	F354	RN staff	3.38
39	F406	Rehab	3.38
40	F282	Assessment by qualified staff	2.53

TABLE IV-4 (CONTINUED)

MOST FREQUENTLY CITED DEFICIENCIES, 1997: NEVADA

Rank	Tag	Requirement	% of Facilities Cited
1	F371	Food sanitation	60.00
2	F221	Physical restraints	53.33
3	F272	Comprehensive assessments	53.33
4	F279	Comprehensive care plan	51.11
5	F241	Dignity	40.00
6	F452	Tag does not exist	37.78
7	F225	Criminal staff/abuse	35.56
8	F250	Social services	35.56
9	F309	Highest practicable care	35.56
10	F246	Accommodate needs	31.11
11	F253	Housekeeping	31.11
12	F276	Assessment review	31.11
13	F248	Activities program	28.89
14	F324	Accident prevention	28.89
15	F329	Drugs	28.89
16	F514	Records complete	28.89
17	F156	Notice of rights/services	24.44
18	F167	Examine survey results	22.22
19	F278	Accuracy of assessments	22.22
20	F312	ADL services	22.22
21	F157	Notice of changes	20.00
22	F280	Plan requirements	20.00
23	F314	Pressure sores	20.00
24	F323	Hazard-free environment	20.00
25	F164	Privacy/confidentiality	17.78
26	F224	Staff treatment of residents	17.78
27	F316	Bladder treatment	17.78
28	F353	Sufficient staff	17.78
29	F441	Infection control	17.78
30	F166	Resolve grievances	15.56
31	F252	Environment-safe, clean	15.56
32	F325	Nutrition	15.56
33	F368	Food schedule	15.56
34	F318	Range of motion treatment	13.33
35	F319	Mental/psychosocial services	13.33
36	F363	Menus/nutritional adequacy	13.33
37	F364	Food quality	13.33
38	F469	Pest control	13.33
39	F154	Informed of medical condition	11.11
40	F222	Chemical restraints	11.11

Table IV-4 (continued)

Most Frequently Cited Deficiencies, 1997: New Hampshire

Rank	Tag	Requirement	% of Facilities Cited
1	F279	Comprehensive care plan	55.56
2	F272	Comprehensive assessments	38.27
3	F314	Pressure sores	23.46
4	F278	Accuracy of assessments	22.22
5	F329	Drugs	18.52
6	F281	Professional standards	16.05
7	F324	Accident prevention	16.05
8	F274	Assessment-condition change	14.81
9	F309	Highest practicable care	14.81
10	F157	Notice of changes	12.35
11	F514	Records complete	12.35
12	F325	Nutrition	9.88
13	F246	Accommodate needs	8.64
14	F253	Housekeeping	8.64
15	F316	Bladder treatment	8.64
16	F371	Food sanitation	8.64
17	F241	Dignity	7.41
18	F441	Infection control	7.41
19	F225	Criminal staff/abuse	6.17
20	F311	Appropriate ADL treatment	6.17
21	F221	Physical restraints	4.94
22	F318	Range of motion treatment	4.94
23	F319	Mental/psychosocial services	4.94
24	F323	Hazard-free environment	4.94
25	F332	Medication errors >5%	4.94
26	F387	Physician visits	4.94
27	F497	N.A. in-service	4.94
28	F273	Assessment 14 days after adm.	3.70
29	F386	Physician documentation	3.70
30	F458	Square footage	3.70
31	F154	Informed of medical condition	2.47
32	F222	Chemical restraints	2.47
33	F252	Environment-safe, clean	2.47
34	F256	Adequate lighting	2.47
35	F312	ADL services	2.47
36	F322	NG treatment	2.47
37	F328	Special treatments	2.47
38	F368	Food schedule	2.47
39	F425	Provide drugs	2.47
40	F444	Hand washing	2.47

Table IV-4 (continued)

Most Frequently Cited Deficiencies, 1997: New Jersey

Rank	Tag	Requirement	% of Facilities Cited
1	F454	Facil.is designed/maintained safely	21.75
2	F279	Comprehensive care plan	18.13
3	F272	Comprehensive assessments	15.41
4	F241	Dignity	14.20
5	F463	Call system in rooms	12.08
6	F281	Professional standards	11.18
7	F248	Activities program	10.57
8	F371	Food sanitation	10.27
9	F309	Highest practicable care	9.97
10	F221	Physical restraints	8.46
11	F329	Drugs	8.46
12	F332	Medication errors >5%	8.46
13	F364	Food quality	8.16
14	F253	Housekeeping	7.85
15	F310	ADLs don't diminish	7.85
16	F325	Nutrition	7.55
17	F314	Pressure sores	6.95
18	F458	Square footage	6.95
19	F246	Accommodate needs	6.34
20	F252	Environment-safe, clean	6.34
21	F497	N.A.in-service	6.34
22	F324	Accident prevention	5.74
23	F166	Resolve grievances	4.53
24	F323	Hazard-free environment	4.53
25	F494	N.A.s are trained	4.53
26	F164	Privacy/confidentiality	4.23
27	F225	Criminal staff/abuse	4.23
28	F278	Accuracy of assessments	4.23
29	F156	Notice of rights/services	3.93
30	F441	Infection control	3.93
31	F167	Examine survey results	3.63
32	F159	Manage funds-facility	3.32
33	F368	Food schedule	3.32
34	F521	Q.A. committee meets/plans	3.32
35	F316	Bladder treatment	3.02
36	F274	Assessment-condition change	2.72
37	F465	Other environment	2.72
38	F276	Assessment review	2.42
39	F311	Appropriate ADL treatment	2.42
40	F406	Rehab	2.42

TABLE IV-4 (CONTINUED)

MOST FREQUENTLY CITED DEFICIENCIES, 1997: NEW MEXICO

Rank	Tag	Requirement	% of Facilities Cited
1	F221	Physical restraints	16.47
2	F314	Pressure sores	14.12
3	F281	Professional standards	12.94
4	F371	Food sanitation	12.94
5	F241	Dignity	11.76
6	F272	Comprehensive assessments	11.76
7	F279	Comprehensive care plan	10.59
8	F323	Hazard-free environment	10.59
9	F246	Accommodate needs	9.41
10	F248	Activities program	8.24
11	F250	Social services	8.24
12	F312	ADL services	8.24
13	F441	Infection control	8.24
14	F325	Nutrition	7.06
15	F332	Medication errors >5%	7.06
16	F364	Food quality	7.06
17	F309	Highest practicable care	5.88
18	F274	Assessment-condition change	4.71
19	F445	Handle linens	4.71
20	F497	N.A. in-service	4.71
21	F500	Outside services	4.71
22	F164	Privacy/confidentiality	3.53
23	F203	Transfer notice	3.53
24	F252	Environment-safe, clean	3.53
25	F284	Post-discharge plan of care	3.53
26	F311	Appropriate ADL treatment	3.53
27	F316	Bladder treatment	3.53
28	F333	Significant medication errors	3.53
29	F365	Food form	3.53
30	F432	Act on drug reports	3.53
31	F514	Records complete	3.53
32	F521	Q.A. committee meets/plans	3.53
33	F151	Rights	2.35
34	F166	Resolve grievances	2.35
35	F278	Accuracy of assessments	2.35
36	F319	Mental/psychosocial services	2.35
37	F324	Accident prevention	2.35
38	F329	Drugs	2.35
39	F361	Qualified dietitian	2.35
40	F406	Rehab	2.35

TABLE IV-4 (CONTINUED)

MOST FREQUENTLY CITED DEFICIENCIES, 1997: NEW YORK

Rank	Tag	Requirement	% of Facilities Cited
1	F241	Dignity	16.43
2	F221	Physical restraints	13.85
3	F314	Pressure sores	13.85
4	F279	Comprehensive care plan	13.04
5	F323	Hazard-free environment	12.72
6	F318	Range of motion treatment	11.59
7	F371	Food sanitation	11.27
8	F441	Infection control	11.11
9	F324	Accident prevention	10.47
10	F253	Housekeeping	10.31
11	F280	Plan requirements	9.50
12	F309	Highest practicable care	9.50
13	F386	Physician documentation	7.89
14	F248	Activities program	7.57
15	F310	ADLs don't diminish	7.09
16	F252	Environment-safe, clean	5.96
17	F272	Comprehensive assessments	5.80
18	F325	Nutrition	5.80
19	F329	Drugs	5.48
20	F312	ADL services	4.83
21	F164	Privacy/confidentiality	4.51
22	F282	Assessment by qualified staff	4.51
23	F250	Social services	4.35
24	F276	Assessment review	4.35
25	F322	NG treatment	4.19
26	F166	Resolve grievances	4.03
27	F278	Accuracy of assessments	4.03
28	F319	Mental/psychosocial services	3.86
29	F327	Hydration	3.86
30	F167	Examine survey results	3.38
31	F364	Food quality	3.38
32	F465	Other environment	3.38
33	F246	Accommodate needs	3.06
34	F368	Food schedule	3.06
35	F316	Bladder treatment	2.74
36	F311	Appropriate ADL treatment	2.58
37	F518	Staff training	2.42
38	F156	Notice of rights/services	2.09
39	F498	N.A. proficiency	2.09
40	F514	Records complete	2.09

Table IV-4 (continued)

Most Frequently Cited Deficiencies, 1997: North Carolina

Rank	Tag	Requirement	% of Facilities Cited
1	F241	Dignity	29.60
2	F309	Highest practicable care	20.65
3	F371	Food sanitation	20.65
4	F272	Comprehensive assessments	18.91
5	F312	ADL services	17.16
6	F316	Bladder treatment	16.67
7	F329	Drugs	16.67
8	F253	Housekeeping	15.17
9	F364	Food quality	14.43
10	F324	Accident prevention	13.93
11	F242	Self determination	13.68
12	F279	Comprehensive care plan	12.44
13	F323	Hazard-free environment	11.19
14	F164	Privacy/confidentiality	10.20
15	F221	Physical restraints	10.20
16	F246	Accommodate needs	9.95
17	F281	Professional standards	9.70
18	F314	Pressure sores	8.71
19	F318	Range of motion treatment	8.21
20	F429	Drug records	7.21
21	F278	Accuracy of assessments	6.72
22	F311	Appropriate ADL treatment	6.72
23	F167	Examine survey results	5.72
24	F224	Staff treatment of residents	5.72
25	F353	Sufficient staff	5.72
26	F166	Resolve grievances	5.47
27	F274	Assessment-condition change	5.47
28	F248	Activities program	4.73
29	F325	Nutrition	4.73
30	F368	Food schedule	4.73
31	F225	Criminal staff/abuse	4.48
32	F252	Environment-safe, clean	4.48
33	F258	Comfortable sound	4.23
34	F332	Medication errors >5%	4.23
35	F469	Pest control	3.98
36	F156	Notice of rights/services	3.73
37	F208	Admissions policy	3.48
38	F276	Assessment review	3.48
39	F322	NG treatment	3.48
40	F372	Garbage	3.48

Table IV-4 (continued)

Most Frequently Cited Deficiencies, 1997: North Dakota

Rank	Tag	Requirement	% of Facilities Cited
1	F452	Tag does not exist	37.50
2	F444	Hand washing	26.14
3	F253	Housekeeping	25.00
4	F371	Food sanitation	23.86
5	F241	Dignity	22.73
6	F280	Plan requirements	22.73
7	F281	Professional standards	22.73
8	F282	Assessment by qualified staff	22.73
9	F314	Pressure sores	22.73
10	F441	Infection control	22.73
11	F272	Comprehensive assessments	20.45
12	F316	Bladder treatment	20.45
13	F221	Physical restraints	19.32
14	F312	ADL services	19.32
15	F279	Comprehensive care plan	18.18
16	F521	Q.A. committee meets/plans	14.77
17	F225	Criminal staff/abuse	13.64
18	F250	Social services	13.64
19	F311	Appropriate ADL treatment	12.50
20	F329	Drugs	12.50
21	F465	Other environment	12.50
22	F164	Privacy/confidentiality	11.36
23	F157	Notice of changes	10.23
24	F246	Accommodate needs	10.23
25	F156	Notice of rights/services	9.09
26	F248	Activities program	9.09
27	F324	Accident prevention	9.09
28	F325	Nutrition	9.09
29	F364	Food quality	9.09
30	F327	Hydration	7.95
31	F328	Special treatments	7.95
32	F242	Self determination	6.82
33	F309	Highest practicable care	6.82
34	F322	NG treatment	6.82
35	F514	Records complete	6.82
36	F353	Sufficient staff	5.68
37	F432	Act on drug reports	5.68
38	F445	Handle linens	5.68
39	F498	N.A. proficiency	5.68
40	F166	Resolve grievances	4.55

TABLE IV-4 (CONTINUED)

MOST FREQUENTLY CITED DEFICIENCIES, 1997: OHIO

Rank	Tag	Requirement	% of Facilities Cited
1	F323	Hazard-free environment	28.40
2	F272	Comprehensive assessments	25.94
3	F371	Food sanitation	22.78
4	F314	Pressure sores	22.39
5	F279	Comprehensive care plan	17.75
6	F324	Accident prevention	14.40
7	F221	Physical restraints	14.30
8	F281	Professional standards	12.03
9	F316	Bladder treatment	12.03
10	F312	ADL services	11.74
11	F241	Dignity	10.65
12	F309	Highest practicable care	10.16
13	F246	Accommodate needs	9.96
14	F364	Food quality	9.96
15	F318	Range of motion treatment	9.76
16	F458	Square footage	9.76
17	F157	Notice of changes	9.57
18	F253	Housekeeping	9.57
19	F441	Infection control	8.88
20	F250	Social services	8.58
21	F278	Accuracy of assessments	8.58
22	F329	Drugs	8.38
23	F325	Nutrition	7.89
24	F248	Activities program	7.79
25	F311	Appropriate ADL treatment	7.40
26	F164	Privacy/confidentiality	6.31
27	F363	Menus/nutritional adequacy	5.82
28	F497	N.A. in-service	5.72
29	F280	Plan requirements	5.62
30	F159	Manage funds-facility	5.42
31	F276	Assessment review	5.42
32	F252	Environment-safe, clean	5.13
33	F444	Hand washing	5.13
34	F225	Criminal staff/abuse	4.64
35	F514	Records complete	4.24
36	F274	Assessment-condition change	3.65
37	F365	Food form	3.55
38	F518	Staff training	3.55
39	F322	NG treatment	2.96
40	F457	Four to a room	2.86

TABLE IV-4 (CONTINUED)

MOST FREQUENTLY CITED DEFICIENCIES, 1997: OKLAHOMA

Rank	Tag	Requirement	% of Facilities Cited
1	F514	Records complete	30.99
2	F371	Food sanitation	26.39
3	F221	Physical restraints	23.73
4	F441	Infection control	19.61
5	F272	Comprehensive assessments	19.37
6	F312	ADL services	18.89
7	F279	Comprehensive care plan	17.92
8	F325	Nutrition	16.46
9	F332	Medication errors >5%	15.74
10	F314	Pressure sores	15.50
11	F354	RN staff	15.01
12	F318	Range of motion treatment	14.77
13	F253	Housekeeping	13.56
14	F363	Menus/nutritional adequacy	11.86
15	F164	Privacy/confidentiality	10.41
16	F311	Appropriate ADL treatment	9.44
17	F364	Food quality	9.44
18	F280	Plan requirements	9.20
19	F465	Other environment	8.96
20	F248	Activities program	8.47
21	F241	Dignity	7.75
22	F252	Environment-safe, clean	7.75
23	F456	Equipment maintenance	7.75
24	F323	Hazard-free environment	7.51
25	F432	Act on drug reports	6.54
26	F464	Dining/activity rooms	6.30
27	F276	Assessment review	5.81
28	F469	Pest control	5.57
29	F246	Accommodate needs	5.33
30	F316	Bladder treatment	5.33
31	F426	Pharmacy procedures	4.84
32	F275	Annual assessments	4.60
33	F494	N.A.s are trained	3.87
34	F254	Clean linens	3.63
35	F310	ADLs don't diminish	3.63
36	F431	Report drug irregularities	3.63
37	F250	Social services	3.39
38	F322	NG treatment	3.39
39	F273	Assessment 14 days after adm.	3.15
40	F329	Drugs	3.15

TABLE IV-4 (CONTINUED)

MOST FREQUENTLY CITED DEFICIENCIES, 1997: OREGON

Rank	Tag	Requirement	% of Facilities Cited
1	F309	Highest practicable care	44.79
2	F272	Comprehensive assessments	44.17
3	F324	Accident prevention	25.77
4	F314	Pressure sores	23.31
5	F276	Assessment review	22.70
6	F323	Hazard-free environment	17.79
7	F225	Criminal staff/abuse	17.18
8	F241	Dignity	16.56
9	F311	Appropriate ADL treatment	15.95
10	F248	Activities program	15.34
11	F312	ADL services	15.34
12	F441	Infection control	14.72
13	F221	Physical restraints	12.88
14	F279	Comprehensive care plan	12.88
15	F318	Range of motion treatment	12.27
16	F371	Food sanitation	11.66
17	F316	Bladder treatment	11.04
18	F329	Drugs	11.04
19	F252	Environment-safe, clean	9.82
20	F253	Housekeeping	9.82
21	F246	Accommodate needs	9.20
22	F280	Plan requirements	9.20
23	F325	Nutrition	9.20
24	F387	Physician visits	9.20
25	F164	Privacy/confidentiality	8.59
26	F274	Assessment-condition change	8.59
27	F250	Social services	7.98
28	F444	Hand washing	7.98
29	F498	N.A. proficiency	7.98
30	F319	Mental/psychosocial services	6.13
31	F521	Q.A. committee meets/plans	5.52
32	F364	Food quality	4.91
33	F278	Accuracy of assessments	4.29
34	F332	Medication errors >5%	4.29
35	F156	Notice of rights/services	3.68
36	F353	Sufficient staff	3.68
37	F469	Pest control	3.68
38	F503	Lab/blood bank services	3.68
39	F514	Records complete	3.68
40	F224	Staff treatment of residents	3.07

Table IV-4 (continued)

Most Frequently Cited Deficiencies, 1997: Pennsylvania

Rank	Tag	Requirement	% of Facilities Cited
1	F279	Comprehensive care plan	21.21
2	F221	Physical restraints	19.82
3	F324	Accident prevention	18.06
4	F514	Records complete	16.29
5	F309	Highest practicable care	14.02
6	F323	Hazard-free environment	13.38
7	F329	Drugs	13.01
8	F314	Pressure sores	12.88
9	F371	Food sanitation	12.75
10	F281	Professional standards	11.11
11	F250	Social services	10.10
12	F325	Nutrition	9.09
13	F241	Dignity	8.84
14	F248	Activities program	8.46
15	F316	Bladder treatment	7.58
16	F465	Other environment	7.58
17	F318	Range of motion treatment	7.32
18	F441	Infection control	7.32
19	F280	Plan requirements	6.57
20	F246	Accommodate needs	6.31
21	F253	Housekeeping	5.93
22	F364	Food quality	5.56
23	F225	Criminal staff/abuse	5.30
24	F157	Notice of changes	4.92
25	F272	Comprehensive assessments	4.92
26	F274	Assessment-condition change	4.55
27	F386	Physician documentation	4.29
28	F312	ADL services	3.79
29	F282	Assessment by qualified staff	3.66
30	F310	ADLs don't diminish	3.66
31	F252	Environment-safe, clean	3.54
32	F319	Mental/psychosocial services	3.54
33	F311	Appropriate ADL treatment	3.41
34	F156	Notice of rights/services	3.28
35	F278	Accuracy of assessments	3.28
36	F430	Act on pharmacist's report	3.28
37	F167	Examine survey results	3.16
38	F315	Catheter use	3.03
39	F327	Hydration	3.03
40	F332	Medication errors >5%	2.78

TABLE IV-4 (CONTINUED)

MOST FREQUENTLY CITED DEFICIENCIES, 1997: RHODE ISLAND

Rank	Tag	Requirement	% of Facilities Cited
1	F272	Comprehensive assessments	26.00
2	F371	Food sanitation	22.00
3	F221	Physical restraints	15.00
4	F281	Professional standards	15.00
5	F159	Manage funds-facility	12.00
6	F329	Drugs	12.00
7	F441	Infection control	12.00
8	F253	Housekeeping	11.00
9	F314	Pressure sores	11.00
10	F323	Hazard-free environment	11.00
11	F252	Environment-safe, clean	9.00
12	F324	Accident prevention	9.00
13	F274	Assessment-condition change	8.00
14	F318	Range of motion treatment	8.00
15	F458	Square footage	8.00
16	F167	Examine survey results	7.00
17	F174	Telephone access	7.00
18	F279	Comprehensive care plan	7.00
19	F311	Appropriate ADL treatment	7.00
20	F364	Food quality	7.00
21	F276	Assessment review	6.00
22	F280	Plan requirements	6.00
23	F312	ADL services	6.00
24	F460	Privacy	6.00
25	F225	Criminal staff/abuse	5.00
26	F248	Activities program	5.00
27	F309	Highest practicable care	5.00
28	F332	Medication errors >5%	5.00
29	F442	Isolate residents	4.00
30	F445	Handle linens	4.00
31	F156	Notice of rights/services	3.00
32	F164	Privacy/confidentiality	3.00
33	F170	Mail service	3.00
34	F176	Self-administration of drugs	3.00
35	F241	Dignity	3.00
36	F275	Annual assessments	3.00
37	F313	Vision/hearing	3.00
38	F367	Therapeutic diets	3.00
39	F368	Food schedule	3.00
40	F432	Act on drug reports	3.00

TABLE IV-4 (CONTINUED)

MOST FREQUENTLY CITED DEFICIENCIES, 1997: SOUTH CAROLINA

Rank	Tag	Requirement	% of Facilities Cited
1	F371	Food sanitation	43.18
2	F316	Bladder treatment	38.07
3	F279	Comprehensive care plan	35.23
4	F241	Dignity	29.55
5	F444	Hand washing	28.41
6	F309	Highest practicable care	25.00
7	F272	Comprehensive assessments	24.43
8	F329	Drugs	24.43
9	F314	Pressure sores	23.86
10	F323	Hazard-free environment	23.86
11	F328	Special treatments	21.02
12	F322	NG treatment	19.89
13	F164	Privacy/confidentiality	18.75
14	F221	Physical restraints	17.05
15	F368	Food schedule	14.20
16	F318	Range of motion treatment	12.50
17	F514	Records complete	11.93
18	F176	Self-administration of drugs	11.36
19	F248	Activities program	11.36
20	F441	Infection control	11.36
21	F274	Assessment-condition change	10.80
22	F325	Nutrition	10.23
23	F324	Accident prevention	9.66
24	F225	Criminal staff/abuse	9.09
25	F253	Housekeeping	9.09
26	F432	Act on drug reports	9.09
27	F353	Sufficient staff	8.52
28	F502	Provide or obtain lab services	8.52
29	F174	Telephone access	7.95
30	F280	Plan requirements	7.95
31	F330	Antipsychotic drug use	7.39
32	F332	Medication errors >5%	7.39
33	F372	Garbage	6.82
34	F445	Handle linens	6.82
35	F223	Abuse	6.25
36	F246	Accommodate needs	6.25
37	F250	Social services	6.25
38	F252	Environment-safe, clean	6.25
39	F278	Accuracy of assessments	6.25
40	F281	Professional standards	6.25

Table IV-4 (continued)

Most Frequently Cited Deficiencies, 1997: South Dakota

Rank	Tag	Requirement	% of Facilities Cited
1	F272	Comprehensive assessments	41.23
2	F329	Drugs	36.84
3	F323	Hazard-free environment	29.82
4	F221	Physical restraints	28.07
5	F279	Comprehensive care plan	24.56
6	F371	Food sanitation	21.05
7	F429	Drug records	18.42
8	F444	Hand washing	14.04
9	F314	Pressure sores	13.16
10	F325	Nutrition	13.16
11	F248	Activities program	12.28
12	F252	Environment-safe, clean	11.40
13	F274	Assessment-condition change	11.40
14	F467	Outside ventilation	7.89
15	F241	Dignity	7.02
16	F246	Accommodate needs	6.14
17	F316	Bladder treatment	6.14
18	F324	Accident prevention	6.14
19	F353	Sufficient staff	6.14
20	F460	Privacy	6.14
21	F253	Housekeeping	5.26
22	F332	Medication errors >5%	5.26
23	F521	Q.A. committee meets/plans	5.26
24	F164	Privacy/confidentiality	4.39
25	F281	Professional standards	4.39
26	F309	Highest practicable care	4.39
27	F310	ADLs don't diminish	4.39
28	F318	Range of motion treatment	4.39
29	F250	Social services	3.51
30	F282	Assessment by qualified staff	3.51
31	F312	ADL services	3.51
32	F441	Infection control	3.51
33	F490	Administration	3.51
34	F494	N.A.s are trained	3.51
35	F176	Self-administration of drugs	2.63
36	F275	Annual assessments	2.63
37	F431	Report drug irregularities	2.63
38	F456	Equipment maintenance	2.63
39	F498	N.A. proficiency	2.63
40	F156	Notice of rights/services	1.75

TABLE IV-4 (CONTINUED)

MOST FREQUENTLY CITED DEFICIENCIES, 1997: TENNESSEE

Rank	Tag	Requirement	% of Facilities Cited
1	F272	Comprehensive assessments	29.02
2	F371	Food sanitation	26.44
3	F279	Comprehensive care plan	21.55
4	F253	Housekeeping	16.38
5	F314	Pressure sores	14.94
6	F323	Hazard-free environment	14.08
7	F329	Drugs	12.07
8	F309	Highest practicable care	10.63
9	F432	Act on drug reports	9.48
10	F241	Dignity	9.20
11	F221	Physical restraints	8.62
12	F514	Records complete	8.62
13	F246	Accommodate needs	8.33
14	F319	Mental/psychosocial services	7.18
15	F441	Infection control	6.90
16	F322	NG treatment	6.61
17	F492	Compliance with laws	6.03
18	F274	Assessment-condition change	5.75
19	F372	Garbage	5.75
20	F469	Pest control	5.75
21	F164	Privacy/confidentiality	5.46
22	F325	Nutrition	5.46
23	F156	Notice of rights/services	5.17
24	F166	Resolve grievances	5.17
25	F311	Appropriate ADL treatment	5.17
26	F252	Environment-safe, clean	4.60
27	F316	Bladder treatment	4.60
28	F312	ADL services	4.31
29	F318	Range of motion treatment	4.31
30	F328	Special treatments	4.31
31	F367	Therapeutic diets	4.31
32	F497	N.A. in-service	4.31
33	F157	Notice of changes	3.74
34	F327	Hydration	3.74
35	F431	Report drug irregularities	3.74
36	F444	Hand washing	3.74
37	F248	Activities program	3.16
38	F254	Clean linens	2.87
39	F278	Accuracy of assessments	2.87
40	F324	Accident prevention	2.59

Table IV-4 (continued)

Most Frequently Cited Deficiencies, 1997: Texas

Rank	Tag	Requirement	% of Facilities Cited
1	F371	Food sanitation	27.38
2	F253	Housekeeping	26.23
3	F309	Highest practicable care	16.92
4	F441	Infection control	16.38
5	F323	Hazard-free environment	14.77
6	F332	Medication errors >5%	14.15
7	F314	Pressure sores	13.38
8	F426	Pharmacy procedures	12.08
9	F279	Comprehensive care plan	11.85
10	F312	ADL services	11.00
11	F514	Records complete	10.46
12	F364	Food quality	9.77
13	F465	Other environment	9.46
14	F221	Physical restraints	8.85
15	F246	Accommodate needs	8.38
16	F458	Square footage	8.00
17	F324	Accident prevention	7.85
18	F325	Nutrition	7.85
19	F252	Environment-safe, clean	7.62
20	F498	N.A. proficiency	7.54
21	F469	Pest control	7.46
22	F241	Dignity	7.08
23	F250	Social services	6.62
24	F272	Comprehensive assessments	6.54
25	F248	Activities program	6.38
26	F318	Range of motion treatment	5.54
27	F456	Equipment maintenance	5.46
28	F329	Drugs	5.08
29	F353	Sufficient staff	5.08
30	F322	NG treatment	4.92
31	F333	Significant medication errors	4.92
32	F157	Notice of changes	4.85
33	F497	N.A. in-service	4.77
34	F368	Food schedule	4.38
35	F316	Bladder treatment	4.31
36	F354	RN staff	4.31
37	F502	Provide or obtain lab services	4.15
38	F363	Menus/nutritional adequacy	4.00
39	F463	Call system in rooms	3.69
40	F278	Accuracy of assessments	3.54

Table IV-4 (continued)

Most Frequently Cited Deficiencies, 1997: Utah

Rank	Tag	Requirement	% of Facilities Cited
1	F323	Hazard-free environment	34.38
2	F371	Food sanitation	30.21
3	F309	Highest practicable care	18.75
4	F241	Dignity	16.67
5	F312	ADL services	16.67
6	F460	Privacy	16.67
7	F364	Food quality	14.58
8	F368	Food schedule	14.58
9	F246	Accommodate needs	12.50
10	F252	Environment-safe, clean	11.46
11	F329	Drugs	11.46
12	F365	Food form	11.46
13	F164	Privacy/confidentiality	10.42
14	F314	Pressure sores	10.42
15	F240	Promote quality of life	9.38
16	F253	Housekeeping	9.38
17	F326	Therapeutic diet	9.38
18	F281	Professional standards	8.33
19	F248	Activities program	7.29
20	F258	Comfortable sound	7.29
21	F157	Notice of changes	6.25
22	F318	Range of motion treatment	6.25
23	F325	Nutrition	6.25
24	F242	Self determination	5.21
25	F316	Bladder treatment	5.21
26	F372	Garbage	5.21
27	F426	Pharmacy procedures	5.21
28	F221	Physical restraints	4.17
29	F279	Comprehensive care plan	4.17
30	F310	ADLs don't diminish	4.17
31	F363	Menus/nutritional adequacy	4.17
32	F156	Notice of rights/services	3.13
33	F166	Resolve grievances	3.13
34	F167	Examine survey results	3.13
35	F272	Comprehensive assessments	3.13
36	F280	Plan requirements	3.13
37	F311	Appropriate ADL treatment	3.13
38	F366	Food substitutions	3.13
39	F432	Act on drug reports	3.13
40	F441	Infection control	3.13

Table IV-4 (continued)

Most Frequently Cited Deficiencies, 1997: Vermont

Rank	Tag	Requirement	% of Facilities Cited
1	F272	Comprehensive assessments	29.55
2	F221	Physical restraints	20.45
3	F314	Pressure sores	20.45
4	F281	Professional standards	18.18
5	F241	Dignity	13.64
6	F329	Drugs	13.64
7	F332	Medication errors >5%	13.64
8	F164	Privacy/confidentiality	11.36
9	F312	ADL services	11.36
10	F322	NG treatment	11.36
11	F354	RN staff	11.36
12	F248	Activities program	9.09
13	F319	Mental/psychosocial services	9.09
14	F325	Nutrition	9.09
15	F246	Accommodate needs	6.82
16	F311	Appropriate ADL treatment	6.82
17	F323	Hazard-free environment	6.82
18	F324	Accident prevention	6.82
19	F225	Criminal staff/abuse	4.55
20	F274	Assessment-condition change	4.55
21	F279	Comprehensive care plan	4.55
22	F282	Assessment by qualified staff	4.55
23	F309	Highest practicable care	4.55
24	F310	ADLs don't diminish	4.55
25	F316	Bladder treatment	4.55
26	F328	Special treatments	4.55
27	F353	Sufficient staff	4.55
28	F363	Menus/nutritional adequacy	4.55
29	F371	Food sanitation	4.55
30	F430	Act on pharmacist's report	4.55
31	F432	Act on drug reports	4.55
32	F441	Infection control	4.55
33	F458	Square footage	4.55
34	F498	N.A. proficiency	4.55
35	F521	Q.A. committee meets/plans	4.55
36	F157	Notice of changes	2.27
37	F159	Manage funds-facility	2.27
38	F240	Promote quality of life	2.27
39	F250	Social services	2.27
40	F278	Accuracy of assessments	2.27

TABLE IV-4 (CONTINUED)

MOST FREQUENTLY CITED DEFICIENCIES, 1997: VIRGINIA

Rank	Tag	Requirement	% of Facilities Cited
1	F279	Comprehensive care plan	25.46
2	F309	Highest practicable care	21.77
3	F221	Physical restraints	16.97
4	F371	Food sanitation	16.61
5	F314	Pressure sores	14.76
6	F246	Accommodate needs	13.28
7	F323	Hazard-free environment	13.28
8	F469	Pest control	12.18
9	F521	Q.A. committee meets/plans	12.18
10	F441	Infection control	11.44
11	F241	Dignity	10.33
12	F312	ADL services	9.96
13	F493	Governing body	9.96
14	F157	Notice of changes	9.59
15	F490	Administration	9.59
16	F224	Staff treatment of residents	9.23
17	F324	Accident prevention	8.86
18	F225	Criminal staff/abuse	8.49
19	F250	Social services	8.49
20	F164	Privacy/confidentiality	7.75
21	F514	Records complete	7.75
22	F248	Activities program	7.38
23	F325	Nutrition	7.01
24	F463	Call system in rooms	7.01
25	F253	Housekeeping	6.27
26	F252	Environment-safe, clean	5.90
27	F353	Sufficient staff	5.90
28	F316	Bladder treatment	5.54
29	F332	Medication errors >5%	5.54
30	F278	Accuracy of assessments	5.17
31	F280	Plan requirements	5.17
32	F282	Assessment by qualified staff	5.17
33	F322	NG treatment	5.17
34	F465	Other environment	5.17
35	F445	Handle linens	4.80
36	F272	Comprehensive assessments	4.06
37	F368	Food schedule	4.06
38	F372	Garbage	4.06
39	F274	Assessment-condition change	3.69
40	F311	Appropriate ADL treatment	3.69

TABLE IV-4 (CONTINUED)

MOST FREQUENTLY CITED DEFICIENCIES, 1997: WASHINGTON

Rank	Tag	Requirement	% of Facilities Cited
1	F309	Highest practicable care	39.30
2	F371	Food sanitation	37.54
3	F314	Pressure sores	36.49
4	F323	Hazard-free environment	30.53
5	F241	Dignity	28.07
6	F253	Housekeeping	26.32
7	F272	Comprehensive assessments	26.32
8	F312	ADL services	24.91
9	F225	Criminal staff/abuse	23.86
10	F316	Bladder treatment	22.46
11	F441	Infection control	22.11
12	F324	Accident prevention	21.75
13	F311	Appropriate ADL treatment	20.70
14	F248	Activities program	20.35
15	F246	Accommodate needs	20.00
16	F276	Assessment review	19.65
17	F465	Other environment	18.95
18	F325	Nutrition	17.54
19	F164	Privacy/confidentiality	17.19
20	F444	Hand washing	16.14
21	F221	Physical restraints	15.44
22	F364	Food quality	15.09
23	F279	Comprehensive care plan	14.39
24	F329	Drugs	14.39
25	F250	Social services	13.68
26	F318	Range of motion treatment	13.68
27	F281	Professional standards	12.28
28	F252	Environment-safe, clean	11.58
29	F458	Square footage	10.53
30	F445	Handle linens	10.18
31	F365	Food form	9.12
32	F154	Informed of medical condition	8.77
33	F322	NG treatment	8.77
34	F319	Mental/psychosocial services	8.07
35	F274	Assessment-condition change	7.37
36	F466	Water supply	7.37
37	F258	Comfortable sound	7.02
38	F151	Rights	6.67
39	F166	Resolve grievances	6.67
40	F278	Accuracy of assessments	6.67

Table IV-4 (continued)

Most Frequently Cited Deficiencies, 1997: West Virginia

Rank	Tag	Requirement	% of Facilities Cited
1	F465	Other environment	50.74
2	F371	Food sanitation	25.74
3	F221	Physical restraints	21.32
4	F246	Accommodate needs	19.85
5	F309	Highest practicable care	19.85
6	F272	Comprehensive assessments	15.44
7	F463	Call system in rooms	14.71
8	F514	Records complete	14.71
9	F250	Social services	13.97
10	F279	Comprehensive care plan	13.97
11	F225	Criminal staff/abuse	13.24
12	F241	Dignity	13.24
13	F278	Accuracy of assessments	13.24
14	F441	Infection control	13.24
15	F312	ADL services	11.76
16	F323	Hazard-free environment	11.03
17	F248	Activities program	10.29
18	F329	Drugs	9.56
19	F363	Menus/nutritional adequacy	9.56
20	F364	Food quality	8.82
21	F455	Private closet space	8.82
22	F314	Pressure sores	8.09
23	F429	Drug records	7.35
24	F445	Handle linens	7.35
25	F152	Resident rights	6.62
26	F157	Notice of changes	6.62
27	F164	Privacy/confidentiality	6.62
28	F274	Assessment-condition change	6.62
29	F456	Equipment maintenance	6.62
30	F252	Environment-safe, clean	5.88
31	F276	Assessment review	5.88
32	F365	Food form	5.88
33	F151	Rights	5.15
34	F242	Self determination	5.15
35	F253	Housekeeping	5.15
36	F316	Bladder treatment	5.15
37	F319	Mental/psychosocial services	5.15
38	F332	Medication errors >5%	5.15
39	F153	Access records	4.41
40	F166	Resolve grievances	4.41

TABLE IV-4 (CONTINUED)

MOST FREQUENTLY CITED DEFICIENCIES, 1997: WISCONSIN

Rank	Tag	Requirement	% of Facilities Cited
1	F272	Comprehensive assessments	42.32
2	F323	Hazard-free environment	17.26
3	F221	Physical restraints	16.31
4	F279	Comprehensive care plan	16.08
5	F309	Highest practicable care	15.13
6	F253	Housekeeping	12.77
7	F514	Records complete	12.77
8	F225	Criminal staff/abuse	12.29
9	F248	Activities program	12.06
10	F324	Accident prevention	11.82
11	F329	Drugs	10.87
12	F364	Food quality	10.40
13	F314	Pressure sores	9.46
14	F371	Food sanitation	8.98
15	F250	Social services	8.51
16	F241	Dignity	8.04
17	F157	Notice of changes	6.86
18	F318	Range of motion treatment	6.86
19	F252	Environment-safe, clean	6.62
20	F156	Notice of rights/services	6.38
21	F312	ADL services	6.38
22	F316	Bladder treatment	5.91
23	F164	Privacy/confidentiality	5.44
24	F246	Accommodate needs	5.20
25	F282	Assessment by qualified staff	5.20
26	F280	Plan requirements	4.96
27	F311	Appropriate ADL treatment	4.96
28	F458	Square footage	3.78
29	F242	Self determination	3.55
30	F492	Compliance with laws	3.55
31	F167	Examine survey results	3.31
32	F444	Hand washing	3.31
33	F332	Medication errors >5%	3.07
34	F465	Other environment	3.07
35	F278	Accuracy of assessments	2.84
36	F274	Assessment-condition change	2.60
37	F441	Infection control	2.36
38	F497	N.A.in-service	2.36
39	F154	Informed of medical condition	2.13
40	F166	Resolve grievances	2.13

TABLE IV-4 (CONTINUED)

MOST FREQUENTLY CITED DEFICIENCIES, 1997: WYOMING

Rank	Tag	Requirement	of Facilities Cited
1	F312	ADL services	60.53
2	F371	Food sanitation	47.37
3	F241	Dignity	42.11
4	F444	Hand washing	36.84
5	F316	Bladder treatment	34.21
6	F248	Activities program	31.58
7	F279	Comprehensive care plan	31.58
8	F441	Infection control	28.95
9	F323	Hazard-free environment	26.32
10	F272	Comprehensive assessments	23.68
11	F164	Privacy/confidentiality	21.05
12	F314	Pressure sores	13.16
13	F319	Mental/psychosocial services	13.16
14	F363	Menus/nutritional adequacy	13.16
15	F221	Physical restraints	10.53
16	F274	Assessment-condition change	10.53
17	F364	Food quality	10.53
18	F281	Professional standards	7.89
19	F309	Highest practicable care	7.89
20	F310	ADLs don't diminish	7.89
21	F317	Range of motion loss	7.89
22	F406	Rehab	7.89
23	F445	Handle linens	7.89
24	F465	Other environment	7.89
25	F223	Abuse	5.26
26	F253	Housekeeping	5.26
27	F258	Comfortable sound	5.26
28	F283	Assessment recap	5.26
29	F284	Post-discharge plan of care	5.26
30	F318	Range of motion treatment	5.26
31	F324	Accident prevention	5.26
32	F325	Nutrition	5.26
33	F327	Hydration	5.26
34	F353	Sufficient staff	5.26
35	F463	Call system in rooms	5.26
36	F521	Q.A. committee meets/plans	5.26
37	F151	Rights	2.63
38	F152	Resident rights	2.63
39	F157	Notice of changes	2.63
40	F205	Bedhold notice	2.63

TABLE IV-5

SCOPE AND SEVERITY CODE UTILIZATION BY STATE, 1997

	% B	% C	% D	% E	% F	% G	% H	% I	% J	% K	% L
UNITED STATES	15.66	10.06	31.29	23.29	6.02	9.90	2.74	0.73	0.09	0.14	0.08
Alabama	13.05	8.68	41.49	23.00	2.81	9.33	1.17	0.40	0.04	0.04	0.00
Alaska	6.85	10.96	43.84	17.81	1.37	17.81	1.37	0.00	0.00	0.00	0.00
Arizona	29.73	7.99	22.91	32.43	1.78	3.75	1.17	0.06	0.00	0.18	0.00
Arkansas	51.21	7.68	25.09	11.09	1.91	2.31	0.64	0.04	0.02	0.00	0.00
California	22.21	7.03	38.02	22.90	2.37	4.81	2.11	0.22	0.09	0.17	0.07
Colorado	13.90	1.16	53.76	22.42	0.99	6.62	1.16	0.00	0.00	0.00	0.00
Connecticut	1.63	2.81	38.57	16.15	4.72	31.58	4.45	0.09	0.00	0.00	0.00
Delaware	18.23	3.65	45.32	21.24	2.54	8.24	0.79	0.00	0.00	0.00	0.00
District of Columbia	60.00	18.00	9.50	4.50	1.50	5.50	0.00	1.00	0.00	0.00	0.00
Florida	6.56	13.20	22.79	32.07	11.26	8.93	3.35	1.59	0.08	0.09	0.09
Georgia	19.17	14.52	14.90	17.97	9.54	12.32	8.63	2.90	0.00	0.00	0.04
Hawaii	19.44	18.52	26.85	12.96	11.11	9.03	0.23	0.93	0.00	0.93	0.00
Idaho	5.09	4.12	24.16	28.28	10.08	24.27	3.68	0.22	0.11	0.00	0.00
Illinois	19.60	15.96	34.38	19.72	3.31	5.74	0.88	0.13	0.11	0.12	0.05
Indiana	13.18	6.74	34.33	25.55	4.42	10.68	4.03	0.74	0.11	0.13	0.08
Iowa	9.65	6.37	34.11	19.97	4.08	23.36	2.43	0.02	0.00	0.00	0.00
Kansas	7.64	9.76	25.09	19.70	9.06	20.10	6.51	1.61	0.25	0.21	0.07
Kentucky	8.13	14.63	18.73	23.76	15.56	7.20	5.03	5.34	0.77	0.31	0.54
Louisiana	44.40	23.96	15.23	11.20	0.91	3.75	0.30	0.08	0.00	0.15	0.03
Maine	13.76	22.57	32.63	14.81	7.76	4.94	0.88	2.65	0.00	0.00	0.00
Maryland	18.79	7.93	29.65	23.17	1.88	11.27	6.89	0.42	0.00	0.00	0.00
Massachusetts	4.66	5.21	27.03	23.45	5.54	23.70	6.94	2.81	0.05	0.58	0.05
Michigan	11.59	4.65	37.74	25.85	6.74	10.72	1.90	0.56	0.08	0.05	0.11
Minnesota	12.33	7.69	31.50	30.01	3.38	13.20	1.72	0.07	0.07	0.03	0.00
Mississippi	19.31	15.35	28.13	17.13	5.83	10.19	3.07	0.71	0.04	0.22	0.00
Missouri	3.26	4.23	27.90	37.06	10.27	11.60	4.67	0.46	0.24	0.30	0.00
Montana	17.97	9.46	23.33	30.78	2.20	14.53	1.63	0.00	0.10	0.00	0.00
Nebraska	6.91	7.47	22.93	25.88	9.80	20.67	5.61	0.45	0.00	0.23	0.06
Nevada	13.51	6.16	30.61	30.97	2.76	12.78	2.85	0.37	0.00	0.00	0.00
New Hampshire	10.67	5.25	41.38	18.72	4.43	13.63	4.11	0.49	0.99	0.00	0.33
New Jersey	16.03	11.93	20.60	22.99	10.13	12.37	4.48	1.36	0.00	0.10	0.00
New Mexico	7.69	4.05	17.00	35.63	19.84	9.31	4.45	1.21	0.00	0.81	0.00
New York	20.90	7.22	38.70	18.45	3.23	9.80	1.46	0.23	0.00	0.00	0.00
North Carolina	15.61	7.24	34.36	17.65	4.64	17.45	2.55	0.33	0.05	0.11	0.00
North Dakota	14.40	7.02	36.01	19.67	2.40	18.37	2.12	0.00	0.00	0.00	0.00
Ohio	7.67	6.01	38.62	27.41	9.16	7.74	2.22	0.88	0.10	0.07	0.11
Oklahoma	14.65	23.10	12.28	35.47	7.35	4.01	2.11	1.03	0.00	0.00	0.00
Oregon	11.70	3.44	27.75	30.10	6.08	12.79	4.42	2.47	0.29	0.75	0.23
Pennsylvania	12.76	10.41	34.91	22.39	4.36	12.37	1.54	0.72	0.03	0.14	0.36

TABLE IV-55: SCOPE AND SEVERITY CODE UTILIZATION BY STATE, 1997 (CONTINUED)

	% B	% C	% D	% E	% F	% G	% H	% I	% J	% K	% L
Rhode Island	6.17	22.47	44.71	9.03	11.01	6.61	0.00	0.00	0.00	0.00	0.00
South Carolina	6.38	4.75	53.26	15.45	7.61	10.22	1.78	0.22	0.18	0.07	0.07
South Dakota	4.21	8.90	31.55	13.75	8.09	28.48	2.91	2.10	0.00	0.00	0.00
Tennessee	5.10	13.28	32.75	27.99	14.90	3.86	1.29	0.55	0.08	0.08	0.11
Texas	20.84	20.43	15.03	20.16	9.96	7.67	3.84	1.39	0.08	0.32	0.28
Utah	23.20	3.18	29.92	30.04	1.30	7.42	3.42	0.59	0.00	0.94	0.00
Vermont	13.90	8.49	36.29	18.53	0.39	18.15	3.86	0.00	0.39	0.00	0.00
Virginia	6.39	6.11	31.81	18.82	19.65	9.93	4.93	2.15	0.07	0.14	0.00
Washington	9.83	8.65	34.23	20.82	4.98	17.71	3.13	0.52	0.10	0.04	0.00
West Virginia	14.70	31.20	24.51	12.25	11.88	2.73	1.60	1.13	0.00	0.00	0.00
Wisconsin	10.42	9.29	38.23	28.74	3.49	8.92	0.82	0.00	0.00	0.09	0.00
Wyoming	9.37	5.23	33.33	30.28	7.84	10.89	2.83	0.22	0.00	0.00	0.00

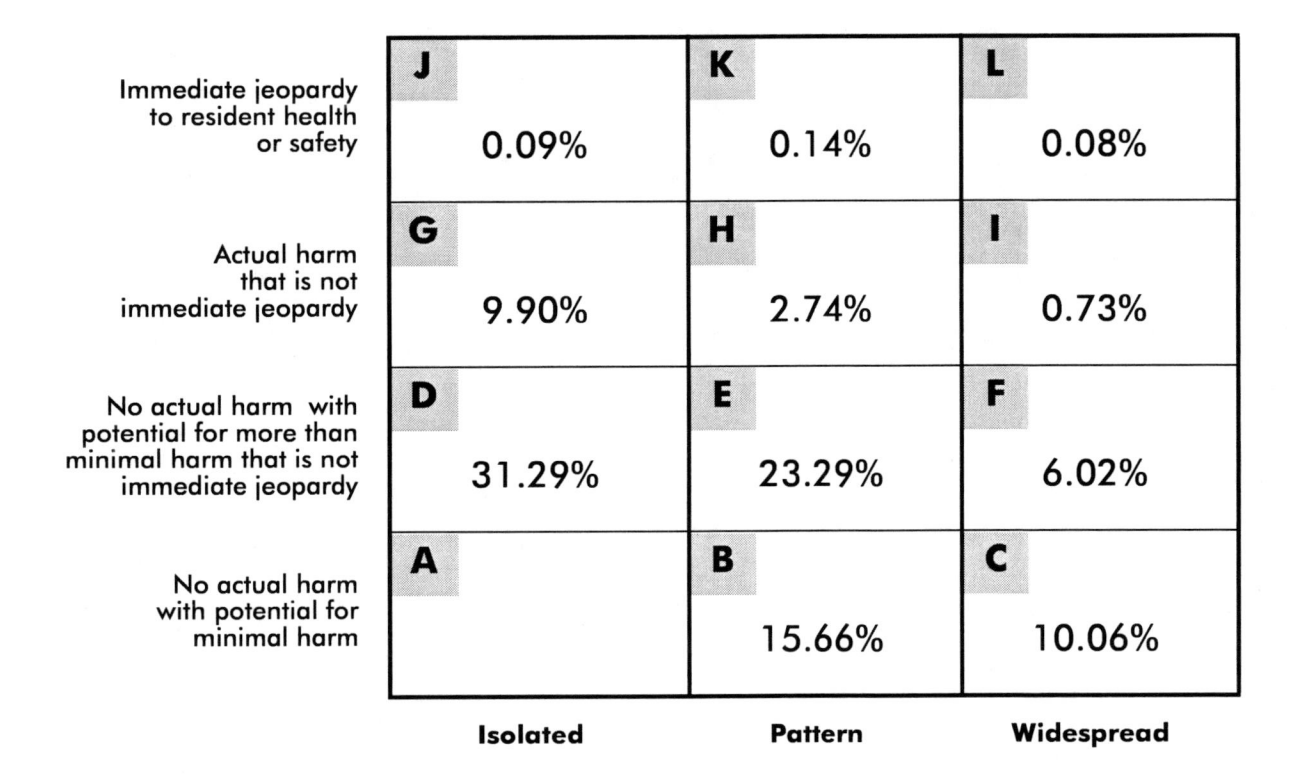

	Isolated	Pattern	Widespread
Immediate jeopardy to resident health or safety	**J** 0.09%	**K** 0.14%	**L** 0.08%
Actual harm that is not immediate jeopardy	**G** 9.90%	**H** 2.74%	**I** 0.73%
No actual harm with potential for more than minimal harm that is not immediate jeopardy	**D** 31.29%	**E** 23.29%	**F** 6.02%
No actual harm with potential for minimal harm	**A**	**B** 15.66%	**C** 10.06%

FIG. IV-B: SCOPE AND SEVERITY CODE UTILIZATION, UNITED STATES, 1997

SECTION V

FACILITY CHARACTERISTICS

Table V-1

Facilities by Type of Certification and State, 1997

	Dually Certified	Medicaid Only	Medicare Only	Total
UNITED STATES	13,183	2,478	1,460	17,121
Alabama	207	5	12	224
Alaska	15	0	1	16
Arizona	136	2	27	165
Arkansas	165	65	31	261
California	1,170	111	138	1,419
Colorado	169	21	35	225
Connecticut	244	10	6	260
Delaware	34	4	5	43
District of Columbia	21	0	0	21
Florida	603	9	85	697
Georgia	303	40	11	354
Hawaii	37	5	1	43
Idaho	77	0	9	86
Illinois	540	236	90	866
Indiana	450	75	52	577
Iowa	250	208	11	469
Kansas	250	140	33	423
Kentucky	284	0	31	315
Louisiana	162	120	57	339
Maine	130	0	5	135
Maryland	216	20	12	248
Massachusetts	505	46	12	563
Michigan	373	60	11	444
Minnesota	419	22	8	449
Mississippi	114	53	36	203
Missouri	422	91	57	570
Montana	95	2	6	103
Nebraska	150	83	4	237
Nevada	34	2	9	45
New Hampshire	61	18	2	81
New Jersey	255	59	17	331
New Mexico	64	12	9	85
New York	619	2	0	621
North Carolina	389	4	9	402
North Dakota	84	0	4	88
Ohio	768	165	81	1,014
Oklahoma	175	200	38	413
Oregon	126	34	3	163
Pennsylvania	635	26	131	792

Table V-1: Facilities by Type of Certification and State, 1997 (Continued)

	Dually Certified	Medicaid Only	Medicare Only	Total
Rhode Island	100	0	0	100
South Carolina	148	0	28	176
South Dakota	82	31	1	114
Tennessee	222	78	48	348
Texas	845	222	233	1,300
Utah	68	15	13	96
Vermont	40	4	0	44
Virginia	202	59	10	271
Washington	266	11	8	285
West Virginia	83	38	15	136
Wisconsin	345	65	13	423
Wyoming	31	5	2	38

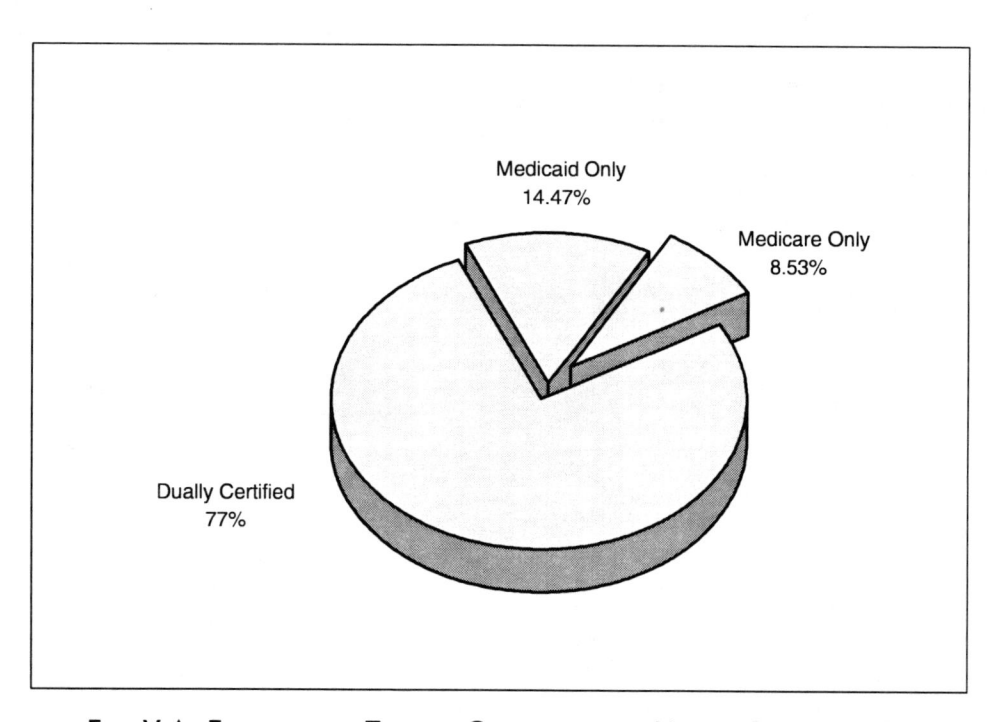

Fig. V-A: Facilities by Type of Certification, United States, 1997

- Medicaid Only 14.47%
- Medicare Only 8.53%
- Dually Certified 77%

TABLE V-2

FACILITIES BY CLASS OF OWNERSHIP AND STATE, 1997

	For Profit	Non-Profit	Government	Total
UNITED STATES	11,240	4,754	1,127	17,121
Alabama	172	30	22	224
Alaska	1	9	6	16
Arizona	103	58	4	165
Arkansas	207	41	13	261
California	1,052	305	62	1,419
Colorado	142	61	22	225
Connecticut	203	55	2	260
Delaware	19	20	4	43
District of Columbia	7	12	2	21
Florida	533	148	16	697
Georgia	272	59	23	354
Hawaii	18	14	11	43
Idaho	52	14	20	86
Illinois	555	262	49	866
Indiana	431	131	15	577
Iowa	255	191	23	469
Kansas	223	143	57	423
Kentucky	206	99	10	315
Louisiana	252	61	26	339
Maine	98	32	5	135
Maryland	143	97	8	248
Massachusetts	409	139	15	563
Michigan	280	121	43	444
Minnesota	147	237	65	449
Mississippi	137	35	31	203
Missouri	375	147	48	570
Montana	37	46	20	103
Nebraska	107	76	54	237
Nevada	35	5	5	45
New Hampshire	43	25	13	81
New Jersey	212	99	20	331
New Mexico	49	28	8	85
New York	296	272	53	621
North Carolina	295	89	18	402
North Dakota	10	76	2	88
Ohio	742	240	32	1,014
Oklahoma	334	54	25	413
Oregon	124	33	6	163
Pennsylvania	326	420	46	792

Table V-2: Facilities by Class of Ownership and State, 1997 (Continued)

	For Profit	Non-Profit	Government	Total
Rhode Island	76	24	0	100
South Carolina	133	22	21	176
South Dakota	40	69	5	114
Tennessee	240	78	30	348
Texas	1,056	206	38	1,300
Utah	77	15	4	96
Vermont	33	10	1	44
Virginia	173	86	12	271
Washington	197	66	22	285
West Virginia	90	32	14	136
Wisconsin	205	156	62	423
Wyoming	18	6	14	38

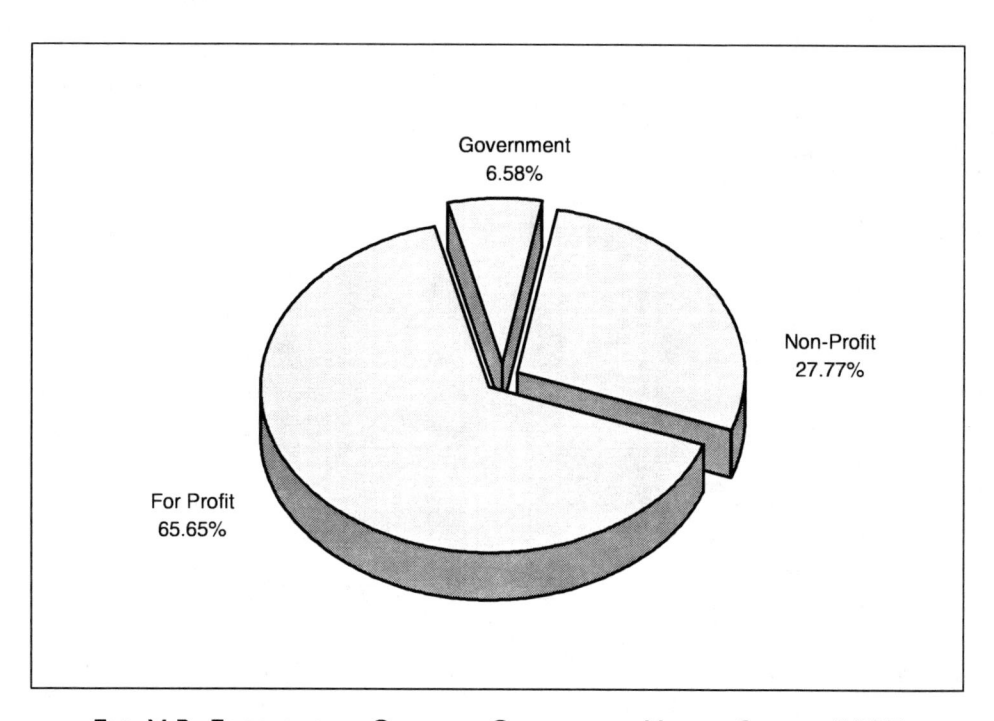

Fig. V-B: Facilities by Class of Ownership, United States, 1997

- Government 6.58%
- Non-Profit 27.77%
- For Profit 65.65%

Section V: Facility Characteristics

TABLE V-3

FACILITIES BY SIZE CATEGORY AND STATE, 1997

	< 61 Beds	61–120 Beds	> 120 Beds	Total
UNITED STATES	4,752	7,380	4,989	17,121
Alabama	37	100	87	224
Alaska	12	3	1	16
Arizona	44	58	63	165
Arkansas	14	166	81	261
California	484	611	324	1,419
Colorado	90	93	42	225
Connecticut	42	112	106	260
Delaware	6	25	12	43
District of Columbia	8	2	11	21
Florida	175	359	163	697
Georgia	51	198	105	354
Hawaii	18	15	10	43
Idaho	38	36	12	86
Illinois	169	349	348	866
Indiana	174	208	195	577
Iowa	148	242	79	469
Kansas	236	152	35	423
Kentucky	126	140	49	315
Louisiana	66	129	144	339
Maine	56	70	9	135
Maryland	55	72	121	248
Massachusetts	136	204	223	563
Michigan	84	194	166	444
Minnesota	104	229	116	449
Mississippi	96	79	28	203
Missouri	193	273	104	570
Montana	51	39	13	103
Nebraska	102	108	27	237
Nevada	18	12	15	45
New Hampshire	21	43	17	81
New Jersey	54	103	174	331
New Mexico	27	48	10	85
New York	62	193	366	621
North Carolina	104	198	100	402
North Dakota	41	35	12	88
Ohio	247	430	337	1,014
Oklahoma	129	226	58	413
Oregon	47	90	26	163
Pennsylvania	231	237	324	792

TABLE V-3: FACILITIES BY SIZE CATEGORY AND STATE, 1997 (CONTINUED)

	< 61 Beds	61–120 Beds	> 120 Beds	Total
Rhode Island	34	33	33	100
South Carolina	43	79	54	176
South Dakota	53	54	7	114
Tennessee	78	138	132	348
Texas	362	638	300	1,300
Utah	39	45	12	96
Vermont	18	15	11	44
Virginia	104	77	90	271
Washington	70	139	76	285
West Virginia	48	70	18	136
Wisconsin	89	198	136	423
Wyoming	18	13	7	38

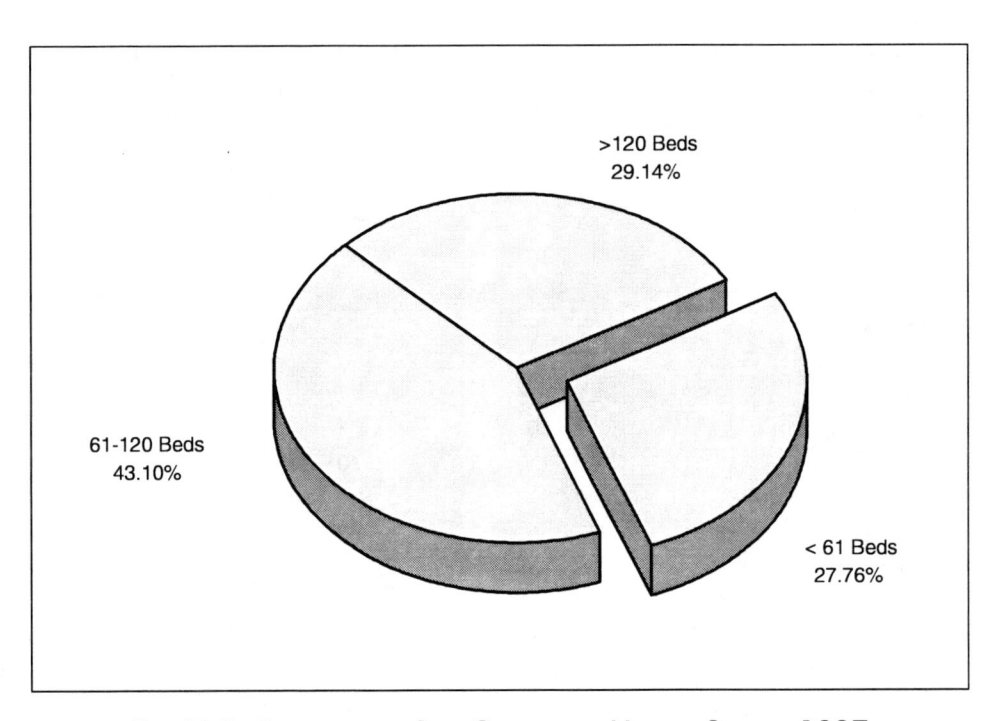

FIG. V-C: FACILITIES BY SIZE CATEGORY, UNITED STATES, 1997

>120 Beds 29.14%
61-120 Beds 43.10%
< 61 Beds 27.76%

SECTION V: FACILITY CHARACTERISTICS

TABLE V-4

BEDS BY TYPE OF CERTIFICATION AND STATE, 1997

	Medicare Only	Medicaid Only	Dually Certified	Uncertified	Total
UNITED STATES	**56,245**	**1,032,389**	**615,082**	**123,899**	**1,827,615**
Alabama	356	15,077	9,023	331	24,787
Alaska	16	241	476	95	828
Arizona	662	12,184	3,610	1,305	17,761
Arkansas	870	21,106	2,485	6,627	31,088
California	4,837	71,810	50,748	13,442	140,837
Colorado	934	13,511	4,396	1,309	20,150
Connecticut	318	10,796	20,626	941	32,681
Delaware	527	2,280	1,570	513	4,890
District of Columbia	58	1,471	1,561	7	3,097
Florida	5,977	45,535	20,483	5,683	77,678
Georgia	472	25,035	12,806	703	39,016
Hawaii	101	699	2,998	32	3,830
Idaho	270	2,489	2,772	984	6,515
Illinois	3,796	81,914	12,786	9,910	108,406
Indiana	2,283	44,129	8,497	7,177	62,086
Iowa	335	22,053	12,486	10,485	45,359
Kansas	590	20,429	6,517	2,002	29,538
Kentucky	1,225	11,300	11,505	1,252	25,282
Louisiana	1,449	30,794	3,952	1,848	38,043
Maine	1,202	5,789	2,302	70	9,363
Maryland	820	16,375	12,289	1,367	30,851
Massachusetts	354	32,224	24,262	934	57,774
Michigan	1,669	28,998	18,255	2,365	51,287
Minnesota	402	9,559	34,769	541	45,271
Mississippi	865	13,304	2,556	301	17,026
Missouri	2,029	41,631	6,794	5,018	55,472
Montana	128	3,460	3,881	52	7,521
Nebraska	228	11,811	5,370	818	18,227
Nevada	787	281	3,101	9	4,178
New Hampshire	123	5,015	2,722	247	8,107
New Jersey	1,276	28,775	18,543	808	49,402
New Mexico	157	5,249	1,543	296	7,245
New York	0	194	109,170	174	109,538
North Carolina	809	23,970	14,453	276	39,508
North Dakota	163	235	6,710	0	7,108
Ohio	2,617	59,155	32,067	27,491	121,330
Oklahoma	820	29,983	2,690	967	34,460
Oregon	291	10,268	3,170	301	14,030
Pennsylvania	4,190	52,761	38,460	1,015	96,426

TABLE V-4: BEDS BY TYPE OF CERTIFICATION AND STATE, 1997 (CONTINUED)

	Medicare Only	Medicaid Only	Dually Certified	Uncertified	Total
Rhode Island	10	5,766	4,203	211	10,190
South Carolina	1,197	7,260	7,928	1,078	17,463
South Dakota	45	3,365	4,656	14	8,080
Tennessee	1,200	28,361	8,768	680	39,009
Texas	6,578	90,670	16,955	11,675	125,878
Utah	1,539	5,581	322	126	7,568
Vermont	60	1,860	1,814	5	3,739
Virginia	522	23,309	5,020	1,064	29,915
Washington	291	18,405	7,982	978	27,656
West Virginia	417	7,420	3,247	119	11,203
Wisconsin	347	26,639	20,571	241	47,798
Wyoming	33	1,863	1,212	12	3,120

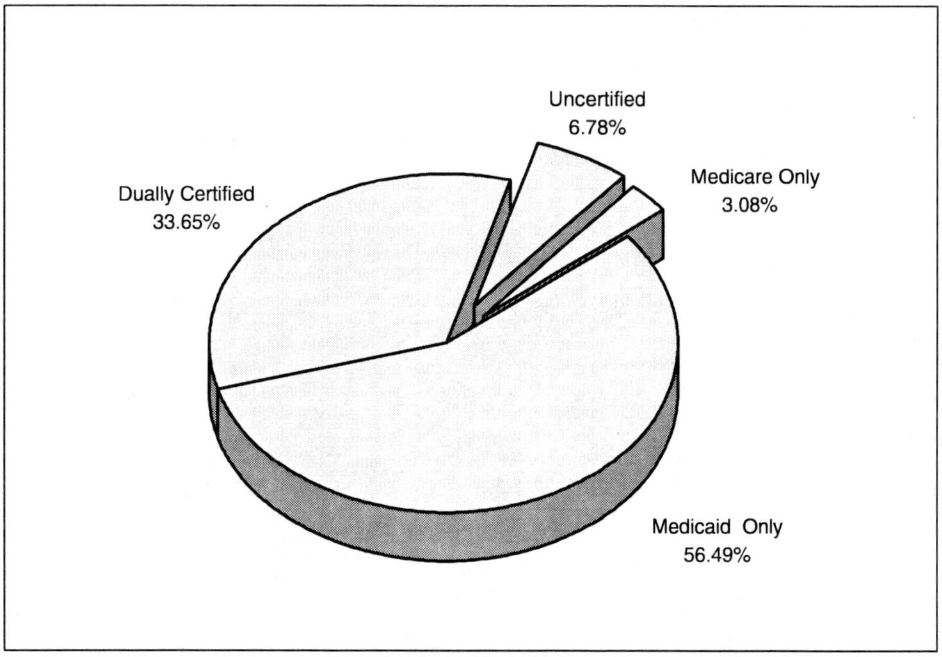

FIG. V-D: BEDS BY TYPE OF CERTIFICATION, UNITED STATES, 1997

- Uncertified 6.78%
- Medicare Only 3.08%
- Medicaid Only 56.49%
- Dually Certified 33.65%

SECTION V: FACILITY CHARACTERISTICS

Table V-5
Dedicated Special Care Units and Beds by State, 1997

	Rehabilitation Units	Rehabilitation Beds	Hospice Units	Hospice Beds	AIDS Units	AIDS Beds	Head Trauma Units	Head Trauma Beds	Disabled Children & Young Adults Units	Disabled Children & Young Adults Beds	Respiratory Units	Respiratory Beds	Dialysis Units	Dialysis Beds	Alzheimer's Units	Alzheimer's Beds	Huntington's Disease Units	Huntington's Disease Beds
UNITED STATES	601	20,119	216	3,858	70	2,416	64	1,665	72	2,698	337	6,234	38	394	2,275	73,832	25	489
Alabama	11	355	3	58	0	0	0	0	2	112	3	63	0	0	14	429	0	0
Alaska	0	0	0	0	0	0	0	0	0	0	0	0	0	0	0	0	0	0
Arizona	9	263	5	84	2	157	1	126	2	131	7	153	1	60	50	1,773	1	126
Arkansas	6	122	4	19	0	0	0	0	0	0	3	14	0	0	17	381	2	3
California	63	3,138	16	420	9	235	3	23	4	171	50	1,282	4	56	98	4,752	2	2
Colorado	14	315	8	78	1	10	1	10	0	0	4	56	2	22	70	1,949	1	10
Connecticut	35	1,322	4	42	3	84	1	30	0	0	5	133	1	4	33	1,318	3	85
Delaware	1	59	0	0	0	0	0	0	1	10	2	34	0	0	11	324	0	0
District of Columbia	0	0	1	9	0	0	0	0	0	0	0	0	0	0	1	36	0	0
Florida	46	1,668	15	148	6	108	3	44	2	47	28	473	2	5	116	4,107	1	1
Georgia	5	169	2	3	0	0	0	0	2	72	2	32	0	0	29	941	0	0
Hawaii	2	22	2	88	0	0	0	0	0	0	0	0	0	0	2	88	0	0
Idaho	7	135	2	14	0	0	0	0	1	42	2	12	0	0	23	478	0	0
Illinois	30	1,561	19	83	2	44	5	31	1	42	25	382	3	23	130	4,354	1	1
Indiana	14	747	9	191	2	58	1	19	3	226	8	126	1	19	93	2,810	1	19
Iowa	6	173	8	66	0	0	3	44	2	55	2	31	2	14	64	1,228	0	0
Kansas	7	168	2	2	0	0	0	0	0	0	0	1	8	0	64	1,646	0	0
Kentucky	5	122	3	99	2	14	1	22	1	46	3	104	0	0	12	547	0	0
Louisiana	17	279	3	11	2	36	3	58	1	12	7	136	0	0	44	1,066	0	0
Maine	8	163	1	3	1	9	3	61	2	13	1	25	1	9	29	839	1	9
Maryland	14	515	3	22	4	173	0	0	0	0	10	138	2	34	38	1,467	0	0
Massachusetts	24	807	1	58	0	0	5	280	4	256	6	171	0	0	66	2,826	1	51
Michigan	6	205	2	23	0	0	1	32	1	1	5	106	1	1	35	1,130	0	0

Table V-5: Dedicated Special Care Units and Beds by State, 1997 (Continued)

	Rehabilitation Units	Rehabilitation Beds	Hospice Units	Hospice Beds	AIDS Units	AIDS Beds	Head Trauma Units	Head Trauma Beds	Disabled Children & Young Adults Units	Disabled Children & Young Adults Beds	Respiratory Units	Respiratory Beds	Dialysis Units	Dialysis Beds	Alzheimer's Units	Alzheimer's Beds	Huntington's Disease Units	Huntington's Disease Beds
Minnesota	20	871	9	31	2	37	1	8	5	155	3	47	0	0	85	3,007	1	50
Mississippi	4	70	1	2	0	0	0	0	0	0	0	0	0	0	9	209	0	0
Missouri	7	154	5	137	1	4	4	58	1	10	7	63	1	16	140	3,363	1	4
Montana	3	35	1	1	0	0	1	19	0	0	0	0	0	0	19	432	0	0
Nebraska	8	184	4	18	0	0	1	29	2	27	4	63	1	2	48	855	0	0
Nevada	1	24	1	2	0	0	0	0	1	7	2	145	0	0	8	274	0	0
New Hampshire	4	116	1	50	0	0	1	15	2	97	2	72	1	50	25	713	0	0
New Jersey	10	312	2	8	2	69	6	188	5	259	13	194	1	3	19	687	2	21
New Mexico	0	0	0	0	0	0	0	0	0	0	0	0	0	0	12	281	0	0
New York	26	1,058	7	46	19	1,182	6	153	8	311	17	286	4	11	75	3,393	1	24
North Carolina	13	334	1	62	1	8	1	72	0	0	13	203	0	0	56	1,405	0	0
North Dakota	0	0	0	0	0	0	0	0	0	0	0	0	0	0	6	127	0	0
Ohio	37	940	20	531	2	41	2	59	2	20	38	828	2	27	133	4,730	2	56
Oklahoma	10	182	6	247	0	0	0	0	1	60	3	26	1	1	38	1,140	0	0
Oregon	5	75	5	77	0	0	0	0	3	80	3	10	0	0	31	869	0	0
Pennsylvania	33	922	10	258	2	34	2	38	3	79	20	288	2	4	129	5,277	1	1
Rhode Island	4	126	0	0	0	0	0	0	0	0	0	0	0	0	10	515	0	0
South Carolina	7	160	0	0	0	0	0	0	0	0	0	0	0	0	19	734	0	0
South Dakota	2	79	0	0	0	0	0	0	0	0	1	36	0	0	15	260	1	16
Tennessee	3	71	1	9	1	9	1	9	1	9	3	40	1	9	7	255	1	9
Texas	14	268	8	268	0	0	0	0	4	177	9	162	0	0	112	3,571	0	0
Utah	6	128	2	8	0	0	0	0	1	1	0	0	0	0	21	591	0	0
Vermont	2	140	0	0	0	0	0	0	0	0	0	0	0	0	7	187	0	0
Virginia	16	343	2	5	2	15	1	34	2	46	12	138	0	0	24	848	0	0
Washington	15	359	11	280	3	87	3	157	1	120	6	78	2	13	78	2,179	0	0
West Virginia	0	0	0	0	0	0	0	0	0	0	0	0	0	0	0	0	0	0
Wisconsin	20	831	5	296	1	2	3	46	1	4	7	76	2	11	95	3,105	1	1
Wyoming	1	29	1	1	0	0	0	0	0	0	0	0	0	0	15	336	0	0

TABLE V-6

OCCUPANCY RATE AS A PERCENT BY STATE, 1994–1997

	1994	1995	1996	1997
UNITED STATES	**85.48**	**84.48**	**83.09**	**82.24**
Alabama	94.07	92.88	92.04	91.70
Alaska	67.20	77.89	75.51	74.76
Arizona	80.23	76.61	79.55	77.78
Arkansas	72.19	69.52	65.33	65.89
California	78.05	78.32	77.62	76.77
Colorado	85.96	85.65	87.22	83.78
Connecticut	90.42	91.23	93.43	92.15
Delaware	75.99	80.59	82.53	79.04
District of Columbia	86.34	80.35	87.81	94.83
Florida	88.97	85.12	83.96	83.85
Georgia	93.56	94.32	93.71	91.86
Hawaii	94.70	96.02	85.03	91.59
Idaho	83.08	81.73	79.99	73.37
Illinois	82.06	81.08	78.78	78.46
Indiana	74.30	74.45	73.71	72.03
Iowa	68.13	68.84	65.84	67.30
Kansas	86.03	83.76	82.25	81.28
Kentucky	90.62	89.13	88.50	88.16
Louisiana	86.11	86.03	82.43	81.28
Maine	94.90	92.90	89.38	88.05
Maryland	87.92	87.05	86.50	84.39
Massachusetts	92.20	91.26	90.03	89.18
Michigan	88.40	87.46	86.26	85.90
Minnesota	93.79	93.84	92.40	92.30
Mississippi	96.68	94.94	93.09	93.18
Missouri	76.99	75.72	74.04	73.50
Montana	90.96	88.97	87.17	83.01
Nebraska	88.43	88.98	87.37	85.81
Nevada	87.71	91.17	87.75	90.31
New Hampshire	93.73	92.78	91.80	90.47
New Jersey	92.06	91.88	92.59	91.20
New Mexico	87.47	86.83	84.50	84.56
New York	95.45	95.97	95.53	94.90
North Carolina	91.55	92.66	93.19	93.85
North Dakota	96.31	96.39	95.43	95.26
Ohio	78.39	73.94	69.27	68.75
Oklahoma	79.79	77.77	76.20	73.69
Oregon	84.02	84.07	80.90	80.57
Pennsylvania	91.35	91.60	90.35	90.26

TABLE V-6: OCCUPANCY RATE BY STATE, 1996–1997 (CONTINUED)

	1994	1995	1996	1997
Rhode Island	95.08	91.79	93.74	92.24
South Carolina	88.39	87.33	87.30	85.69
South Dakota	95.06	95.54	94.53	94.91
Tennessee	93.95	91.52	90.68	89.60
Texas	74.55	72.61	71.53	69.57
Utah	81.94	82.13	82.57	78.01
Vermont	95.13	96.24	94.62	94.92
Virginia	92.82	93.51	92.26	90.55
Washington	88.99	87.67	85.09	82.91
West Virginia	93.77	93.70	93.89	92.32
Wisconsin	91.36	90.24	90.59	88.63
Wyoming	83.88	87.68	83.52	84.62

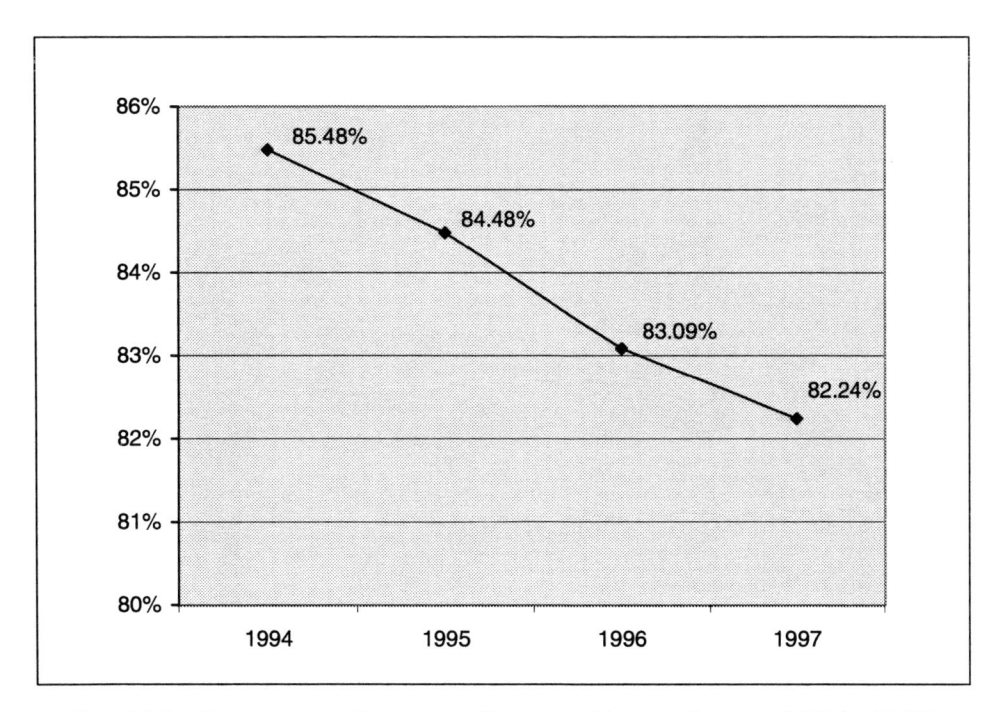

FIG. V-A: OCCUPANCY RATE AS A PERCENT, UNITED STATES, 1994–1997

Table V-7

Facilities by Type of Certification and HSA, 1997

HSA	Medicare Only	Medicaid Only	Dually Certified	Total
1	1	2	15	18
2	2	0	14	16
3	2	0	25	27
4	1	2	85	88
5	1	4	11	16
6	1	4	30	35
7	1	3	14	18
8	1	3	28	32
9	0	0	33	33
10	0	1	28	29
11	0	0	7	7
12	3	1	22	26
13	0	1	7	8
14	1	8	22	31
15	1	3	16	20
16	6	13	102	121
17	3	0	25	28
18	2	0	30	32
19	0	0	18	18
20	0	0	113	113
21	0	0	12	12
22	10	27	259	296
23	1	6	41	48
24	2	4	16	22
25	1	10	10	21
26	7	0	12	19
27	1	0	8	9
28	55	5	159	219
29	3	0	13	16
30	0	3	7	10
31	2	2	12	16
32	0	5	47	52
33	0	7	33	40
34	2	7	10	19
35	0	0	19	19
36	5	14	40	59
37	1	0	5	6
38	0	0	25	25
39	1	3	8	12
40	1	0	4	5

Table V-7: Facilities by Type of Certification and HSA, 1997 (Continued)

HSA	Medicare Only	Medicaid Only	Dually Certified	Total
41	0	0	57	57
42	27	1	102	130
43	2	2	43	47
44	0	0	11	11
45	1	0	18	19
46	3	4	16	23
47	2	1	20	23
48	1	1	27	29
49	0	2	7	9
50	1	2	5	8
51	1	0	11	12
52	2	0	8	10
53	1	0	8	9
54	0	0	105	105
55	0	3	3	6
56	0	0	26	26
57	3	2	25	30
58	0	0	13	13
59	0	0	25	25
60	1	3	10	14
61	3	1	78	82
62	0	0	8	8
63	0	3	4	7
64	0	2	17	19
65	0	0	12	12
66	3	17	62	82
67	1	0	5	6
68	0	3	48	51
69	3	1	23	27
70	2	6	4	12
71	0	3	3	6
72	1	4	17	22
73	0	1	5	6
74	3	13	68	84
75	4	5	27	36
76	0	0	8	8
77	0	0	5	5
78	2	0	32	34
79	0	1	5	6
80	0	0	15	15
81	0	0	11	11
82	0	0	6	6
83	0	0	117	117
84	7	2	28	37

TABLE V-7: FACILITIES BY TYPE OF CERTIFICATION AND HSA, 1997 (CONTINUED)

HSA	Medicare Only	Medicaid Only	Dually Certified	Total
85	4	8	95	107
86	0	0	14	14
87	2	4	18	24
88	0	0	20	20
89	1	0	11	12
90	0	0	12	12
91	0	7	33	40
92	2	4	6	12
93	2	3	6	11
94	0	1	62	63
95	0	0	21	21
96	0	0	9	9
97	1	2	5	8
98	1	0	19	20
99	0	5	11	16
100	2	0	22	24
101	0	1	78	79
102	0	0	2	2
103	0	1	9	10
104	0	0	2	2
105	0	0	8	8
106	3	1	30	34
107	0	1	9	10
108	3	10	54	67
109	1	0	4	5
110	0	1	10	11
111	0	1	0	1
112	0	1	27	28
113	0	0	48	48
114	0	0	5	5
115	1	2	7	10
116	1	0	3	4
117	1	1	6	8
119	0	0	4	4
120	0	0	1	1
121	1	0	44	45
122	0	1	3	4
123	0	0	1	1
124	1	0	2	3
125	0	0	2	2
126	1	2	13	16
127	0	1	4	5
128	0	0	3	3
129	2	2	7	11

TABLE V-7: FACILITIES BY TYPE OF CERTIFICATION AND HSA, 1997 (CONTINUED)

HSA	Medicare Only	Medicaid Only	Dually Certified	Total
130	0	0	3	3
131	0	0	5	5
132	0	0	6	6
133	0	0	9	9
135	0	1	5	6
136	1	0	12	13
137	0	1	3	4
138	0	3	2	5
139	4	0	13	17
140	6	2	27	35
141	4	0	20	24
142	8	1	82	91
143	7	1	20	28
144	0	0	9	9
145	0	0	4	4
146	6	10	28	44
147	4	7	22	33
148	15	9	24	48
149	1	0	27	28
150	7	0	46	53
151	2	4	14	20
152	1	2	26	29
153	6	4	49	59
154	0	0	17	17
155	0	1	13	14
156	0	2	10	12
157	0	1	11	12
158	3	1	50	54
159	2	0	20	22
160	3	0	17	20
161	3	1	25	29
162	0	0	11	11
163	5	1	25	31
164	0	1	11	12
165	5	0	24	29
166	0	0	12	12
167	1	0	26	27
168	0	0	12	12
169	3	5	10	18
170	0	1	19	20
171	0	2	16	18
172	0	2	12	14
173	1	1	5	7
174	0	0	5	5

TABLE V-7: FACILITIES BY TYPE OF CERTIFICATION AND HSA, 1997 (CONTINUED)

HSA	Medicare Only	Medicaid Only	Dually Certified	Total
175	0	0	8	8
176	0	0	7	7
177	0	0	13	13
178	0	1	6	7
179	1	0	12	13
180	0	1	7	8
181	1	3	5	9
182	7	0	26	33
183	0	1	20	21
184	2	0	16	18
185	0	0	6	6
186	1	0	39	40
187	0	0	9	9
188	1	13	13	27
189	0	3	4	7
190	1	2	20	23
191	2	0	17	19
192	0	0	7	7
193	0	6	21	27
194	0	0	7	7
195	0	0	10	10
196	1	0	7	8
197	0	0	10	10
198	1	0	25	26
199	1	0	5	6
200	7	1	71	79
201	0	3	5	8
202	2	0	28	30
203	1	0	11	12
204	0	0	4	4
205	0	0	12	12
206	0	1	13	14
207	0	0	15	15
208	1	2	8	11
209	0	0	7	7
210	1	0	13	14
211	0	2	11	13
212	2	0	16	18
213	7	1	28	36
214	0	0	15	15
215	2	3	6	11
216	0	0	4	4
217	1	2	5	8
218	0	0	23	23

Table V-7: Facilities by Type of Certification and HSA, 1997 (Continued)

HSA	Medicare Only	Medicaid Only	Dually Certified	Total
219	0	0	14	14
220	0	1	2	3
221	13	1	60	74
222	0	1	10	11
223	2	2	3	7
224	0	0	15	15
225	1	1	36	38
226	0	2	13	15
227	28	1	125	154
228	0	0	4	4
229	1	1	15	17
230	0	0	4	4
231	3	3	10	16
232	0	3	3	6
233	0	0	17	17
234	1	2	5	8
235	0	0	17	17
236	0	0	2	2
237	2	0	21	23
238	0	1	11	12
239	0	0	8	8
240	0	0	4	4
241	0	0	6	6
242	0	0	11	11
243	1	0	6	7
244	2	0	5	7
245	0	5	1	6
246	2	0	8	10
247	0	0	4	4
248	0	3	5	8
249	2	0	4	6
250	0	3	3	6
251	2	0	10	12
252	1	2	5	8
253	0	2	2	4
254	0	2	2	4
256	0	0	4	4
257	0	0	7	7
258	0	0	3	3
259	0	0	2	2
260	0	0	3	3
261	0	0	2	2
262	0	0	12	12
263	0	0	2	2

TABLE V-7: FACILITIES BY TYPE OF CERTIFICATION AND HSA, 1997 (CONTINUED)

HSA	Medicare Only	Medicaid Only	Dually Certified	Total
264	0	0	4	4
266	1	1	11	13
267	0	0	6	6
268	0	0	1	1
269	0	1	4	5
270	14	33	97	144
271	0	1	12	13
272	11	0	58	69
273	2	6	30	38
274	9	24	122	155
275	9	18	83	110
276	7	9	45	61
277	5	11	28	44
278	0	2	21	23
279	3	7	19	29
280	9	5	71	85
281	8	10	57	75
282	0	3	19	22
283	0	3	11	14
284	0	5	9	14
285	1	2	16	19
286	2	6	53	61
287	48	58	208	314
288	16	17	116	149
289	0	4	40	44
290	0	6	26	32
291	2	11	21	34
292	3	7	30	40
293	0	3	8	11
294	0	0	9	9
295	6	4	50	60
296	0	1	13	14
297	0	0	7	7
298	0	3	19	22
299	4	8	23	35
300	2	4	16	22
301	1	4	41	46
302	0	14	10	24
303	0	5	14	19
304	4	5	36	45
305	2	10	9	21
306	1	6	23	30
307	3	5	10	18
308	4	6	27	37

Table V-7: Facilities by Type of Certification and HSA, 1997 (Continued)

HSA	Medicare Only	Medicaid Only	Dually Certified	Total
309	0	3	33	36
310	1	6	19	26
311	3	4	20	27
312	1	4	22	27
313	1	2	12	15
314	0	1	3	4
315	0	5	11	16
316	1	0	13	14
317	0	0	4	4
318	3	13	18	34
319	0	3	6	9
320	1	0	16	17
321	3	3	12	18
322	0	4	15	19
323	1	2	16	19
324	2	6	8	16
325	1	6	29	36
326	0	3	10	13
327	0	3	11	14
328	0	5	14	19
329	0	0	9	9
330	0	1	9	10
331	1	12	10	23
332	1	4	13	18
333	1	2	10	13
334	1	4	13	18
335	1	5	2	8
336	4	10	14	28
337	0	8	19	27
338	2	7	15	24
339	1	0	10	11
340	0	8	6	14
341	2	2	11	15
342	0	3	11	14
343	1	6	8	15
344	1	6	19	26
345	6	2	47	55
346	3	2	16	21
347	3	20	48	71
348	0	0	16	16
349	3	1	17	21
350	0	3	5	8
351	1	1	5	7
352	5	6	45	56

TABLE V-7: FACILITIES BY TYPE OF CERTIFICATION AND HSA, 1997 (CONTINUED)

HSA	Medicare Only	Medicaid Only	Dually Certified	Total
353	1	8	17	26
354	0	3	22	25
355	1	4	16	21
356	2	2	12	16
357	0	1	7	8
358	1	2	7	10
359	0	1	5	6
360	0	2	9	11
361	0	12	9	21
362	1	0	11	12
363	1	1	7	9
364	3	0	12	15
365	1	2	10	13
366	4	7	37	48
367	0	4	7	11
368	1	4	17	22
369	0	3	16	19
370	0	0	21	21
371	0	2	4	6
372	1	1	9	11
373	2	5	20	27
374	0	7	3	10
375	0	0	19	19
376	1	1	9	11
377	2	7	15	24
378	1	1	8	10
379	0	1	5	6
380	0	6	14	20
381	0	0	11	11
382	0	4	14	18
383	0	5	1	6
384	0	5	6	11
385	2	1	13	16
386	0	0	12	12
387	0	0	12	12
388	0	6	14	20
389	3	3	14	20
390	2	3	18	23
391	0	1	4	5
392	0	0	6	6
394	0	1	6	7
395	0	2	1	3
396	0	0	6	6
398	1	1	4	6

TABLE V-7: FACILITIES BY TYPE OF CERTIFICATION AND HSA, 1997 (CONTINUED)

HSA	Medicare Only	Medicaid Only	Dually Certified	Total
399	0	0	2	2
400	0	0	2	2
401	0	0	5	5
402	1	0	5	6
403	12	14	29	55
404	4	6	26	36
405	3	9	18	30
406	5	11	18	34
407	1	3	5	9
408	46	20	64	130
409	2	1	8	11
410	18	12	59	89
411	7	11	15	33
412	3	5	10	18
413	8	3	30	41
414	9	30	22	61
415	4	0	10	14
416	6	18	24	48
417	12	30	36	78
418	1	4	7	12
419	8	15	17	40
420	1	4	27	32
421	3	14	14	31
422	0	4	1	5
423	2	3	4	9
424	6	14	12	32
425	11	16	29	56
426	2	12	8	22
427	3	3	13	19
428	3	9	20	32
429	3	15	6	24
430	2	7	14	23
431	3	3	3	9
432	10	10	27	47
433	2	2	19	23
434	24	6	64	94
435	1	2	6	9
436	4	7	22	33
437	7	5	25	37
438	0	4	8	12
439	1	6	7	14
440	1	3	3	7
441	4	6	27	37
442	1	4	3	8

TABLE V-7: FACILITIES BY TYPE OF CERTIFICATION AND HSA, 1997 (CONTINUED)

HSA	Medicare Only	Medicaid Only	Dually Certified	Total
443	3	12	16	31
444	1	3	6	10
445	0	11	14	25
446	7	9	13	29
447	3	4	12	19
448	2	6	11	19
449	3	4	11	18
450	3	14	17	34
451	0	11	12	23
452	5	9	15	29
453	31	9	80	120
454	4	5	20	29
455	1	4	2	7
456	3	2	7	12
457	0	0	7	7
458	0	1	3	4
459	1	3	1	5
460	1	2	4	7
461	1	1	5	7
462	1	7	34	42
463	3	6	4	13
464	1	3	10	14
465	1	4	9	14
466	1	8	6	15
467	2	2	8	12
468	1	4	10	15
469	1	7	2	10
470	5	7	9	21
471	1	0	5	6
472	2	7	3	12
473	1	5	11	17
474	1	5	9	15
475	0	3	5	8
476	1	8	4	13
477	2	0	7	9
478	0	9	6	15
479	0	0	4	4
480	1	0	5	6
481	0	1	6	7
482	2	4	4	10
483	0	3	4	7
484	0	1	5	6
485	2	1	10	13
486	1	1	9	11

Table V-7: Facilities by Type of Certification and HSA, 1997 (Continued)

HSA	Medicare Only	Medicaid Only	Dually Certified	Total
487	2	5	7	14
488	2	2	3	7
489	1	2	9	12
490	1	3	6	10
491	0	0	4	4
492	3	4	2	9
493	1	7	11	19
494	1	2	5	8
495	5	2	20	27
496	0	3	4	7
497	1	7	3	11
498	1	1	4	6
499	2	2	6	10
500	5	2	11	18
501	0	1	3	4
502	1	0	3	4
503	0	3	4	7
504	0	0	2	2
505	3	0	16	19
506	4	4	9	17
507	0	2	7	9
508	1	1	5	7
509	2	5	14	21
510	2	2	8	12
511	1	0	5	6
512	0	1	3	4
513	0	0	5	5
514	0	0	3	3
515	2	11	3	16
516	0	0	5	5
517	0	1	3	4
518	1	1	2	4
519	0	0	2	2
520	3	3	9	15
521	0	0	2	2
522	0	0	2	2
523	0	3	0	3
524	0	1	0	1
525	0	0	1	1
526	0	1	0	1
527	0	1	5	6
528	1	0	3	4
529	0	7	2	9
530	0	1	1	2

TABLE V-7: FACILITIES BY TYPE OF CERTIFICATION AND HSA, 1997 (CONTINUED)

HSA	Medicare Only	Medicaid Only	Dually Certified	Total
531	0	0	1	1
532	3	2	7	12
533	1	0	1	2
534	0	0	2	2
535	0	1	0	1
536	0	1	2	3
537	0	2	1	3
538	2	0	3	5
539	2	2	19	23
540	5	9	99	113
541	14	13	103	130
542	3	15	36	54
543	2	0	14	16
544	0	5	31	36
545	1	24	20	45
546	1	27	43	71
547	2	1	30	33
548	16	16	68	100
549	2	5	51	58
550	0	0	11	11
551	1	8	3	12
552	1	4	33	38
553	2	6	20	28
554	1	14	39	54
555	0	7	6	13
556	1	10	12	23
557	2	9	25	36
558	1	2	10	13
559	0	2	3	5
560	1	15	25	41
561	1	11	19	31
562	0	4	0	4
563	6	6	38	50
564	0	3	8	11
565	0	8	4	12
566	1	6	4	11
567	1	3	8	12
568	0	2	7	9
569	1	5	9	15
570	0	6	12	18
571	1	7	19	27
572	0	2	13	15
573	0	0	14	14
574	1	0	19	20

Table V-7: Facilities by Type of Certification and HSA, 1997 (Continued)

HSA	Medicare Only	Medicaid Only	Dually Certified	Total
575	0	6	1	7
576	11	21	40	72
577	0	1	12	13
578	0	6	15	21
579	0	0	4	4
580	0	8	12	20
581	2	6	23	31
582	0	0	14	14
583	0	2	7	9
584	0	1	21	22
585	1	4	9	14
586	0	0	3	3
587	1	3	1	5
588	0	3	16	19
589	0	7	9	16
590	0	2	6	8
591	0	9	14	23
592	0	0	14	14
593	0	2	5	7
594	0	3	3	6
595	0	1	3	4
596	0	5	21	26
597	0	0	7	7
598	1	3	11	15
599	5	1	11	17
600	0	2	3	5
601	1	2	17	20
602	0	1	15	16
603	0	0	6	6
604	0	0	5	5
605	0	0	3	3
606	1	15	9	25
607	1	3	6	10
608	0	0	8	8
609	0	0	8	8
610	0	1	5	6
611	0	1	3	4
612	0	1	12	13
613	0	3	2	5
614	0	4	5	9
615	0	5	6	11
616	0	4	4	8
617	0	3	3	6
618	0	3	2	5

TABLE V-7: FACILITIES BY TYPE OF CERTIFICATION AND HSA, 1997 (CONTINUED)

HSA	Medicare Only	Medicaid Only	Dually Certified	Total
619	0	1	14	15
621	5	1	14	20
622	0	2	3	5
623	0	4	2	6
624	7	6	31	44
625	1	9	1	11
626	0	1	6	7
627	1	3	9	13
628	0	1	3	4
629	0	1	2	3
630	0	5	10	15
631	0	0	3	3
632	0	0	5	5
633	0	7	7	14
634	0	3	5	8
635	0	4	4	8
636	0	0	2	2
637	0	5	2	7
638	0	0	4	4
639	1	1	5	7
640	0	0	4	4
641	1	8	7	16
642	1	4	5	10
643	0	2	0	2
644	0	6	3	9
645	0	1	1	2
646	0	0	7	7
647	0	0	5	5
648	0	2	1	3
649	0	2	4	6
650	1	4	5	10
651	0	1	5	6
652	0	6	2	8
654	0	3	0	3
655	0	0	3	3
656	1	7	6	14
657	0	2	4	6
658	0	5	2	7
659	0	2	2	4
660	0	3	3	6
661	0	4	2	6
662	0	0	3	3
663	0	0	2	2
664	0	1	0	1

Table V-7: Facilities by Type of Certification and HSA, 1997 (Continued)

HSA	Medicare Only	Medicaid Only	Dually Certified	Total
665	0	3	2	5
666	1	0	6	7
667	0	1	2	3
668	0	0	1	1
669	0	0	2	2
670	0	0	1	1
671	0	2	2	4
672	0	3	3	6
673	0	0	4	4
674	1	5	3	9
675	0	1	2	3
676	1	0	3	4
678	0	2	2	4
679	1	6	3	10
680	0	0	3	3
681	0	1	2	3
682	0	2	0	2
683	0	3	0	3
684	0	0	3	3
685	1	0	3	4
686	0	3	1	4
687	0	0	1	1
688	22	6	61	89
689	4	20	65	89
690	1	0	7	8
691	1	0	16	17
692	0	0	12	12
693	3	0	23	26
694	1	1	10	12
695	1	0	9	10
696	1	0	8	9
697	2	0	19	21
698	0	3	29	32
699	21	1	90	112
700	4	1	33	38
701	3	0	16	19
702	1	0	5	6
703	1	5	14	20
704	2	3	12	17
705	0	5	17	22
707	6	3	21	30
708	7	7	26	40
709	3	5	55	63
710	1	1	11	13

TABLE V-7: FACILITIES BY TYPE OF CERTIFICATION AND HSA, 1997 (CONTINUED)

HSA	Medicare Only	Medicaid Only	Dually Certified	Total
711	2	5	7	14
712	0	0	4	4
713	3	0	14	17
714	0	0	7	7
715	1	0	4	5
716	4	0	22	26
717	1	1	9	11
718	0	7	41	48
719	0	3	4	7
720	0	0	1	1
721	1	0	5	6
722	1	0	6	7
723	45	35	441	521
724	0	0	7	7
725	0	2	4	6
726	0	0	4	4
727	0	0	8	8
728	0	0	9	9
729	0	1	4	5
730	0	0	3	3
731	0	0	6	6
732	2	1	6	9
733	0	0	2	2
734	1	0	12	13
735	0	0	2	2
736	4	1	110	115
737	0	5	26	31
738	0	1	6	7
739	0	1	19	20
740	0	1	11	12
741	1	2	5	8
742	1	1	5	7
743	0	0	3	3
744	2	1	17	20
745	1	2	5	8
746	3	3	26	32
747	0	3	13	16
748	0	0	4	4
749	0	0	5	5
750	2	1	31	34
751	9	10	65	84
752	0	0	13	13
753	1	1	7	9
754	2	1	23	26

TABLE V-7: FACILITIES BY TYPE OF CERTIFICATION AND HSA, 1997 (CONTINUED)

HSA	Medicare Only	Medicaid Only	Dually Certified	Total
755	0	1	1	2
756	0	0	2	2
757	4	3	40	47
758	1	0	20	21
759	0	1	4	5
760	1	0	12	13
761	1	0	12	13
763	0	2	3	5
764	11	4	30	45
765	0	1	3	4
766	21	11	91	123
767	0	0	5	5
768	10	7	93	110
769	0	0	3	3
770	0	1	2	3
771	0	1	4	5
772	2	2	5	9
773	0	0	5	5
774	15	12	71	98
775	0	0	2	2
777	1	0	5	6
778	0	0	2	2
779	0	0	3	3
780	0	0	6	6
781	5	0	26	31
782	0	1	17	18
783	0	0	4	4
784	0	0	6	6
785	0	1	5	6
786	0	0	1	1
787	1	0	4	5
788	0	0	2	2
789	0	1	15	16
790	2	1	20	23
792	0	0	1	1
793	0	1	2	3
794	0	1	23	24
795	3	0	7	10
796	1	0	12	13
797	0	1	0	1
799	0	0	2	2
800	0	1	6	7
801	1	1	3	5
802	1	3	11	15

TABLE V-7: FACILITIES BY TYPE OF CERTIFICATION AND HSA, 1997 (CONTINUED)

HSA	Medicare Only	Medicaid Only	Dually Certified	Total
803	1	0	5	6
804	0	0	1	1
805	0	0	1	1
806	0	1	0	1
807	2	0	19	21
808	0	0	1	1
809	2	0	3	5
810	0	1	2	3
811	0	0	6	6
812	0	2	4	6
813	0	0	1	1
814	0	0	1	1
815	0	0	11	11
816	0	0	2	2
817	0	0	3	3
818	0	0	2	2
819	0	0	3	3
820	1	0	7	8
821	1	4	23	28
822	0	1	4	5
823	0	0	10	10

TABLE V-8

BEDS BY TYPE OF CERTIFICATION AND HSA, 1997

HSA	Medicare Only	Medicaid Only	Dually Certified	Uncertified	Total
1	66	675	917	2	1,660
2	170	742	691	174	1,777
3	128	1,505	1,805	78	3,516
4	88	3,821	7,309	244	11,462
5	5	1,612	300	62	1,979
6	36	3,506	960	107	4,609
7	36	1,287	444	4	1,771
8	15	2,597	1,175	0	3,787
9	213	1,482	863	0	2,558
10	0	216	3,747	4	3,967
11	0	230	251	0	481
12	142	1,178	733	82	2,135
13	0	575	231	0	806
14	108	2,855	564	96	3,623
15	56	1,090	677	0	1,823
16	405	8,241	5,387	879	14,912
17	513	1,097	131	28	1,769
18	140	1,086	1,415	126	2,767
19	0	413	2,311	2	2,726
20	10	6,271	5,399	301	11,981
21	0	0	1,346	0	1,346
22	317	16,533	12,470	522	29,842
23	127	4,480	3,055	10	7,672
24	49	889	846	212	1,996
25	31	1,271	196	7	1,505
26	140	1,163	584	116	2,003
27	25	322	283	40	670
28	2,079	14,659	9,741	655	27,134
29	38	618	441	44	1,141
30	0	616	126	38	780
31	129	625	534	0	1,288
32	0	3,637	2,324	76	6,037
33	26	3,750	804	256	4,836
34	43	1,097	359	26	1,525
35	0	378	1,436	0	1,814
36	512	5,167	3,791	552	10,022
37	16	234	249	0	499
38	156	948	417	11	1,532
39	25	803	180	0	1,008
40	16	261	137	0	414

TABLE V-8: BEDS BY TYPE OF CERTIFICATION AND HSA, 1997 (CONTINUED)

HSA	Medicare Only	Medicaid Only	Dually Certified	Uncertified	Total
41	0	0	8,960	4	8,964
42	775	7,967	6,797	75	15,614
43	37	2,976	2,951	0	5,964
44	0	920	571	0	1,491
45	24	765	717	14	1,520
46	68	1,075	682	242	2,067
47	42	1,687	966	0	2,695
48	23	1,945	2,064	95	4,127
49	60	488	352	0	900
50	25	152	427	0	604
51	23	386	556	0	965
52	26	664	322	0	1,012
53	16	358	395	28	797
54	0	0	14,831	2	14,833
55	0	525	46	0	571
56	0	0	4,373	2	4,375
57	56	1,892	1,465	4	3,417
58	0	0	1,514	1	1,515
59	0	0	2,968	3	2,971
60	11	910	307	0	1,228
61	341	6,344	4,458	264	11,407
62	5	231	364	12	612
63	0	750	198	0	948
64	0	1,378	1,247	0	2,625
65	0	0	1,450	2	1,452
66	144	7,775	4,553	118	12,590
67	20	141	149	0	310
68	0	2,929	2,477	27	5,433
69	236	2,492	642	390	3,760
70	29	700	92	0	821
71	0	481	53	0	534
72	18	1,534	1,367	47	2,966
73	0	455	70	0	525
74	57	4,454	3,360	216	8,087
75	429	1,748	1,213	491	3,881
76	0	0	910	0	910
77	0	292	112	24	428
78	31	1,932	1,867	0	3,830
79	0	552	137	0	689
80	0	0	1,765	0	1,765
81	0	0	1,016	1	1,017
82	7	283	204	0	494
83	0	0	24,824	119	24,943
84	210	3,421	2,196	113	5,940

Table V-8: Beds by Type of Certification and HSA, 1997 (Continued)

HSA	Medicare Only	Medicaid Only	Dually Certified	Uncertified	Total
85	150	4,202	7,305	607	12,264
86	0	0	2,061	0	2,061
87	82	2,447	989	64	3,582
88	0	0	3,211	0	3,211
89	15	406	351	40	812
90	0	513	400	0	913
91	47	2,626	1,372	213	4,258
92	42	683	112	0	837
93	50	689	306	37	1,082
94	0	136	17,762	32	17,930
95	127	1,195	395	27	1,744
96	0	462	324	6	792
97	22	390	154	0	566
98	26	813	712	0	1,551
99	11	1,107	193	61	1,372
100	58	1,363	889	0	2,310
101	0	4,687	3,277	107	8,071
102	0	0	121	2	123
103	0	280	297	5	582
104	0	4	132	0	136
105	0	0	955	2	957
106	78	1,723	2,275	7	4,083
107	0	852	426	0	1,278
108	265	5,169	3,442	27	8,903
109	19	277	124	17	437
110	0	458	489	0	947
111	0	45	0	0	45
112	0	1,057	1,919	0	2,976
113	0	0	11,368	0	11,368
114	28	152	178	30	388
115	10	958	282	0	1,250
116	10	80	166	0	256
117	32	538	333	0	903
119	0	54	115	51	220
120	0	25	61	20	106
121	80	1,954	4,613	0	6,647
122	0	345	109	0	454
123	0	86	66	0	152
124	36	49	112	35	232
125	0	60	198	0	258
126	96	1,104	855	0	2,055
127	0	566	305	0	871
128	0	118	150	0	268
129	45	610	271	0	926

TABLE V-8: BEDS BY TYPE OF CERTIFICATION AND HSA, 1997 (CONTINUED)

HSA	Medicare Only	Medicaid Only	Dually Certified	Uncertified	Total
130	0	222	40	0	262
131	0	0	243	0	243
132	30	762	107	0	899
133	0	0	1,713	0	1,713
135	0	511	100	0	611
136	167	470	136	4	777
137	0	328	26	0	354
138	0	330	90	0	420
139	141	1,682	1,027	12	2,862
140	286	2,181	1,815	29	4,311
141	76	2,027	895	0	2,998
142	597	6,651	2,172	769	10,189
143	197	1,586	621	161	2,565
144	0	44	1,036	0	1,080
145	0	283	167	0	450
146	366	3,702	1,580	188	5,836
147	99	3,192	990	0	4,281
148	386	3,106	1,204	270	4,966
149	49	1,711	913	68	2,741
150	259	3,748	1,809	133	5,949
151	65	1,665	407	44	2,181
152	31	1,688	1,062	150	2,931
153	338	5,375	1,981	441	8,135
154	0	1,246	516	0	1,762
155	106	640	808	120	1,674
156	0	1,024	482	0	1,506
157	0	677	614	0	1,291
158	222	3,706	1,842	219	5,989
159	96	1,440	749	9	2,294
160	240	1,169	1,302	237	2,948
161	63	1,947	906	129	3,045
162	0	778	742	0	1,520
163	140	2,123	853	146	3,262
164	0	772	284	2	1,058
165	275	1,574	518	421	2,788
166	0	1,160	448	0	1,608
167	30	1,879	1,089	6	3,004
168	43	474	689	0	1,206
169	56	1,258	291	6	1,611
170	139	1,335	663	2	2,139
171	0	1,601	590	0	2,191
172	52	512	822	0	1,386
173	12	688	146	0	846
174	0	186	437	0	623

TABLE V-8: BEDS BY TYPE OF CERTIFICATION AND HSA, 1997 (CONTINUED)

HSA	Medicare Only	Medicaid Only	Dually Certified	Uncertified	Total
175	0	253	414	0	667
176	0	322	291	0	613
177	0	852	525	0	1,377
178	0	242	344	0	586
179	28	756	530	0	1,314
180	0	608	212	0	820
181	40	695	173	0	908
182	291	1,373	1,268	197	3,129
183	227	899	1,048	83	2,257
184	49	348	1,156	0	1,553
185	0	593	172	5	770
186	91	2,342	1,569	0	4,002
187	118	447	370	160	1,095
188	13	2,298	440	0	2,751
189	0	511	201	0	712
190	19	1,902	615	98	2,634
191	53	588	1,069	63	1,773
192	0	513	193	0	706
193	0	2,152	660	0	2,812
194	0	276	270	0	546
195	0	798	394	0	1,192
196	18	406	229	0	653
197	0	687	447	0	1,134
198	54	1,674	1,085	102	2,915
199	13	62	323	0	398
200	1,028	5,368	2,930	1,107	10,433
201	0	674	188	0	862
202	288	2,073	1,017	77	3,455
203	30	874	308	0	1,212
204	0	448	98	0	546
205	37	490	540	0	1,067
206	0	856	559	0	1,415
207	37	421	756	0	1,214
208	20	753	278	4	1,055
209	64	313	287	0	664
210	6	963	634	64	1,667
211	0	1,016	372	0	1,388
212	95	1,168	524	172	1,959
213	396	2,503	765	428	4,092
214	41	801	388	0	1,230
215	24	824	179	0	1,027
216	0	331	319	0	650
217	15	795	179	163	1,152
218	22	1,206	832	42	2,102

TABLE V-8: BEDS BY TYPE OF CERTIFICATION AND HSA, 1997 (CONTINUED)

HSA	Medicare Only	Medicaid Only	Dually Certified	Uncertified	Total
219	0	755	565	0	1,320
220	0	152	122	0	274
221	947	3,510	2,532	1,213	8,202
222	0	644	358	0	1,002
223	30	475	82	0	587
224	0	1,113	809	0	1,922
225	60	2,190	969	28	3,247
226	0	1,468	413	3	1,884
227	1,211	10,843	3,477	671	16,202
228	0	104	275	0	379
229	15	892	678	0	1,585
230	0	129	196	0	325
231	43	1,149	319	40	1,551
232	0	490	99	0	589
233	62	1,446	522	20	2,050
234	29	622	119	0	770
235	8	1,197	588	5	1,798
236	0	58	183	0	241
237	242	1,504	588	276	2,610
238	2	1,039	231	0	1,272
239	0	492	317	0	809
240	0	265	110	0	375
241	0	380	241	0	621
242	0	871	324	4	1,199
243	27	436	94	0	557
244	51	177	368	37	633
245	0	476	25	0	501
246	77	552	238	49	916
247	0	101	264	0	365
248	0	706	186	0	892
249	48	88	346	32	514
250	0	377	90	0	467
251	31	647	230	43	951
252	18	646	185	0	849
253	0	206	28	0	234
254	0	245	42	0	287
256	8	248	161	0	417
257	35	655	146	4	840
258	0	209	51	0	260
259	0	158	31	0	189
260	0	146	97	0	243
261	0	110	110	0	220
262	11	469	599	0	1,079
263	0	118	34	0	152

Table V-8: Beds by Type of Certification and HSA, 1997 (Continued)

HSA	Medicare Only	Medicaid Only	Dually Certified	Uncertified	Total
264	8	256	206	0	470
266	74	781	470	77	1,402
267	0	492	239	0	731
268	0	93	24	0	117
269	0	337	146	1	484
270	322	7,823	4,179	5,442	17,766
271	56	393	761	0	1,210
272	456	2,240	2,335	528	5,559
273	98	3,263	659	40	4,060
274	1,355	13,945	4,851	1,634	21,785
275	487	7,948	1,683	1,773	11,891
276	229	4,301	1,435	2,009	7,974
277	289	3,417	503	596	4,805
278	0	1,358	786	10	2,154
279	46	2,151	459	241	2,897
280	247	6,623	5,628	122	12,620
281	165	4,543	2,712	729	8,149
282	0	1,499	1,194	0	2,693
283	20	936	207	54	1,217
284	0	621	450	0	1,071
285	33	1,094	1,008	155	2,290
286	166	2,208	4,774	183	7,331
287	2,168	38,309	6,056	5,775	52,308
288	776	10,123	5,269	7,277	23,445
289	6	852	3,384	16	4,258
290	0	1,055	1,994	11	3,060
291	140	2,899	466	649	4,154
292	58	2,049	859	1,231	4,197
293	0	345	614	0	959
294	0	325	513	0	838
295	225	3,738	2,186	1,819	7,968
296	0	731	747	0	1,478
297	40	663	298	0	1,001
298	0	1,128	1,070	0	2,198
299	168	2,352	393	205	3,118
300	84	1,576	283	309	2,252
301	41	2,125	2,116	56	4,338
302	0	1,552	363	1,383	3,298
303	45	2,340	284	230	2,899
304	105	3,736	652	628	5,121
305	69	1,647	323	15	2,054
306	24	2,101	1,293	51	3,469
307	97	1,528	199	244	2,068
308	190	3,325	618	270	4,403

TABLE V-8: BEDS BY TYPE OF CERTIFICATION AND HSA, 1997 (CONTINUED)

HSA	Medicare Only	Medicaid Only	Dually Certified	Uncertified	Total
309	76	1,663	1,995	244	3,978
310	34	1,765	376	222	2,397
311	77	2,136	379	226	2,818
312	62	2,315	488	352	3,217
313	72	1,238	131	198	1,639
314	0	169	138	0	307
315	0	752	749	0	1,501
316	52	685	333	62	1,132
317	12	231	205	8	456
318	96	2,578	376	281	3,331
319	0	724	159	24	907
320	8	974	581	7	1,570
321	125	940	337	37	1,439
322	0	705	1,000	0	1,705
323	65	1,273	374	259	1,971
324	77	1,031	123	176	1,407
325	126	3,368	643	234	4,371
326	0	954	707	0	1,661
327	0	886	607	0	1,493
328	16	1,383	578	200	2,177
329	25	710	170	107	1,012
330	0	629	325	88	1,042
331	13	1,671	314	73	2,071
332	19	1,236	159	798	2,212
333	59	1,070	227	40	1,396
334	29	1,314	187	7	1,537
335	30	486	63	0	579
336	122	1,904	301	208	2,535
337	0	1,432	577	126	2,135
338	32	1,659	236	138	2,065
339	39	957	141	99	1,236
340	0	743	209	114	1,066
341	96	1,019	283	118	1,516
342	0	731	592	0	1,323
343	42	1,382	100	72	1,596
344	20	1,565	1,208	0	2,793
345	209	2,813	2,658	1,295	6,975
346	71	1,161	767	837	2,836
347	62	4,849	2,103	760	7,774
348	0	859	837	0	1,696
349	67	1,650	279	210	2,206
350	0	389	241	0	630
351	14	521	88	20	643
352	194	3,827	1,491	2,187	7,699

Table V-8: Beds by Type of Certification and HSA, 1997 (Continued)

HSA	Medicare Only	Medicaid Only	Dually Certified	Uncertified	Total
353	20	2,104	210	279	2,613
354	14	1,303	615	11	1,943
355	15	1,953	581	0	2,549
356	45	818	370	81	1,314
357	0	492	287	0	779
358	6	802	145	0	953
359	0	77	365	0	442
360	28	467	307	359	1,161
361	0	1,451	200	387	2,038
362	55	848	151	16	1,070
363	13	671	175	0	859
364	91	1,121	198	163	1,573
365	87	890	157	177	1,311
366	123	3,025	1,377	799	5,324
367	0	735	149	100	984
368	24	892	694	129	1,739
369	16	1,043	486	33	1,578
370	0	315	1,407	0	1,722
371	0	381	114	29	524
372	12	303	365	138	818
373	105	2,211	301	384	3,001
374	0	487	216	0	703
375	73	925	891	0	1,889
376	18	609	525	130	1,282
377	64	1,181	833	1,092	3,170
378	54	941	137	52	1,184
379	0	569	120	0	689
380	10	937	403	264	1,614
381	0	680	438	0	1,118
382	0	1,596	759	0	2,355
383	0	406	98	0	504
384	0	894	85	0	979
385	88	954	170	56	1,268
386	0	707	447	66	1,220
387	0	705	573	0	1,278
388	0	781	973	119	1,873
389	75	1,588	243	543	2,449
390	114	1,807	325	230	2,476
391	0	112	214	0	326
392	0	316	177	0	493
394	40	518	79	54	691
395	0	223	12	50	285
396	0	146	400	0	546
398	10	241	179	120	550

TABLE V-8: BEDS BY TYPE OF CERTIFICATION AND HSA, 1997 (CONTINUED)

HSA	Medicare Only	Medicaid Only	Dually Certified	Uncertified	Total
399	0	222	75	0	297
400	0	237	94	0	331
401	7	600	58	294	959
402	17	426	121	0	564
403	494	4,893	1,179	204	6,770
404	111	2,611	462	76	3,260
405	161	1,426	527	338	2,452
406	155	1,846	259	148	2,408
407	35	617	118	162	932
408	1,138	8,615	1,350	1,708	12,811
409	59	759	253	0	1,071
410	565	6,070	985	1,484	9,104
411	143	2,478	361	24	3,006
412	52	1,160	293	8	1,513
413	243	2,641	730	246	3,860
414	213	4,972	257	130	5,572
415	145	901	261	100	1,407
416	132	4,205	467	536	5,340
417	310	6,037	496	205	7,048
418	36	957	116	10	1,119
419	174	3,718	774	225	4,891
420	87	2,223	481	230	3,021
421	81	2,814	154	930	3,979
422	0	307	20	0	327
423	26	777	78	16	897
424	101	3,004	131	127	3,363
425	300	3,958	452	922	5,632
426	40	1,466	123	57	1,686
427	89	1,321	258	99	1,767
428	107	1,907	437	207	2,658
429	33	1,605	44	23	1,705
430	55	1,719	106	326	2,206
431	35	538	44	68	685
432	199	3,483	505	2,205	6,392
433	54	1,632	481	95	2,262
434	564	6,714	1,146	1,602	10,026
435	15	579	109	14	717
436	97	2,602	295	94	3,088
437	157	2,990	430	191	3,768
438	24	1,336	134	2	1,496
439	12	1,214	143	116	1,485
440	16	389	54	0	459
441	227	2,593	483	299	3,602
442	10	693	34	160	897

Table V-8: Beds by Type of Certification and HSA, 1997 (Continued)

HSA	Medicare Only	Medicaid Only	Dually Certified	Uncertified	Total
443	165	2,841	209	120	3,335
444	33	767	112	40	952
445	0	2,013	222	0	2,235
446	211	2,059	204	863	3,337
447	60	1,192	208	49	1,509
448	67	1,352	170	433	2,022
449	58	1,419	166	41	1,684
450	70	3,173	293	142	3,678
451	0	1,259	153	0	1,412
452	93	1,835	593	233	2,754
453	903	8,908	1,492	1,547	12,850
454	132	2,301	322	318	3,073
455	25	566	48	0	639
456	91	838	162	63	1,154
457	32	822	99	0	953
458	0	400	37	1	438
459	14	359	28	0	401
460	24	412	53	14	503
461	33	474	60	20	587
462	108	3,016	1,053	226	4,403
463	54	1,306	62	77	1,499
464	9	1,415	327	16	1,767
465	20	1,100	118	81	1,319
466	16	828	186	8	1,038
467	28	1,130	123	41	1,322
468	40	846	306	45	1,237
469	14	399	156	8	577
470	100	2,018	144	168	2,430
471	76	375	69	0	520
472	26	824	22	0	872
473	37	1,503	143	525	2,208
474	30	915	135	101	1,181
475	0	634	64	0	698
476	11	881	48	0	940
477	39	496	149	0	684
478	0	1,182	44	173	1,399
479	0	311	73	0	384
480	7	361	88	73	529
481	0	480	69	1	550
482	22	488	76	0	586
483	0	491	125	0	616
484	0	248	249	0	497
485	16	950	251	48	1,265
486	53	646	359	327	1,385

TABLE V-8: BEDS BY TYPE OF CERTIFICATION AND HSA, 1997 (CONTINUED)

HSA	Medicare Only	Medicaid Only	Dually Certified	Uncertified	Total
487	44	929	166	0	1,139
488	33	376	40	0	449
489	32	803	203	18	1,056
490	14	803	65	99	981
491	80	153	94	30	357
492	65	555	36	52	708
493	28	1,265	153	1	1,447
494	24	611	66	160	861
495	111	1,652	473	102	2,338
496	12	586	59	0	657
497	16	874	26	0	916
498	20	378	66	0	464
499	36	875	79	257	1,247
500	83	1,367	309	32	1,791
501	0	346	60	44	450
502	14	319	58	0	391
503	0	410	91	0	501
504	0	52	68	0	120
505	44	1,385	332	156	1,917
506	109	988	130	107	1,334
507	0	634	225	0	859
508	34	424	50	0	508
509	30	1,452	321	100	1,903
510	15	835	147	21	1,018
511	14	370	55	108	547
512	0	262	38	4	304
513	0	353	76	32	461
514	0	206	28	32	266
515	32	1,058	26	0	1,116
516	12	384	46	36	478
517	12	561	34	58	665
518	18	258	34	29	339
519	0	157	16	4	177
520	100	1,131	162	39	1,432
521	6	234	16	0	256
522	0	171	27	0	198
523	0	279	0	20	299
524	0	84	0	0	84
525	0	90	15	0	105
526	0	56	0	0	56
527	5	445	47	21	518
528	10	329	40	2	381
529	0	680	23	0	703
530	0	230	8	8	246

Table V-8: Beds by Type of Certification and HSA, 1997 (Continued)

HSA	Medicare Only	Medicaid Only	Dually Certified	Uncertified	Total
531	0	94	6	0	100
532	108	839	176	49	1,172
533	10	156	24	0	190
534	0	153	31	0	184
535	0	62	0	0	62
536	29	283	16	83	411
537	0	308	10	0	318
538	53	317	46	14	430
539	39	1,593	336	16	1,984
540	164	4,027	9,179	290	13,660
541	973	9,890	1,957	3,334	16,154
542	147	3,836	1,017	319	5,319
543	45	0	1,176	0	1,221
544	0	887	1,832	0	2,719
545	42	2,215	832	1,293	4,382
546	37	3,304	1,886	1,595	6,822
547	118	187	2,585	0	2,890
548	390	7,843	1,008	795	10,036
549	135	4,757	741	192	5,825
550	0	61	798	0	859
551	9	344	208	25	586
552	64	637	2,555	8	3,264
553	65	1,768	289	133	2,255
554	7	3,136	811	456	4,410
555	14	585	157	75	831
556	30	954	941	392	2,317
557	64	1,178	1,349	1,171	3,762
558	44	341	483	8	876
559	0	150	122	0	272
560	40	1,810	1,079	920	3,849
561	47	1,680	845	244	2,816
562	0	183	0	0	183
563	163	3,126	613	21	3,923
564	0	603	176	23	802
565	0	489	164	18	671
566	20	760	32	23	835
567	18	646	136	56	856
568	0	277	377	0	654
569	26	506	288	26	846
570	0	548	515	35	1,098
571	45	2,410	277	368	3,100
572	0	332	686	3	1,021
573	0	162	937	0	1,099
574	16	1,582	275	148	2,021

TABLE V-8: BEDS BY TYPE OF CERTIFICATION AND HSA, 1997 (CONTINUED)

HSA	Medicare Only	Medicaid Only	Dually Certified	Uncertified	Total
575	0	408	17	12	437
576	251	3,642	1,273	396	5,562
577	0	370	553	0	923
578	0	517	801	17	1,335
579	0	0	338	0	338
580	0	736	808	9	1,553
581	24	1,952	273	0	2,249
582	0	30	1,097	5	1,132
583	0	534	122	26	682
584	0	71	1,638	0	1,709
585	12	625	450	238	1,325
586	0	0	294	0	294
587	11	181	81	9	282
588	0	667	1,177	2	1,846
589	0	497	682	261	1,440
590	0	150	351	0	501
591	10	1,792	223	110	2,135
592	0	230	1,129	0	1,359
593	0	330	173	6	509
594	0	329	73	0	402
595	0	45	196	0	241
596	0	850	1,107	665	2,622
597	0	65	462	0	527
598	20	430	644	121	1,215
599	96	1,067	219	110	1,492
600	0	223	146	0	369
601	12	642	341	64	1,059
602	2	119	1,030	0	1,151
603	0	219	516	0	735
604	0	33	393	0	426
605	0	0	339	0	339
606	19	1,371	611	398	2,399
607	12	642	92	38	784
608	0	76	766	0	842
609	0	88	442	0	530
610	0	81	298	0	379
611	0	234	126	0	360
612	0	384	1,082	0	1,466
613	0	266	71	16	353
614	0	728	90	10	828
615	1	308	439	0	748
616	0	215	206	21	442
617	0	285	149	53	487
618	0	180	102	21	303

TABLE V-8: BEDS BY TYPE OF CERTIFICATION AND HSA, 1997 (CONTINUED)

HSA	Medicare Only	Medicaid Only	Dually Certified	Uncertified	Total
619	0	74	793	0	867
621	127	957	401	110	1,595
622	0	315	30	10	355
623	0	186	99	22	307
624	87	2,957	426	392	3,862
625	21	652	88	160	921
626	0	185	418	0	603
627	16	676	151	51	894
628	0	263	27	42	332
629	0	164	43	0	207
630	0	907	130	0	1,037
631	0	0	165	0	165
632	0	0	458	0	458
633	0	666	286	126	1,078
634	0	326	229	0	555
635	0	300	122	29	451
636	0	0	103	0	103
637	0	397	18	12	427
638	0	0	294	0	294
639	10	466	64	0	540
640	0	0	267	0	267
641	44	1,407	104	333	1,888
642	9	351	112	53	525
643	0	60	0	0	60
644	0	527	127	9	663
645	0	51	79	0	130
646	0	0	759	39	798
647	0	72	288	0	360
648	0	211	24	0	235
649	0	36	333	101	470
650	9	528	112	0	649
651	0	263	208	0	471
652	0	360	92	33	485
654	0	171	0	0	171
655	0	0	288	0	288
656	13	876	93	91	1,073
657	0	364	97	11	472
658	20	321	84	1	426
659	0	142	76	20	238
660	0	433	32	5	470
661	0	236	99	24	359
662	0	90	53	56	199
663	0	189	24	0	213
664	0	60	0	0	60

TABLE V-8: BEDS BY TYPE OF CERTIFICATION AND HSA, 1997 (CONTINUED)

HSA	Medicare Only	Medicaid Only	Dually Certified	Uncertified	Total
665	0	223	86	0	309
666	26	577	80	7	690
667	0	143	16	0	159
668	0	0	68	0	68
669	0	0	89	0	89
670	0	0	25	0	25
671	0	224	21	0	245
672	0	236	124	78	438
673	0	271	49	0	320
674	4	380	245	50	679
675	0	135	22	0	157
676	23	258	32	0	313
678	0	258	17	0	275
679	26	880	173	588	1,667
680	0	80	170	0	250
681	0	111	114	25	250
682	0	61	0	0	61
683	0	303	0	1	304
684	0	0	193	0	193
685	14	188	50	2	254
686	0	261	14	34	309
687	0	0	110	2	112
688	628	5,917	1,550	861	8,956
689	229	5,041	1,799	356	7,425
690	6	418	186	167	777
691	49	646	582	41	1,318
692	0	412	629	0	1,041
693	33	1,755	488	276	2,552
694	32	382	349	127	890
695	31	250	351	116	748
696	9	173	274	97	553
697	41	892	614	277	1,824
698	0	1,908	1,015	15	2,938
699	491	8,300	2,472	1,130	12,393
700	132	2,866	878	175	4,051
701	314	0	1,432	0	1,746
702	21	343	92	10	466
703	213	919	157	3	1,292
704	56	1,139	339	0	1,534
705	10	1,443	377	73	1,903
707	563	544	1,655	9	2,771
708	700	2,430	112	91	3,333
709	46	3,390	2,929	137	6,502
710	17	696	401	391	1,505

TABLE V-8: BEDS BY TYPE OF CERTIFICATION AND HSA, 1997 (CONTINUED)

HSA	Medicare Only	Medicaid Only	Dually Certified	Uncertified	Total
711	59	870	76	11	1,016
712	0	7	289	0	296
713	33	519	419	0	971
714	0	188	170	0	358
715	40	266	82	0	388
716	106	958	679	557	2,300
717	14	691	167	0	872
718	128	821	3,131	43	4,123
719	45	343	77	0	465
720	10	21	66	0	97
721	12	217	167	0	396
722	35	381	119	0	535
723	1,878	29,713	17,140	3,491	52,222
724	0	573	94	0	667
725	16	301	112	0	429
726	0	269	238	4	511
727	0	596	141	0	737
728	0	277	512	1	790
729	12	230	146	0	388
730	0	51	129	0	180
731	0	109	198	0	307
732	30	444	284	8	766
733	0	0	126	0	126
734	45	321	605	87	1,058
735	0	48	62	0	110
736	137	8,156	3,561	425	12,279
737	18	1,225	1,276	80	2,599
738	0	373	151	0	524
739	0	1,251	472	0	1,723
740	17	755	130	34	936
741	12	553	101	0	666
742	12	535	89	0	636
743	0	183	94	0	277
744	409	1,365	0	32	1,806
745	12	287	177	0	476
746	43	2,016	826	2,321	5,206
747	0	753	366	29	1,148
748	0	356	54	0	410
749	0	75	385	0	460
750	58	1,975	1,017	559	3,609
751	152	5,024	2,063	274	7,513
752	17	949	369	8	1,343
753	17	319	289	152	777
754	83	1,365	579	127	2,154

TABLE V-8: BEDS BY TYPE OF CERTIFICATION AND HSA, 1997 (CONTINUED)

HSA	Medicare Only	Medicaid Only	Dually Certified	Uncertified	Total
755	13	62	0	0	75
756	0	101	76	0	177
757	126	1,395	4,340	324	6,185
758	28	1,039	579	293	1,939
759	0	202	118	0	320
760	20	1,005	243	0	1,268
761	4	558	404	38	1,004
763	0	183	119	0	302
764	318	2,098	1,206	1,527	5,149
765	0	250	57	0	307
766	654	4,361	3,867	672	9,554
767	22	71	233	0	326
768	363	5,891	3,398	1,172	10,824
769	0	242	38	0	280
770	0	260	24	0	284
771	0	214	86	8	308
772	28	537	125	0	690
773	0	147	195	0	342
774	512	6,024	3,225	1,199	10,960
775	0	102	18	0	120
777	21	271	91	0	383
778	0	0	67	0	67
779	0	0	214	10	224
780	0	131	100	20	251
781	102	1,234	986	211	2,533
782	54	1,171	463	65	1,753
783	0	236	56	0	292
784	0	240	179	0	419
785	0	359	97	0	456
786	0	101	11	0	112
787	20	410	109	0	539
788	0	52	24	0	76
789	55	246	1,294	298	1,893
790	198	1,166	748	0	2,112
792	0	54	6	0	60
793	0	143	266	8	417
794	27	2,311	634	5	2,977
795	35	641	241	142	1,059
796	37	741	234	96	1,108
797	0	43	0	0	43
799	0	89	71	0	160
800	0	380	168	10	558
801	16	320	20	0	356
802	40	892	307	0	1,239

Table V-8: Beds by Type of Certification and HSA, 1997 (Continued)

HSA	Medicare Only	Medicaid Only	Dually Certified	Uncertified	Total
803	19	383	95	0	497
804	0	0	51	0	51
805	9	0	90	0	99
806	0	52	0	0	52
807	42	1,007	874	2	1,925
808	0	0	25	0	25
809	61	168	0	0	229
810	0	288	89	0	377
811	0	253	135	115	503
812	0	384	128	0	512
813	0	0	40	0	40
814	0	35	6	4	45
815	0	624	364	0	988
816	0	39	39	0	78
817	0	0	74	19	93
818	0	0	49	19	68
819	0	0	176	0	176
820	16	241	177	57	491
821	41	498	2,145	32	2,716
822	0	36	229	0	265
823	60	165	624	0	849

TABLE V-9
DEDICATED SPECIAL CARE UNITS AND BEDS BY HSA, 1997

HSA	Rehabilitation Units	Rehabilitation Beds	Hospice Units	Hospice Beds	AIDS Units	AIDS Beds	Head Trauma Units	Head Trauma Beds	Disabled Children & Young Adults Units	Disabled Children & Young Adults Beds	Respiratory Units	Respiratory Beds	Dialysis Units	Dialysis Beds	Alzheimer's Units	Alzheimer's Beds	Huntington's Disease Units	Huntington's Disease Beds
1	0	0	1	1	0	0	0	0	0	0	1	4	0	0	0	0	0	0
2	1	42	0	0	0	0	0	0	0	0	0	0	0	0	2	68	0	0
3	1	44	0	0	0	0	0	0	0	0	2	34	0	0	6	167	0	0
4	18	683	3	38	1	24	0	0	0	0	1	5	0	0	16	577	1	25
5	0	0	0	0	0	0	0	0	0	0	0	0	0	0	2	73	0	0
6	1	38	0	0	0	0	1	34	0	0	4	44	0	0	3	72	0	0
7	0	0	0	0	0	0	0	0	0	0	0	0	0	0	0	0	0	0
8	0	0	0	0	0	0	0	0	0	0	0	0	0	0	4	192	0	0
9	1	17	0	0	0	0	0	0	0	0	0	0	0	0	8	268	0	0
10	1	72	0	0	0	0	0	0	1	58	0	0	0	0	4	180	0	0
11	0	0	0	0	0	0	0	0	0	0	0	0	0	0	0	0	0	0
12	0	0	0	0	0	0	0	0	0	0	0	0	0	0	0	0	0	0
13	0	0	0	0	0	0	0	0	0	0	0	0	0	0	0	0	0	0
14	5	97	1	2	1	5	0	0	1	8	2	35	0	0	3	146	0	0
15	0	0	0	0	0	0	0	0	0	0	0	0	0	0	4	124	0	0
16	3	95	1	20	3	123	0	0	0	0	5	91	1	10	17	769	0	0
17	3	64	1	3	1	9	2	21	1	9	1	25	1	9	6	195	1	9
18	1	16	3	99	0	0	0	0	0	0	0	0	0	0	2	42	0	0
19	0	0	0	0	0	0	0	0	0	0	0	0	0	0	5	218	0	0
20	7	259	0	0	1	30	0	0	0	0	1	30	0	0	12	607	1	30
21	0	0	0	0	0	0	0	0	0	0	2	41	0	0	2	65	0	0
22	10	311	1	58	0	0	4	168	3	213	3	118	0	0	32	1,414	1	51
23	2	72	1	2	1	9	2	33	1	107	2	36	1	3	5	150	1	1
24	0	0	0	0	0	0	0	0	0	0	0	0	0	0	0	0	0	0
25	1	7	0	0	0	0	0	0	0	0	0	0	0	0	0	0	0	0
26	1	20	1	6	0	0	0	0	0	0	0	0	0	0	4	138	0	0
27	0	0	0	0	0	0	0	0	0	0	0	0	0	0	0	0	0	0
28	10	266	2	176	2	34	1	20	3	79	10	150	1	3	26	1,083	1	1

Table V-9: Dedicated Special Care Units and Beds by HSA, 1997 (Continued)

HSA	Rehabilitation Units	Rehabilitation Beds	Hospice Units	Hospice Beds	AIDS Units	AIDS Beds	Head Trauma Units	Head Trauma Beds	Disabled Children & Young Adults Units	Disabled Children & Young Adults Beds	Respiratory Units	Respiratory Beds	Dialysis Units	Dialysis Beds	Alzheimer's Units	Alzheimer's Beds	Huntington's Disease Units	Huntington's Disease Beds
29	0	0	0	0	0	0	0	0	0	0	0	0	0	0	1	60	0	0
30	0	0	0	0	0	0	0	0	0	0	0	0	0	0	0	0	0	0
31	0	0	0	0	0	0	0	0	0	0	0	0	0	0	0	0	0	0
32	5	246	0	0	0	0	0	0	1	43	0	0	0	0	7	302	0	0
33	2	50	0	0	0	0	0	0	0	0	0	0	0	0	4	128	0	0
34	0	0	0	0	0	0	0	0	0	0	1	9	0	0	1	18	0	0
35	0	0	0	0	0	0	0	0	0	0	0	0	0	0	0	0	0	0
36	0	0	1	6	0	0	0	0	1	66	3	37	0	0	3	199	0	0
37	0	0	0	0	0	0	0	0	0	0	0	0	0	0	0	0	0	0
38	1	10	0	0	0	0	0	0	0	0	0	0	0	0	2	56	0	0
39	2	25	0	0	0	0	0	0	0	0	1	4	0	0	0	0	0	0
40	0	0	0	0	0	0	0	0	0	0	0	0	0	0	0	0	0	0
41	3	93	1	3	1	20	1	10	2	64	3	35	0	0	13	478	0	0
42	8	229	1	8	0	0	0	0	0	0	6	83	0	0	19	822	0	0
43	0	0	0	0	0	0	1	18	0	0	2	23	0	0	12	360	0	0
44	0	0	0	0	0	0	0	0	0	0	0	0	0	0	4	111	0	0
45	0	0	0	0	0	0	0	0	0	0	0	0	0	0	0	0	0	0
46	0	0	0	0	0	0	0	0	0	0	0	0	0	0	1	60	0	0
47	0	0	0	0	0	0	0	0	0	0	0	0	0	0	5	252	0	0
48	2	75	1	12	0	0	0	0	0	0	1	20	0	0	9	340	0	0
49	2	140	0	0	0	0	0	0	0	0	0	0	0	0	1	50	0	0
50	0	0	0	0	0	0	0	0	0	0	0	0	0	0	0	0	0	0
51	0	0	0	0	0	0	0	0	0	0	0	0	0	0	0	0	0	0
52	0	0	0	0	0	0	0	0	0	0	0	0	0	0	0	0	0	0
53	0	0	0	0	0	0	0	0	0	0	0	0	0	0	0	0	0	0
54	8	156	2	3	3	28	1	10	1	12	0	0	0	0	13	543	0	0
55	0	0	0	0	0	0	0	0	0	0	0	0	0	0	1	13	0	0
56	2	65	0	0	1	10	1	20	0	0	1	5	0	0	3	111	0	0

SECTION V: FACILITY CHARACTERISTICS

TABLE V-9: DEDICATED SPECIAL CARE UNITS AND BEDS BY HSA, 1997 (CONTINUED)

HSA	Rehabilitation Units	Rehabilitation Beds	Hospice Units	Hospice Beds	AIDS Units	AIDS Beds	Head Trauma Units	Head Trauma Beds	Disabled Children & Young Adults Units	Disabled Children & Young Adults Beds	Respiratory Units	Respiratory Beds	Dialysis Units	Dialysis Beds	Alzheimer's Units	Alzheimer's Beds	Huntington's Disease Units	Huntington's Disease Beds
57	2	55	0	0	0	0	0	0	0	0	0	0	0	0	6	305	0	0
58	0	0	0	0	0	0	0	0	0	0	0	0	0	0	1	38	0	0
59	0	0	0	0	0	0	0	0	1	40	2	15	0	0	3	122	0	0
60	0	0	0	0	0	0	0	0	0	0	0	0	0	0	0	0	0	0
61	9	346	2	10	1	50	0	0	0	0	2	19	1	24	14	499	0	0
62	0	0	0	0	0	0	0	0	0	0	1	60	0	0	0	0	0	0
63	0	0	0	0	0	0	0	0	0	0	2	20	0	0	1	12	0	0
64	2	69	0	0	0	0	1	16	0	0	1	16	0	0	3	89	0	0
65	0	0	0	0	0	0	0	0	0	0	0	0	0	0	0	0	0	0
66	4	119	0	0	1	60	2	89	1	27	3	37	0	0	3	72	1	20
67	0	0	0	0	0	0	0	0	0	0	0	0	0	0	0	0	0	0
68	1	30	0	0	0	0	0	0	0	0	0	0	0	0	6	220	0	0
69	2	66	0	0	1	10	0	0	1	38	1	24	0	0	6	264	0	0
70	0	0	1	3	0	0	0	0	0	0	0	0	0	0	1	30	0	0
71	0	0	0	0	0	0	0	0	0	0	0	0	0	0	0	0	0	0
72	0	0	0	0	0	0	0	0	0	0	0	0	0	0	8	274	0	0
73	0	0	0	0	0	0	0	0	0	0	0	0	0	0	0	0	0	0
74	4	121	1	50	0	0	1	112	1	50	1	50	1	50	11	349	0	0
75	2	89	0	0	0	0	0	0	1	10	1	4	0	0	7	204	0	0
76	0	0	0	0	0	0	0	0	0	0	0	0	0	0	0	0	0	0
77	0	0	0	0	0	0	0	0	0	0	0	0	0	0	0	0	0	0
78	1	20	0	0	0	0	0	0	0	0	0	0	0	0	1	60	0	0
79	0	0	0	0	0	0	0	0	0	0	0	0	0	0	0	0	0	0
80	0	0	0	0	0	0	0	0	0	0	0	0	0	0	0	0	0	0
81	1	8	0	0	0	0	0	0	0	0	0	0	0	0	1	15	0	0
82	0	0	0	0	0	0	0	0	0	0	0	0	0	0	0	0	0	0
83	4	252	1	6	4	156	1	20	1	76	4	65	3	10	13	559	0	0
84	3	110	1	1	0	0	0	0	0	0	1	22	1	1	9	444	0	0

TABLE V-9: DEDICATED SPECIAL CARE UNITS AND BEDS BY HSA, 1997 (CONTINUED)

HSA	Rehabilitation Units	Rehabilitation Beds	Hospice Units	Hospice Beds	AIDS Units	AIDS Beds	Head Trauma Units	Head Trauma Beds	Disabled Children & Young Adults Units	Disabled Children & Young Adults Beds	Respiratory Units	Respiratory Beds	Dialysis Units	Dialysis Beds	Alzheimer's Units	Alzheimer's Beds	Huntington's Disease Units	Huntington's Disease Beds
85	9	251	1	4	1	30	1	30	0	0	2	90	0	0	8	352	1	30
86	0	0	0	0	0	0	0	0	0	0	0	0	0	0	0	0	0	0
87	0	0	0	0	0	0	0	0	1	35	1	17	0	0	1	60	0	0
88	0	0	0	0	0	0	1	72	0	0	0	0	0	0	0	0	0	0
89	0	0	0	0	0	0	0	0	0	0	0	0	0	0	0	0	0	0
90	0	0	0	0	0	0	0	0	0	0	0	0	0	0	2	70	0	0
91	1	26	0	0	0	0	1	15	1	47	1	22	0	0	14	429	0	0
92	0	0	0	0	0	0	0	0	0	0	0	0	0	0	0	0	0	0
93	0	0	0	0	0	0	0	0	0	0	0	0	0	0	0	0	0	0
94	3	228	1	4	9	848	0	0	1	29	1	22	1	1	7	474	1	24
95	2	41	0	0	0	0	0	0	1	4	0	0	0	0	8	199	0	0
96	0	0	0	0	0	0	0	0	0	0	0	0	0	0	0	0	0	0
97	1	43	0	0	0	0	0	0	0	0	0	0	0	0	0	0	0	0
98	1	20	0	0	0	0	1	40	0	0	0	0	0	0	5	122	0	0
99	1	14	0	0	0	0	0	0	0	0	1	8	0	0	0	0	0	0
100	1	60	1	2	0	0	0	0	0	0	1	10	0	0	3	139	0	0
101	6	169	0	0	0	0	0	0	0	0	2	13	0	0	11	389	0	0
102	0	0	0	0	0	0	0	0	0	0	0	0	0	0	0	0	0	0
103	0	0	0	0	0	0	0	0	0	0	0	0	0	0	1	27	0	0
104	0	0	0	0	0	0	0	0	0	0	0	0	0	0	0	0	0	0
105	2	52	0	0	0	0	0	0	0	0	0	0	0	0	2	80	0	0
106	2	30	0	0	0	0	0	0	0	0	0	0	0	0	4	118	0	0
107	0	0	0	0	0	0	0	0	0	0	0	0	0	0	1	42	0	0
108	2	52	0	0	0	0	1	50	1	24	3	51	0	0	2	86	0	0
109	0	0	0	0	0	0	0	0	0	0	0	0	0	0	1	60	0	0
110	0	0	0	0	0	0	0	0	0	0	0	0	0	0	0	0	0	0
111	0	0	0	0	0	0	0	0	0	0	0	0	0	0	0	0	0	0
112	0	0	0	0	0	0	0	0	0	0	2	70	0	0	4	235	0	0

TABLE V-9: DEDICATED SPECIAL CARE UNITS AND BEDS BY HSA, 1997 (CONTINUED)

HSA	Rehabilitation Units	Rehabilitation Beds	Hospice Units	Hospice Beds	AIDS Units	AIDS Beds	Head Trauma Units	Head Trauma Beds	Disabled Children & Young Adults Units	Disabled Children & Young Adults Beds	Respiratory Units	Respiratory Beds	Dialysis Units	Dialysis Beds	Alzheimer's Units	Alzheimer's Beds	Huntington's Disease Units	Huntington's Disease Beds
113	2	132	2	30	1	120	1	21	1	32	3	73	0	0	7	457	0	0
114	0	0	0	0	0	0	0	0	0	0	0	0	0	0	0	0	0	0
115	0	0	0	0	0	0	0	0	0	0	0	0	0	0	0	0	0	0
116	0	0	0	0	0	0	0	0	0	0	0	0	0	0	0	0	0	0
117	0	0	0	0	0	0	0	0	0	0	0	0	0	0	3	142	0	0
119	0	0	0	0	0	0	0	0	0	0	0	0	0	0	0	0	0	0
120	0	0	0	0	0	0	0	0	0	0	0	0	0	0	0	0	0	0
121	5	255	0	0	0	0	0	0	0	0	1	8	1	4	7	297	0	0
122	0	0	0	0	0	0	0	0	0	0	0	0	0	0	1	18	0	0
123	0	0	0	0	0	0	0	0	0	0	0	0	0	0	0	0	0	0
124	0	0	0	0	0	0	0	0	0	0	0	0	0	0	1	17	0	0
125	0	0	0	0	0	0	0	0	0	0	0	0	0	0	0	0	0	0
126	0	0	0	0	0	0	0	0	0	0	0	0	0	0	2	31	0	0
127	0	0	0	0	0	0	0	0	0	0	0	0	0	0	0	0	0	0
128	0	0	0	0	0	0	0	0	0	0	0	0	0	0	0	0	0	0
129	0	0	0	0	0	0	0	0	0	0	0	0	0	0	1	62	0	0
130	0	0	0	0	0	0	0	0	0	0	0	0	0	0	0	0	0	0
131	0	0	0	0	0	0	0	0	0	0	0	0	0	0	0	0	0	0
132	0	0	0	0	0	0	0	0	0	0	0	0	0	0	1	20	0	0
133	0	0	0	0	0	0	0	0	0	0	0	0	0	0	3	113	0	0
135	0	0	0	0	0	0	0	0	0	0	0	0	0	0	1	30	0	0
136	1	31	0	0	0	0	0	0	0	0	0	0	0	0	1	19	0	0
137	0	0	0	0	0	0	0	0	0	0	0	0	0	0	1	20	0	0
138	0	0	0	0	0	0	0	0	0	0	0	0	0	0	1	19	0	0
139	3	57	1	50	0	0	0	0	0	0	0	0	0	0	5	162	0	0
140	0	0	1	1	0	0	0	0	0	0	0	0	0	0	8	326	0	0
141	0	0	0	0	0	0	0	0	0	0	0	0	0	0	0	0	0	0
142	5	104	2	3	1	10	0	0	0	0	5	87	0	0	12	463	0	0

TABLE V-9: DEDICATED SPECIAL CARE UNITS AND BEDS BY HSA, 1997 (CONTINUED)

HSA	Rehabilitation Units	Rehabilitation Beds	Hospice Units	Hospice Beds	AIDS Units	AIDS Beds	Head Trauma Units	Head Trauma Beds	Disabled Children & Young Adults Units	Disabled Children & Young Adults Beds	Respiratory Units	Respiratory Beds	Dialysis Units	Dialysis Beds	Alzheimer's Units	Alzheimer's Beds	Huntington's Disease Units	Huntington's Disease Beds
143	0	0	0	0	0	0	0	0	0	0	0	0	0	0	3	38	0	0
144	0	0	1	1	0	0	0	0	0	0	0	0	0	0	2	34	0	0
145	0	0	0	0	0	0	0	0	0	0	0	0	0	0	0	0	0	0
146	1	22	0	0	0	0	0	0	0	0	1	3	0	0	0	0	0	0
147	0	0	0	0	0	0	0	0	0	0	0	0	0	0	0	0	0	0
148	0	0	0	0	0	0	0	0	0	0	1	28	0	0	2	79	0	0
149	0	0	0	0	0	0	0	0	0	0	1	10	0	0	1	19	0	0
150	5	245	0	0	0	0	0	0	0	0	2	37	0	0	5	168	0	0
151	1	3	0	0	0	0	0	0	0	0	1	3	0	0	0	0	0	0
152	0	0	0	0	0	0	0	0	0	0	0	0	0	0	5	166	0	0
153	2	79	0	0	0	0	0	0	1	71	2	32	0	0	10	494	0	0
154	0	0	0	0	0	0	0	0	0	0	0	0	0	0	2	27	0	0
155	0	0	0	0	0	0	0	0	0	0	0	0	0	0	2	84	0	0
156	0	0	0	0	0	0	0	0	0	0	0	0	0	0	0	0	0	0
157	0	0	0	0	0	0	0	0	0	0	0	0	0	0	0	0	0	0
158	2	120	1	18	0	0	0	0	0	0	1	11	0	0	10	362	0	0
159	1	30	0	0	0	0	0	0	0	0	0	0	0	0	7	170	0	0
160	1	30	0	0	0	0	0	0	0	0	0	0	0	0	6	174	0	0
161	4	68	2	28	0	0	0	0	0	0	0	0	0	0	2	32	0	0
162	0	0	0	0	0	0	0	0	0	0	0	0	0	0	1	50	0	0
163	3	62	0	0	0	0	0	0	0	0	0	0	0	0	5	139	0	0
164	0	0	0	0	0	0	0	0	0	0	0	0	0	0	0	0	0	0
165	3	86	1	35	0	0	0	0	0	0	1	18	0	0	8	293	0	0
166	1	32	0	0	0	0	0	0	0	0	0	0	0	0	1	50	0	0
167	4	124	0	0	0	0	0	0	0	0	2	25	0	0	6	221	0	0
168	2	77	0	0	0	0	0	0	0	0	0	0	0	0	1	22	0	0
169	0	0	0	0	0	0	0	0	0	0	0	0	0	0	2	78	0	0
170	0	0	0	0	0	0	1	72	0	0	1	12	0	0	4	81	0	0

Table V-9: Dedicated Special Care Units and Beds by HSA, 1997 (Continued)

HSA	Rehabilitation Units	Rehabilitation Beds	Hospice Units	Hospice Beds	AIDS Units	AIDS Beds	Head Trauma Units	Head Trauma Beds	Disabled Children & Young Adults Units	Disabled Children & Young Adults Beds	Respiratory Units	Respiratory Beds	Dialysis Units	Dialysis Beds	Alzheimer's Units	Alzheimer's Beds	Huntington's Disease Units	Huntington's Disease Beds
171	0	0	0	0	0	0	0	0	2	112	0	0	0	0	2	56	0	0
172	0	0	0	0	0	0	0	0	0	0	0	0	0	0	0	0	0	0
173	0	0	0	0	0	0	0	0	0	0	0	0	0	0	0	0	0	0
174	0	0	0	0	0	0	0	0	0	0	0	0	0	0	0	0	0	0
175	0	0	0	0	0	0	0	0	0	0	0	0	0	0	0	0	0	0
176	0	0	0	0	0	0	0	0	0	0	0	0	0	0	1	44	0	0
177	0	0	0	0	0	0	0	0	0	0	0	0	0	0	0	0	0	0
178	0	0	0	0	0	0	0	0	0	0	0	0	0	0	0	0	0	0
179	0	0	0	0	0	0	0	0	0	0	0	0	0	0	1	50	0	0
180	0	0	0	0	0	0	0	0	0	0	0	0	0	0	1	28	0	0
181	1	40	0	0	0	0	0	0	0	0	0	0	0	0	0	0	0	0
182	2	40	0	0	0	0	0	0	0	0	0	0	0	0	2	155	0	0
183	1	42	0	0	0	0	0	0	0	0	0	0	0	0	2	50	0	0
184	1	8	0	0	0	0	0	0	0	0	0	0	0	0	1	22	0	0
185	0	0	0	0	0	0	0	0	0	0	0	0	0	0	0	0	0	0
186	0	0	0	0	0	0	0	0	0	0	2	32	0	0	5	109	0	0
187	0	0	0	0	0	0	0	0	0	0	0	0	0	0	1	20	0	0
188	0	0	0	0	0	0	0	0	0	0	0	0	0	0	0	0	0	0
189	0	0	0	0	0	0	0	0	0	0	0	0	0	0	1	22	0	0
190	1	33	0	0	0	0	0	0	0	0	0	0	0	0	2	60	0	0
191	1	44	0	0	0	0	0	0	0	0	0	0	0	0	0	0	0	0
192	0	0	0	0	0	0	0	0	0	0	2	53	0	0	1	20	0	0
193	0	0	1	2	0	0	0	0	0	0	0	0	0	0	1	19	0	0
194	0	0	0	0	0	0	0	0	0	0	0	0	0	0	0	0	0	0
195	1	10	0	0	1	8	0	0	0	0	1	8	0	0	2	46	0	0
196	0	0	0	0	0	0	0	0	0	0	0	0	0	0	0	0	0	0
197	0	0	0	0	0	0	0	0	0	0	0	0	0	0	1	49	0	0
198	2	44	0	0	0	0	0	0	0	0	1	20	0	0	7	154	0	0

TABLE V-9: DEDICATED SPECIAL CARE UNITS AND BEDS BY HSA, 1997 (CONTINUED)

HSA	Rehabilitation Units	Rehabilitation Beds	Hospice Units	Hospice Beds	AIDS Units	AIDS Beds	Head Trauma Units	Head Trauma Beds	Disabled Children & Young Adults Units	Disabled Children & Young Adults Beds	Respiratory Units	Respiratory Beds	Dialysis Units	Dialysis Beds	Alzheimer's Units	Alzheimer's Beds	Huntington's Disease Units	Huntington's Disease Beds
199	0	0	0	0	0	0	0	0	0	0	0	0	0	0	0	0	0	0
200	10	404	8	64	3	68	2	29	1	18	8	154	1	3	10	432	1	1
201	0	0	0	0	0	0	0	0	0	0	0	0	0	0	0	0	0	0
202	2	80	1	1	0	0	0	0	0	0	1	16	0	0	4	220	0	0
203	1	22	0	0	0	0	0	0	0	0	0	0	0	0	3	80	0	0
204	0	0	0	0	0	0	0	0	0	0	0	0	0	0	0	0	0	0
205	0	0	0	0	0	0	0	0	0	0	0	0	0	0	3	60	0	0
206	0	0	0	0	0	0	0	0	0	0	0	0	0	0	2	36	0	0
207	0	0	0	0	0	0	0	0	0	0	0	0	0	0	1	15	0	0
208	0	0	0	0	0	0	0	0	0	0	0	0	0	0	0	0	0	0
209	0	0	0	0	0	0	0	0	0	0	0	0	0	0	2	46	0	0
210	0	0	0	0	0	0	0	0	0	0	1	26	0	0	1	30	0	0
211	0	0	0	0	0	0	0	0	0	0	0	0	0	0	0	0	0	0
212	1	18	0	0	0	0	0	0	0	0	0	0	0	0	3	133	0	0
213	2	46	0	0	0	0	0	0	0	0	0	0	0	0	8	223	0	0
214	0	0	0	0	0	0	0	0	0	0	0	0	0	0	3	77	0	0
215	1	9	1	9	1	9	1	9	1	9	1	9	1	9	1	9	1	9
216	0	0	0	0	0	0	0	0	0	0	0	0	0	0	0	0	0	0
217	0	0	0	0	0	0	0	0	0	0	0	0	0	0	0	0	0	0
218	0	0	0	0	0	0	0	0	0	0	0	0	0	0	2	40	0	0
219	1	32	0	0	0	0	0	0	0	0	0	0	0	0	0	0	0	0
220	0	0	0	0	0	0	0	0	0	0	0	0	0	0	0	0	0	0
221	4	132	0	0	1	29	0	0	0	0	3	51	1	2	8	399	0	0
222	0	0	0	0	0	0	0	0	0	0	0	0	0	0	0	0	0	0
223	0	0	0	0	0	0	0	0	0	0	0	0	0	0	0	0	0	0
224	1	10	0	0	0	0	0	0	0	0	0	0	0	0	2	43	0	0
225	0	0	0	0	0	0	0	0	0	0	2	37	0	0	4	159	0	0
226	0	0	0	0	0	0	0	0	0	0	0	0	0	0	1	24	0	0

TABLE V-9: DEDICATED SPECIAL CARE UNITS AND BEDS BY HSA, 1997 (CONTINUED)

HSA	Rehabilitation Units	Rehabilitation Beds	Hospice Units	Hospice Beds	AIDS Units	AIDS Beds	Head Trauma Units	Head Trauma Beds	Disabled Children & Young Adults Units	Disabled Children & Young Adults Beds	Respiratory Units	Respiratory Beds	Dialysis Units	Dialysis Beds	Alzheimer's Units	Alzheimer's Beds	Huntington's Disease Units	Huntington's Disease Beds
227	7	337	1	26	1	1	1	15	1	29	7	96	0	0	29	979	0	0
228	0	0	0	0	0	0	0	0	0	0	0	0	0	0	0	0	0	0
229	0	0	0	0	0	0	0	0	0	0	0	0	0	0	1	30	0	0
230	1	25	0	0	0	0	0	0	0	0	0	0	0	0	0	0	0	0
231	0	0	0	0	0	0	0	0	0	0	0	0	0	0	1	65	0	0
232	0	0	1	1	0	0	0	0	0	0	0	0	0	0	0	0	0	0
233	3	128	0	0	0	0	0	0	0	0	0	0	0	0	6	177	0	0
234	0	0	0	0	0	0	0	0	0	0	0	0	0	0	0	0	0	0
235	1	26	0	0	0	0	0	0	0	0	0	0	0	0	2	40	0	0
236	0	0	0	0	0	0	0	0	0	0	0	0	0	0	0	0	0	0
237	1	30	0	0	0	0	0	0	0	0	1	18	0	0	5	116	0	0
238	0	0	0	0	0	0	0	0	0	0	0	0	0	0	1	20	0	0
239	0	0	0	0	0	0	0	0	0	0	0	0	0	0	0	0	0	0
240	0	0	1	62	0	0	0	0	0	0	0	0	0	0	0	0	0	0
241	0	0	0	0	0	0	0	0	0	0	1	6	0	0	0	0	0	0
242	1	11	0	0	0	0	0	0	0	0	0	0	0	0	2	50	0	0
243	0	0	0	0	0	0	0	0	0	0	0	0	0	0	0	0	0	0
244	0	0	0	0	0	0	0	0	0	0	0	0	0	0	0	0	0	0
245	0	0	0	0	0	0	0	0	1	1	0	0	0	0	0	0	0	0
246	1	20	0	0	0	0	0	0	0	0	0	0	0	0	2	88	0	0
247	0	0	0	0	0	0	0	0	0	0	0	0	0	0	0	0	0	0
248	0	0	0	0	0	0	0	0	0	0	0	0	0	0	0	0	0	0
249	0	0	0	0	0	0	0	0	0	0	0	0	0	0	0	0	0	0
250	0	0	0	0	0	0	0	0	0	0	0	0	0	0	1	16	0	0
251	0	0	0	0	0	0	0	0	0	0	0	0	0	0	0	0	0	0
252	0	0	0	0	0	0	0	0	0	0	0	0	0	0	0	0	0	0
253	0	0	0	0	0	0	0	0	0	0	0	0	0	0	0	0	0	0
254	0	0	0	0	0	0	0	0	0	0	0	0	0	0	0	0	0	0

TABLE V-9: DEDICATED SPECIAL CARE UNITS AND BEDS BY HSA, 1997 (CONTINUED)

HSA	Rehabilitation Units	Rehabilitation Beds	Hospice Units	Hospice Beds	AIDS Units	AIDS Beds	Head Trauma Units	Head Trauma Beds	Disabled Children & Young Adults Units	Disabled Children & Young Adults Beds	Respiratory Units	Respiratory Beds	Dialysis Units	Dialysis Beds	Alzheimer's Units	Alzheimer's Beds	Huntington's Disease Units	Huntington's Disease Beds
256	0	0	0	0	0	0	0	0	0	0	0	0	0	0	1	30	0	0
257	1	37	0	0	0	0	0	0	0	0	0	0	0	0	0	0	0	0
258	0	0	0	0	0	0	0	0	0	0	0	0	0	0	1	20	0	0
259	0	0	0	0	0	0	0	0	0	0	0	0	0	0	0	0	0	0
260	0	0	0	0	0	0	0	0	0	0	0	0	0	0	0	0	0	0
261	0	0	0	0	0	0	0	0	0	0	0	0	0	0	0	0	0	0
262	0	0	0	0	0	0	0	0	0	0	0	0	0	0	1	20	0	0
263	0	0	0	0	0	0	0	0	0	0	0	0	0	0	0	0	0	0
264	0	0	0	0	0	0	0	0	0	0	0	0	0	0	1	26	0	0
266	1	30	0	0	0	0	0	0	0	0	1	22	0	0	0	0	0	0
267	1	20	0	0	0	0	0	0	0	0	0	0	0	0	0	0	0	0
268	0	0	0	0	0	0	0	0	0	0	0	0	0	0	0	0	0	0
269	0	0	0	0	0	0	0	0	0	0	0	0	0	0	0	0	0	0
270	3	102	2	114	0	0	0	0	0	0	2	58	1	3	21	796	0	0
271	1	70	0	0	0	0	0	0	0	0	0	0	0	0	2	87	0	0
272	3	64	0	0	2	14	1	22	1	46	2	44	0	0	4	133	0	0
273	0	0	0	0	0	0	0	0	0	0	0	0	0	0	6	277	0	0
274	2	62	1	20	0	0	0	0	0	0	2	57	0	0	8	323	0	0
275	4	78	4	62	1	39	0	0	0	0	1	4	0	0	19	598	0	0
276	5	84	0	0	0	0	0	0	0	0	4	60	0	0	7	278	0	0
277	0	0	0	0	0	0	0	0	1	42	2	7	0	0	7	185	0	0
278	0	0	0	0	0	0	0	0	0	0	0	0	0	0	7	198	0	0
279	1	16	2	21	0	0	1	9	0	0	1	6	1	20	5	129	0	0
280	9	285	1	8	1	2	1	8	1	4	1	15	1	10	16	786	0	0
281	3	86	1	8	1	20	0	0	1	16	5	78	0	0	10	399	1	32
282	0	0	1	2	0	0	0	0	0	0	0	0	0	0	5	169	0	0
283	1	12	0	0	0	0	0	0	0	0	1	4	0	0	2	38	0	0
284	0	0	0	0	0	0	0	0	0	0	1	8	0	0	4	96	0	0

Table V-9: Dedicated Special Care Units and Beds by HSA, 1997 (Continued)

HSA	Rehabilitation Units	Rehabilitation Beds	Hospice Units	Hospice Beds	AIDS Units	AIDS Beds	Head Trauma Units	Head Trauma Beds	Disabled Children & Young Adults Units	Disabled Children & Young Adults Beds	Respiratory Units	Respiratory Beds	Dialysis Units	Dialysis Beds	Alzheimer's Units	Alzheimer's Beds	Huntington's Disease Units	Huntington's Disease Beds
285	1	21	0	0	0	0	0	0	0	0	0	0	0	0	3	100	0	0
286	6	193	0	0	0	0	0	0	0	0	1	8	1	1	11	339	0	0
287	18	1,302	7	31	1	40	1	6	0	0	14	260	1	2	54	2,316	1	1
288	11	332	4	23	1	21	2	59	0	0	10	351	1	24	17	720	1	24
289	1	22	0	0	0	0	0	0	1	25	0	0	0	0	5	206	0	0
290	2	173	0	0	0	0	0	0	0	0	1	16	0	0	6	135	0	0
291	1	100	0	0	0	0	0	0	0	0	1	39	1	1	6	185	0	0
292	0	0	0	0	0	0	0	0	0	0	1	16	0	0	5	116	0	0
293	0	0	0	0	0	0	0	0	0	0	0	0	0	0	0	0	0	0
294	1	12	0	0	0	0	0	0	0	0	0	0	0	0	2	36	0	0
295	2	35	1	148	0	0	0	0	0	0	1	24	0	0	14	568	0	0
296	0	0	0	0	0	0	0	0	0	0	0	0	0	0	1	50	0	0
297	0	0	0	0	0	0	0	0	0	0	0	0	0	0	1	20	0	0
298	1	58	1	58	0	0	0	0	0	0	2	17	0	0	5	151	0	0
299	3	69	1	1	0	0	0	0	0	0	1	3	0	0	1	28	0	0
300	0	0	0	0	0	0	0	0	0	0	0	0	0	0	3	89	0	0
301	2	59	1	150	0	0	0	0	0	0	0	0	0	0	15	316	0	0
302	1	20	0	0	0	0	0	0	0	0	0	0	0	0	3	54	0	0
303	1	15	0	0	0	0	0	0	0	0	0	0	0	0	6	249	0	0
304	3	51	1	2	0	0	0	0	0	0	0	0	0	0	7	216	0	0
305	1	8	2	8	0	0	0	0	0	0	1	8	0	0	4	137	0	0
306	2	70	1	78	0	0	1	30	0	0	0	0	0	0	7	213	0	0
307	0	0	2	6	0	0	0	0	0	0	0	0	0	0	4	79	0	0
308	0	0	0	0	0	0	0	0	0	0	1	26	0	0	5	187	0	0
309	1	40	0	0	0	0	1	32	0	0	0	0	0	0	5	154	0	0
310	0	0	1	1	0	0	0	0	0	0	0	0	0	0	1	28	0	0
311	1	99	0	0	0	0	0	0	0	0	0	0	0	0	3	71	0	0
312	0	0	1	6	0	0	0	0	0	0	0	0	0	0	4	100	0	0

TABLE V-9: DEDICATED SPECIAL CARE UNITS AND BEDS BY HSA, 1997 (CONTINUED)

HSA	Rehabilitation Units	Rehabilitation Beds	Hospice Units	Hospice Beds	AIDS Units	AIDS Beds	Head Trauma Units	Head Trauma Beds	Disabled Children & Young Adults Units	Disabled Children & Young Adults Beds	Respiratory Units	Respiratory Beds	Dialysis Units	Dialysis Beds	Alzheimer's Units	Alzheimer's Beds	Huntington's Disease Units	Huntington's Disease Beds
313	0	0	0	0	0	0	0	0	0	0	0	0	0	0	3	83	0	0
314	0	0	0	0	0	0	0	0	0	0	0	0	0	0	0	0	0	0
315	0	0	0	0	0	0	0	0	0	0	0	0	0	0	5	110	0	0
316	0	0	0	0	0	0	0	0	0	0	0	0	0	0	2	184	0	0
317	0	0	0	0	0	0	0	0	0	0	0	0	0	0	0	0	0	0
318	0	0	1	2	0	0	1	6	0	0	1	16	0	0	1	16	0	0
319	0	0	0	0	0	0	0	0	0	0	0	0	0	0	1	20	0	0
320	0	0	0	0	0	0	0	0	0	0	0	0	0	0	2	81	0	0
321	1	100	0	0	0	0	0	0	0	0	1	10	0	0	1	32	0	0
322	0	0	0	0	0	0	0	0	0	0	1	10	0	0	0	0	0	0
323	0	0	0	0	0	0	0	0	0	0	0	0	0	0	3	73	0	0
324	0	0	0	0	0	0	0	0	0	0	0	0	0	0	2	47	0	0
325	2	28	2	11	1	4	1	6	0	0	2	21	0	0	4	159	0	0
326	0	0	0	0	0	0	0	0	0	0	0	0	0	0	4	145	0	0
327	0	0	0	0	0	0	0	0	0	0	0	0	0	0	0	0	0	0
328	0	0	0	0	0	0	0	0	0	0	1	22	0	0	2	52	0	0
329	0	0	0	0	0	0	0	0	1	82	1	32	0	0	2	30	0	0
330	0	0	0	0	0	0	0	0	0	0	0	0	0	0	1	28	0	0
331	0	0	0	0	0	0	0	0	0	0	0	0	0	0	1	23	0	0
332	0	0	0	0	0	0	0	0	0	0	0	0	0	0	7	150	0	0
333	0	0	0	0	0	0	0	0	0	0	0	0	0	0	0	0	0	0
334	0	0	0	0	0	0	0	0	0	0	0	0	0	0	0	0	0	0
335	0	0	0	0	0	0	0	0	0	0	0	0	0	0	0	0	0	0
336	1	2	1	2	0	0	0	0	0	0	0	0	0	0	2	36	0	0
337	0	0	0	0	0	0	0	0	0	0	1	28	0	0	0	0	0	0
338	0	0	0	0	0	0	0	0	0	0	1	4	0	0	7	159	0	0
339	0	0	0	0	0	0	0	0	0	0	0	0	0	0	2	53	0	0
340	0	0	0	0	0	0	0	0	0	0	0	0	0	0	1	6	0	0

TABLE V-9: DEDICATED SPECIAL CARE UNITS AND BEDS BY HSA, 1997 (CONTINUED)

HSA	Rehabilitation Units	Rehabilitation Beds	Hospice Units	Hospice Beds	AIDS Units	AIDS Beds	Head Trauma Units	Head Trauma Beds	Disabled Children & Young Adults Units	Disabled Children & Young Adults Beds	Respiratory Units	Respiratory Beds	Dialysis Units	Dialysis Beds	Alzheimer's Units	Alzheimer's Beds	Huntington's Disease Units	Huntington's Disease Beds
341	0	0	0	0	0	0	0	0	0	0	0	0	0	0	2	67	0	0
342	0	0	0	0	0	0	0	0	0	0	0	0	0	0	0	0	0	0
343	0	0	0	0	0	0	0	0	0	0	0	0	0	0	3	64	0	0
344	0	0	0	0	0	0	0	0	0	0	0	0	0	0	4	116	0	0
345	0	0	1	2	0	0	0	0	1	4	4	30	0	0	8	349	0	0
346	0	0	1	1	0	0	0	0	0	0	2	60	0	0	5	180	0	0
347	2	108	1	120	0	0	0	0	0	0	3	47	0	0	7	208	0	0
348	0	0	0	0	0	0	0	0	0	0	0	0	0	0	2	99	0	0
349	0	0	0	0	0	0	0	0	0	0	1	7	0	0	5	146	0	0
350	1	25	0	0	0	0	0	0	0	0	0	0	0	0	1	16	0	0
351	1	103	0	0	0	0	0	0	0	0	0	0	0	0	2	47	0	0
352	3	60	0	0	0	0	0	0	0	0	1	12	0	0	7	369	0	0
353	0	0	0	0	0	0	0	0	0	0	0	0	0	0	8	181	0	0
354	1	25	1	1	0	0	0	0	0	0	0	0	0	0	2	44	0	0
355	1	103	0	0	0	0	0	0	0	0	2	20	0	0	6	261	0	0
356	1	6	0	0	0	0	0	0	0	0	0	0	0	0	1	10	0	0
357	0	0	0	0	0	0	0	0	0	0	0	0	0	0	1	49	0	0
358	0	0	0	0	0	0	0	0	0	0	0	0	0	0	2	44	0	0
359	0	0	0	0	0	0	1	4	0	0	0	0	0	0	0	0	0	0
360	0	0	0	0	0	0	0	0	0	0	0	0	0	0	0	0	0	0
361	0	0	0	0	0	0	0	0	0	0	0	0	0	0	1	20	0	0
362	0	0	0	0	0	0	0	0	0	0	0	0	0	0	2	87	0	0
363	1	5	0	0	0	0	0	0	0	0	1	18	0	0	2	48	0	0
364	0	0	0	0	0	0	0	0	1	8	1	8	0	0	1	28	0	0
365	1	25	0	0	0	0	0	0	0	0	0	0	0	0	1	20	0	0
366	2	50	8	102	0	0	0	0	0	0	0	0	0	0	9	238	0	0
367	0	0	0	0	0	0	0	0	0	0	0	0	0	0	1	38	0	0
368	1	20	0	0	0	0	0	0	0	0	0	0	0	0	2	41	0	0

TABLE V-9: DEDICATED SPECIAL CARE UNITS AND BEDS BY HSA, 1997 (CONTINUED)

HSA	Rehabilitation Units	Rehabilitation Beds	Hospice Units	Hospice Beds	AIDS Units	AIDS Beds	Head Trauma Units	Head Trauma Beds	Disabled Children & Young Adults Units	Disabled Children & Young Adults Beds	Respiratory Units	Respiratory Beds	Dialysis Units	Dialysis Beds	Alzheimer's Units	Alzheimer's Beds	Huntington's Disease Units	Huntington's Disease Beds
369	0	0	0	0	0	0	0	0	0	0	0	0	0	0	5	116	0	0
370	0	0	1	1	0	0	0	0	1	49	0	0	0	0	3	42	0	0
371	0	0	0	0	0	0	0	0	0	0	0	0	0	0	0	0	0	0
372	0	0	0	0	0	0	0	0	0	0	0	0	0	0	0	0	0	0
373	1	16	0	0	0	0	0	0	0	0	0	0	0	0	7	180	0	0
374	0	0	0	0	0	0	0	0	0	0	0	0	0	0	2	43	0	0
375	0	0	1	3	0	0	0	0	1	1	0	0	1	1	3	22	0	0
376	1	8	0	0	0	0	0	0	0	0	0	0	0	0	5	116	0	0
377	0	0	0	0	0	0	0	0	0	0	0	0	0	0	2	34	0	0
378	1	129	0	0	1	19	1	19	0	0	1	19	1	19	3	87	1	19
379	0	0	0	0	0	0	0	0	0	0	0	0	0	0	2	27	0	0
380	0	0	1	1	0	0	0	0	0	0	0	0	0	0	0	0	0	0
381	0	0	0	0	0	0	0	0	0	0	0	0	0	0	0	0	0	0
382	3	83	0	0	0	0	1	8	0	0	0	0	0	0	2	123	0	0
383	0	0	0	0	0	0	0	0	0	0	0	0	0	0	0	0	0	0
384	0	0	0	0	0	0	0	0	0	0	0	0	0	0	1	19	0	0
385	0	0	1	119	0	0	0	0	0	0	0	0	0	0	1	25	0	0
386	0	0	0	0	0	0	0	0	0	0	0	0	0	0	3	110	0	0
387	0	0	0	0	0	0	0	0	0	0	0	0	0	0	1	67	0	0
388	1	12	1	14	0	0	0	0	0	0	2	51	0	0	3	107	0	0
389	0	0	1	1	0	0	0	0	1	136	0	0	0	0	5	150	0	0
390	3	265	0	0	0	0	0	0	0	0	0	0	0	0	5	160	0	0
391	0	0	0	0	0	0	0	0	0	0	0	0	0	0	1	12	0	0
392	0	0	0	0	0	0	0	0	0	0	1	17	0	0	0	0	0	0
394	0	0	0	0	0	0	0	0	0	0	0	0	0	0	1	20	0	0
395	0	0	0	0	0	0	0	0	0	0	0	0	0	0	0	0	0	0
396	0	0	0	0	0	0	0	0	0	0	0	0	0	0	2	62	0	0
398	0	0	0	0	0	0	0	0	0	0	0	0	0	0	1	8	0	0

TABLE V-9: DEDICATED SPECIAL CARE UNITS AND BEDS BY HSA, 1997 (CONTINUED)

HSA	Rehabilitation Units	Rehabilitation Beds	Hospice Units	Hospice Beds	AIDS Units	AIDS Beds	Head Trauma Units	Head Trauma Beds	Disabled Children & Young Adults Units	Disabled Children & Young Adults Beds	Respiratory Units	Respiratory Beds	Dialysis Units	Dialysis Beds	Alzheimer's Units	Alzheimer's Beds	Huntington's Disease Units	Huntington's Disease Beds
399	0	0	0	0	0	0	0	0	0	0	0	0	0	0	1	28	0	0
400	0	0	0	0	0	0	0	0	0	0	0	0	0	0	1	62	0	0
401	0	0	0	0	0	0	0	0	0	0	0	0	0	0	1	20	0	0
402	0	0	0	0	0	0	0	0	0	0	1	20	0	0	1	24	0	0
403	0	0	0	0	1	24	0	0	0	0	2	38	0	0	5	194	0	0
404	2	9	1	1	0	0	0	0	0	0	2	7	0	0	2	48	0	0
405	0	0	0	0	0	0	0	0	0	0	0	0	0	0	3	58	0	0
406	0	0	0	0	0	0	0	0	0	0	1	12	0	0	3	73	0	0
407	0	0	0	0	0	0	0	0	0	0	0	0	0	0	0	0	0	0
408	2	20	4	44	0	0	0	0	0	0	1	16	0	0	14	721	0	0
409	0	0	0	0	0	0	0	0	0	0	0	0	0	0	2	61	0	0
410	2	47	0	0	0	0	0	0	0	0	3	53	0	0	10	432	0	0
411	2	38	0	0	0	0	0	0	0	0	0	0	0	0	2	56	0	0
412	0	0	1	30	0	0	0	0	0	0	0	0	0	0	0	0	0	0
413	1	14	0	0	0	0	0	0	0	0	0	0	0	0	0	0	0	0
414	0	0	0	0	0	0	0	0	0	0	1	6	0	0	4	183	0	0
415	0	0	0	0	0	0	0	0	0	0	0	0	0	0	1	15	0	0
416	2	34	1	3	0	0	0	0	0	0	0	0	0	0	4	100	0	0
417	1	8	2	142	0	0	0	0	0	0	1	14	0	0	9	329	0	0
418	0	0	0	0	0	0	0	0	0	0	0	0	0	0	2	37	0	0
419	3	56	0	0	0	0	0	0	0	0	1	8	0	0	7	153	0	0
420	0	0	0	0	0	0	0	0	0	0	0	0	0	0	3	84	0	0
421	1	22	1	15	0	0	0	0	0	0	1	6	0	0	5	126	1	2
422	0	0	0	0	0	0	0	0	0	0	0	0	0	0	0	0	0	0
423	0	0	0	0	0	0	0	0	0	0	0	0	0	0	0	0	0	0
424	1	12	0	0	0	0	0	0	0	0	0	0	0	0	3	80	0	0
425	0	0	1	200	0	0	0	0	0	0	0	0	0	0	3	76	0	0
426	1	14	0	0	0	0	0	0	0	0	0	0	0	0	1	18	0	0

TABLE V-9: DEDICATED SPECIAL CARE UNITS AND BEDS BY HSA, 1997 (CONTINUED)

HSA	Rehabilitation Units	Rehabilitation Beds	Hospice Units	Hospice Beds	AIDS Units	AIDS Beds	Head Trauma Units	Head Trauma Beds	Disabled Children & Young Adults Units	Disabled Children & Young Adults Beds	Respiratory Units	Respiratory Beds	Dialysis Units	Dialysis Beds	Alzheimer's Units	Alzheimer's Beds	Huntington's Disease Units	Huntington's Disease Beds
427	0	0	0	0	0	0	0	0	0	0	1	20	0	0	0	0	0	0
428	1	13	0	0	0	0	0	0	0	0	0	0	0	0	3	145	0	0
429	1	4	0	0	0	0	0	0	0	0	0	0	0	0	2	24	0	0
430	0	0	0	0	0	0	0	0	0	0	0	0	0	0	3	62	0	0
431	0	0	0	0	0	0	0	0	0	0	0	0	0	0	1	12	0	0
432	1	10	1	2	0	0	0	0	0	0	1	7	0	0	1	42	0	0
433	1	16	0	0	0	0	0	0	0	0	0	0	0	0	0	0	0	0
434	1	30	0	0	0	0	0	0	0	0	0	0	0	0	7	316	0	0
435	0	0	0	0	0	0	0	0	0	0	0	0	0	0	1	22	0	0
436	0	0	0	0	0	0	0	0	0	0	0	0	0	0	4	121	0	0
437	0	0	0	0	0	0	0	0	0	0	0	0	0	0	3	77	0	0
438	1	28	0	0	0	0	0	0	0	0	0	0	0	0	3	94	0	0
439	1	12	0	0	1	12	1	12	0	0	0	0	0	0	3	64	0	0
440	0	0	0	0	0	0	0	0	0	0	0	0	0	0	0	0	0	0
441	0	0	0	0	0	0	0	0	0	0	0	0	0	0	3	56	0	0
442	1	14	0	0	0	0	0	0	0	0	0	0	0	0	0	0	0	0
443	4	43	0	0	0	0	0	0	0	0	1	10	0	0	3	65	0	0
444	0	0	0	0	0	0	0	0	0	0	0	0	0	0	1	16	0	0
445	0	0	0	0	0	0	0	0	0	0	0	0	0	0	3	71	0	0
446	0	0	0	0	0	0	0	0	0	0	0	0	0	0	5	135	0	0
447	1	8	0	0	0	0	0	0	0	0	0	0	0	0	2	30	0	0
448	0	0	0	0	0	0	0	0	0	0	0	0	0	0	2	32	0	0
449	0	0	1	5	0	0	0	0	0	0	0	0	0	0	2	54	0	0
450	3	35	2	8	0	0	0	0	0	0	0	0	0	0	10	212	0	0
451	1	12	1	1	0	0	0	0	0	0	0	0	0	0	3	75	0	0
452	0	0	0	0	0	0	0	0	2	56	0	0	0	0	2	67	0	0
453	0	0	1	7	0	0	0	0	0	0	2	14	0	0	7	177	0	0
454	0	0	0	0	0	0	0	0	1	120	1	47	0	0	4	100	0	0

Table V-9: Dedicated Special Care Units and Beds by HSA, 1997 (Continued)

HSA	Rehabilitation Units	Rehabilitation Beds	Hospice Units	Hospice Beds	AIDS Units	AIDS Beds	Head Trauma Units	Head Trauma Beds	Disabled Children & Young Adults Units	Disabled Children & Young Adults Beds	Respiratory Units	Respiratory Beds	Dialysis Units	Dialysis Beds	Alzheimer's Units	Alzheimer's Beds	Huntington's Disease Units	Huntington's Disease Beds
455	0	0	0	0	0	0	0	0	0	0	0	0	0	0	0	0	0	0
456	0	0	0	0	0	0	0	0	0	0	0	0	0	0	1	21	0	0
457	1	36	1	1	0	0	0	0	0	0	0	0	0	0	4	57	0	0
458	0	0	0	0	0	0	0	0	0	0	0	0	0	0	0	0	0	0
459	0	0	0	0	0	0	0	0	0	0	0	0	0	0	0	0	0	0
460	0	0	0	0	0	0	0	0	0	0	0	0	0	0	0	0	0	0
461	0	0	0	0	0	0	0	0	0	0	0	0	0	0	0	0	0	0
462	0	0	0	0	0	0	0	0	0	0	0	0	0	0	6	158	0	0
463	1	18	0	0	0	0	0	0	0	0	0	0	0	0	1	50	0	0
464	0	0	0	0	0	0	0	0	0	0	0	0	0	0	0	0	0	0
465	0	0	1	31	0	0	0	0	0	0	0	0	0	0	1	42	0	0
466	1	8	0	0	0	0	0	0	0	0	0	0	0	0	1	20	0	0
467	1	44	0	0	0	0	0	0	0	0	1	64	0	0	2	32	0	0
468	0	0	0	0	0	0	0	0	0	0	0	0	0	0	0	0	0	0
469	1	31	1	31	0	0	0	0	0	0	0	0	0	0	1	31	0	0
470	0	0	0	0	0	0	1	1	0	0	0	0	0	0	4	85	0	0
471	0	0	0	0	0	0	0	0	0	0	0	0	0	0	0	0	0	0
472	0	0	0	0	0	0	0	0	0	0	0	0	0	0	0	0	0	0
473	0	0	0	0	0	0	0	0	0	0	0	0	0	0	1	3	1	1
474	0	0	0	0	0	0	0	0	0	0	0	0	0	0	1	16	0	0
475	2	98	1	70	0	0	0	0	1	60	0	0	0	0	2	124	0	0
476	0	0	1	2	0	0	0	0	0	0	0	0	1	1	1	22	0	0
477	0	0	0	0	0	0	0	0	0	0	0	0	0	0	0	0	0	0
478	1	6	0	0	0	0	0	0	0	0	0	0	0	0	0	0	0	0
479	0	0	0	0	0	0	0	0	0	0	0	0	0	0	0	0	0	0
480	0	0	0	0	0	0	0	0	0	0	0	0	0	0	0	0	0	0
481	0	0	0	0	0	0	0	0	0	0	0	0	0	0	0	0	0	0
482	1	10	0	0	0	0	0	0	0	0	0	0	0	0	0	0	0	0

Table V-9: Dedicated Special Care Units and Beds by HSA, 1997 (Continued)

HSA	Rehabilitation Units	Rehabilitation Beds	Hospice Units	Hospice Beds	AIDS Units	AIDS Beds	Head Trauma Units	Head Trauma Beds	Disabled Children & Young Adults Units	Disabled Children & Young Adults Beds	Respiratory Units	Respiratory Beds	Dialysis Units	Dialysis Beds	Alzheimer's Units	Alzheimer's Beds	Huntington's Disease Units	Huntington's Disease Beds
483	1	10	0	0	0	0	0	0	0	0	0	0	0	0	1	10	0	0
484	0	0	0	0	0	0	0	0	0	0	0	0	0	0	0	0	0	0
485	0	0	1	12	0	0	0	0	0	0	0	0	0	0	1	26	0	0
486	0	0	0	0	0	0	0	0	0	0	0	0	0	0	0	0	0	0
487	0	0	0	0	0	0	0	0	0	0	0	0	0	0	0	0	0	0
488	0	0	0	0	0	0	0	0	0	0	0	0	0	0	0	0	0	0
489	0	0	1	12	0	0	0	0	0	0	0	0	0	0	2	32	0	0
490	0	0	0	0	0	0	0	0	1	1	0	0	0	0	3	72	0	0
491	0	0	0	0	0	0	0	0	0	0	0	0	0	0	1	12	0	0
492	0	0	0	0	0	0	0	0	0	0	0	0	0	0	1	34	0	0
493	0	0	0	0	0	0	0	0	0	0	0	0	0	0	1	22	0	0
494	0	0	0	0	0	0	0	0	0	0	0	0	0	0	0	0	0	0
495	1	52	0	0	0	0	0	0	0	0	0	0	0	0	4	99	0	0
496	0	0	0	0	0	0	0	0	0	0	0	0	0	0	0	0	0	0
497	0	0	0	0	0	0	0	0	0	0	0	0	0	0	1	34	0	0
498	0	0	0	0	0	0	0	0	0	0	0	0	0	0	0	0	0	0
499	0	0	0	0	0	0	0	0	0	0	0	0	0	0	1	11	0	0
500	2	47	1	2	0	0	1	45	1	12	2	16	0	0	2	31	0	0
501	0	0	0	0	0	0	0	0	0	0	0	0	0	0	0	0	0	0
502	0	0	0	0	0	0	0	0	0	0	0	0	0	0	0	0	0	0
503	0	0	0	0	0	0	0	0	0	0	0	0	0	0	0	0	0	0
504	0	0	0	0	0	0	0	0	0	0	0	0	0	0	0	0	0	0
505	2	26	0	0	0	0	0	0	0	0	0	0	0	0	3	62	0	0
506	0	0	0	0	0	0	0	0	0	0	0	0	0	0	3	105	0	0
507	0	0	0	0	0	0	0	0	0	0	0	0	0	0	2	28	0	0
508	0	0	0	0	0	0	0	0	0	0	0	0	0	0	1	28	0	0
509	0	0	0	0	0	0	0	0	0	0	0	0	0	0	3	71	0	0
510	0	0	0	0	0	0	0	0	0	0	0	0	0	0	1	30	0	0

Table V-9: Dedicated Special Care Units and Beds by HSA, 1997 (Continued)

HSA	Rehabilitation Units	Rehabilitation Beds	Hospice Units	Hospice Beds	AIDS Units	AIDS Beds	Head Trauma Units	Head Trauma Beds	Disabled Children & Young Adults Units	Disabled Children & Young Adults Beds	Respiratory Units	Respiratory Beds	Dialysis Units	Dialysis Beds	Alzheimer's Units	Alzheimer's Beds	Huntington's Disease Units	Huntington's Disease Beds
511	0	0	0	0	0	0	0	0	0	0	0	0	0	0	0	0	0	0
512	0	0	0	0	0	0	0	0	0	0	0	0	0	0	0	0	0	0
513	0	0	0	0	0	0	0	0	0	0	0	0	0	0	0	0	0	0
514	0	0	0	0	0	0	0	0	0	0	0	0	0	0	0	0	0	0
515	0	0	1	2	0	0	0	0	0	0	0	0	0	0	1	33	0	0
516	0	0	0	0	0	0	0	0	0	0	0	0	0	0	0	0	0	0
517	0	0	0	0	0	0	0	0	0	0	0	0	0	0	2	70	0	0
518	0	0	0	0	0	0	0	0	0	0	0	0	0	0	1	26	0	0
519	0	0	0	0	0	0	0	0	0	0	0	0	0	0	0	0	0	0
520	0	0	0	0	0	0	0	0	0	0	0	0	0	0	0	0	0	0
521	0	0	0	0	0	0	0	0	0	0	0	0	0	0	0	0	0	0
522	0	0	0	0	0	0	0	0	0	0	0	0	0	0	0	0	0	0
523	0	0	0	0	0	0	0	0	0	0	0	0	0	0	0	0	0	0
524	0	0	0	0	0	0	0	0	0	0	0	0	0	0	0	0	0	0
525	0	0	0	0	0	0	0	0	0	0	0	0	0	0	0	0	0	0
526	0	0	0	0	0	0	0	0	0	0	0	0	0	0	0	0	0	0
527	0	0	0	0	0	0	0	0	0	0	0	0	0	0	0	0	0	0
528	0	0	0	0	0	0	0	0	0	0	0	0	0	0	0	0	0	0
529	0	0	0	0	0	0	0	0	0	0	0	0	0	0	1	24	0	0
530	0	0	0	0	0	0	0	0	0	0	0	0	0	0	0	0	0	0
531	0	0	0	0	0	0	0	0	0	0	0	0	0	0	0	0	0	0
532	0	0	0	0	0	0	0	0	0	0	0	0	0	0	0	0	0	0
533	0	0	0	0	0	0	0	0	0	0	0	0	0	0	0	0	0	0
534	0	0	0	0	0	0	0	0	0	0	0	0	0	0	0	0	0	0
535	0	0	0	0	0	0	0	0	0	0	0	0	0	0	0	0	0	0
536	0	0	0	0	0	0	0	0	0	0	0	0	0	0	0	0	0	0
537	0	0	0	0	0	0	0	0	0	0	0	0	0	0	0	0	0	0
538	0	0	0	0	0	0	0	0	0	0	0	0	0	0	0	0	0	0

TABLE V-9: DEDICATED SPECIAL CARE UNITS AND BEDS BY HSA, 1997 (CONTINUED)

HSA	Rehabilitation Units	Rehabilitation Beds	Hospice Units	Hospice Beds	AIDS Units	AIDS Beds	Head Trauma Units	Head Trauma Beds	Disabled Children & Young Adults Units	Disabled Children & Young Adults Beds	Respiratory Units	Respiratory Beds	Dialysis Units	Dialysis Beds	Alzheimer's Units	Alzheimer's Beds	Huntington's Disease Units	Huntington's Disease Beds
539	0	0	1	114	0	0	1	16	0	0	2	32	1	16	10	271	0	0
540	12	617	2	24	2	37	1	8	3	81	2	39	0	0	32	1,557	1	50
541	0	0	0	0	0	0	1	26	0	0	2	20	0	0	26	707	0	0
542	4	96	0	0	0	0	1	29	2	27	1	24	0	0	11	265	0	0
543	0	0	0	0	0	0	0	0	0	0	0	0	0	0	2	35	0	0
544	2	79	0	0	0	0	0	0	0	0	1	36	0	0	5	85	1	16
545	0	0	0	0	0	0	0	0	0	0	0	0	0	0	6	102	0	0
546	1	17	1	1	0	0	1	22	1	33	1	23	0	0	9	185	0	0
547	0	0	0	0	0	0	0	0	0	0	0	0	0	0	4	189	0	0
548	3	84	2	20	1	4	2	16	1	10	2	10	0	0	28	788	1	4
549	3	52	0	0	0	0	0	0	0	0	1	1	0	0	17	362	0	0
550	0	0	0	0	0	0	0	0	0	0	0	0	0	0	0	0	0	0
551	0	0	0	0	0	0	0	0	0	0	0	0	0	0	2	39	0	0
552	0	0	0	0	0	0	0	0	0	0	0	0	0	0	7	150	0	0
553	0	0	0	0	0	0	0	0	0	0	0	0	0	0	9	167	0	0
554	2	40	0	0	0	0	0	0	0	0	0	0	0	0	7	183	0	0
555	2	21	2	3	0	0	0	0	0	0	1	3	1	2	1	10	0	0
556	0	0	0	0	0	0	1	10	0	0	0	0	0	0	5	70	0	0
557	0	0	1	1	0	0	0	0	0	0	0	0	0	0	3	41	0	0
558	0	0	0	0	0	0	0	0	0	0	0	0	0	0	3	47	0	0
559	0	0	0	0	0	0	0	0	0	0	0	0	0	0	1	10	0	0
560	2	65	3	6	0	0	1	12	0	0	1	8	1	4	7	143	0	0
561	2	67	2	15	0	0	0	0	0	0	2	36	0	0	8	136	0	0
562	0	0	0	0	0	0	0	0	0	0	0	0	0	0	2	29	0	0
563	0	0	0	0	0	0	0	0	0	0	0	0	0	0	8	160	0	0
564	0	0	0	0	0	0	0	0	0	0	0	0	0	0	1	21	0	0
565	0	0	0	0	0	0	0	0	0	0	0	0	0	0	0	0	0	0
566	0	0	0	0	0	0	0	0	0	0	0	0	0	0	4	57	0	0

TABLE V-9: DEDICATED SPECIAL CARE UNITS AND BEDS BY HSA, 1997 (CONTINUED)

HSA	Rehabilitation Units	Rehabilitation Beds	Hospice Units	Hospice Beds	AIDS Units	AIDS Beds	Head Trauma Units	Head Trauma Beds	Disabled Children & Young Adults Units	Disabled Children & Young Adults Beds	Respiratory Units	Respiratory Beds	Dialysis Units	Dialysis Beds	Alzheimer's Units	Alzheimer's Beds	Huntington's Disease Units	Huntington's Disease Beds
567	0	0	0	0	0	0	0	0	0	0	0	0	0	0	1	21	0	0
568	0	0	0	0	0	0	0	0	0	0	0	0	0	0	1	14	0	0
569	0	0	1	1	0	0	0	0	0	0	0	0	0	0	3	37	0	0
570	0	0	0	0	0	0	0	0	0	0	0	0	0	0	3	50	0	0
571	0	0	0	0	0	0	0	0	0	0	0	0	0	0	3	68	0	0
572	0	0	0	0	0	0	0	0	0	0	0	0	0	0	2	48	0	0
573	0	0	0	0	0	0	0	0	0	0	0	0	0	0	4	112	0	0
574	1	36	0	0	0	0	0	0	0	0	0	0	0	0	6	136	0	0
575	0	0	0	0	0	0	0	0	0	0	0	0	0	0	1	20	0	0
576	1	60	0	0	0	0	0	0	0	0	1	8	0	0	16	378	0	0
577	0	0	0	0	0	0	0	0	0	0	0	0	0	0	4	62	0	0
578	0	0	0	0	0	0	0	0	0	0	0	0	0	0	1	11	0	0
579	0	0	0	0	0	0	0	0	0	0	0	0	0	0	1	24	0	0
580	0	0	2	2	0	0	0	0	0	0	0	0	0	0	2	41	0	0
581	1	18	0	0	0	0	0	0	0	0	0	0	0	0	6	140	0	0
582	0	0	0	0	0	0	0	0	0	0	0	0	0	0	2	41	0	0
583	0	0	0	0	0	0	0	0	0	0	0	0	0	0	3	58	0	0
584	0	0	0	0	0	0	0	0	0	0	0	0	0	0	3	60	0	0
585	0	0	0	0	0	0	0	0	0	0	0	0	0	0	2	68	0	0
586	0	0	0	0	0	0	0	0	0	0	0	0	0	0	2	50	0	0
587	0	0	0	0	0	0	0	0	0	0	0	0	0	0	0	0	0	0
588	0	0	0	0	0	0	0	0	0	0	0	0	0	0	2	44	0	0
589	0	0	1	1	0	0	0	0	0	0	0	0	1	10	1	20	0	0
590	0	0	0	0	0	0	0	0	0	0	0	0	0	0	0	0	0	0
591	0	0	2	3	0	0	0	0	0	0	0	0	0	0	6	124	0	0
592	0	0	1	1	0	0	0	0	0	0	0	0	0	0	2	39	0	0
593	0	0	0	0	0	0	0	0	0	0	0	0	0	0	3	66	0	0
594	0	0	0	0	0	0	0	0	0	0	0	0	0	0	1	14	0	0

TABLE V-9: DEDICATED SPECIAL CARE UNITS AND BEDS BY HSA, 1997 (CONTINUED)

HSA	Rehabilitation Units	Rehabilitation Beds	Hospice Units	Hospice Beds	AIDS Units	AIDS Beds	Head Trauma Units	Head Trauma Beds	Disabled Children & Young Adults Units	Disabled Children & Young Adults Beds	Respiratory Units	Respiratory Beds	Dialysis Units	Dialysis Beds	Alzheimer's Units	Alzheimer's Beds	Huntington's Disease Units	Huntington's Disease Beds
595	0	0	0	0	0	0	0	0	0	0	0	0	0	0	0	0	0	0
596	0	0	0	0	0	0	0	0	1	22	0	0	0	0	4	71	0	0
597	1	39	0	0	0	0	0	0	0	0	0	0	0	0	0	0	0	0
598	0	0	0	0	0	0	0	0	0	0	0	0	0	0	2	82	0	0
599	0	0	0	0	0	0	0	0	0	0	0	0	0	0	3	47	0	0
600	0	0	0	0	0	0	0	0	0	0	0	0	0	0	0	0	0	0
601	1	10	0	0	0	0	0	0	0	0	0	0	0	0	2	57	0	0
602	0	0	1	1	0	0	0	0	0	0	0	0	0	0	1	22	0	0
603	0	0	0	0	0	0	0	0	0	0	0	0	0	0	2	36	0	0
604	0	0	0	0	0	0	0	0	0	0	0	0	0	0	1	32	0	0
605	0	0	0	0	0	0	0	0	0	0	0	0	0	0	0	0	0	0
606	0	0	0	0	0	0	0	0	0	0	0	0	0	0	4	67	0	0
607	0	0	0	0	0	0	0	0	0	0	0	0	0	0	2	40	0	0
608	0	0	0	0	0	0	0	0	0	0	0	0	0	0	3	68	0	0
609	0	0	0	0	0	0	0	0	0	0	0	0	0	0	0	0	0	0
610	0	0	0	0	0	0	0	0	0	0	0	0	0	0	1	16	0	0
611	0	0	0	0	0	0	0	0	0	0	0	0	0	0	1	19	0	0
612	0	0	1	1	0	0	0	0	0	0	0	0	0	0	1	29	0	0
613	0	0	0	0	0	0	0	0	0	0	0	0	0	0	1	19	0	0
614	0	0	0	0	0	0	0	0	0	0	0	0	0	0	0	0	0	0
615	0	0	0	0	0	0	0	0	0	0	0	0	0	0	0	0	0	0
616	0	0	0	0	0	0	0	0	0	0	0	0	0	0	3	34	0	0
617	0	0	0	0	0	0	0	0	0	0	0	0	0	0	1	10	0	0
618	0	0	0	0	0	0	0	0	0	0	0	0	0	0	0	0	0	0
619	0	0	0	0	0	0	0	0	0	0	0	0	0	0	1	17	0	0
621	0	0	0	0	0	0	0	0	0	0	0	0	0	0	4	188	0	0
622	0	0	0	0	0	0	0	0	0	0	0	0	0	0	0	0	0	0
623	0	0	0	0	0	0	0	0	0	0	0	0	0	0	1	8	0	0

TABLE V-9: DEDICATED SPECIAL CARE UNITS AND BEDS BY HSA, 1997 (CONTINUED)

HSA	Rehabilitation Units	Rehabilitation Beds	Hospice Units	Hospice Beds	AIDS Units	AIDS Beds	Head Trauma Units	Head Trauma Beds	Disabled Children & Young Adults Units	Disabled Children & Young Adults Beds	Respiratory Units	Respiratory Beds	Dialysis Units	Dialysis Beds	Alzheimer's Units	Alzheimer's Beds	Huntington's Disease Units	Huntington's Disease Beds
624	2	32	0	0	0	0	0	0	0	0	0	0	0	0	9	321	0	0
625	0	0	0	0	0	0	0	0	0	0	0	0	0	0	1	10	0	0
626	0	0	0	0	0	0	0	0	0	0	0	0	0	0	3	50	0	0
627	0	0	0	0	0	0	0	0	0	0	0	0	0	0	3	70	0	0
628	0	0	0	0	0	0	0	0	0	0	0	0	0	0	1	16	0	0
629	0	0	0	0	0	0	0	0	0	0	0	0	0	0	0	0	0	0
630	1	26	0	0	0	0	0	0	0	0	0	0	0	0	3	63	0	0
631	0	0	0	0	0	0	0	0	0	0	0	0	0	0	0	0	0	0
632	0	0	0	0	0	0	0	0	0	0	0	0	0	0	0	0	0	0
633	0	0	0	0	0	0	0	0	0	0	0	0	0	0	1	12	0	0
634	0	0	0	0	0	0	0	0	0	0	0	0	0	0	0	0	0	0
635	0	0	0	0	0	0	0	0	0	0	0	0	0	0	0	0	0	0
636	0	0	0	0	0	0	0	0	0	0	0	0	0	0	0	0	0	0
637	0	0	0	0	0	0	0	0	0	0	0	0	0	0	1	12	0	0
638	0	0	1	0	0	0	0	0	0	0	0	0	0	0	0	0	0	0
639	0	0	1	55	0	0	0	0	0	0	0	0	0	0	2	50	0	0
640	0	0	0	0	0	0	0	0	0	0	0	0	0	0	1	8	0	0
641	0	0	0	0	0	0	0	0	0	0	0	0	0	0	5	159	0	0
642	0	0	0	0	0	0	0	0	0	0	0	0	0	0	0	0	0	0
643	0	0	0	0	0	0	0	0	0	0	0	0	0	0	0	0	0	0
644	0	0	0	0	0	0	0	0	0	0	0	0	0	0	0	0	0	0
645	0	0	0	0	0	0	0	0	0	0	0	0	0	0	0	0	0	0
646	0	0	0	0	0	0	0	0	0	0	0	0	0	0	3	64	0	0
647	0	0	0	0	0	0	0	0	0	0	0	0	0	0	1	16	0	0
648	0	0	0	0	0	0	0	0	0	0	0	0	0	0	1	19	0	0
649	1	30	0	0	0	0	0	0	0	0	0	0	0	0	0	0	0	0
650	0	0	0	0	0	0	0	0	0	0	0	0	0	0	1	12	0	0
651	0	0	0	0	0	0	0	0	0	0	0	0	0	0	2	36	0	0

TABLE V-9: DEDICATED SPECIAL CARE UNITS AND BEDS BY HSA, 1997 (CONTINUED)

HSA	Rehabilitation Units	Rehabilitation Beds	Hospice Units	Hospice Beds	AIDS Units	AIDS Beds	Head Trauma Units	Head Trauma Beds	Disabled Children & Young Adults Units	Disabled Children & Young Adults Beds	Respiratory Units	Respiratory Beds	Dialysis Units	Dialysis Beds	Alzheimer's Units	Alzheimer's Beds	Huntington's Disease Units	Huntington's Disease Beds
652	0	0	0	0	0	0	0	0	0	0	0	0	0	0	2	28	0	0
654	0	0	0	0	0	0	0	0	0	0	0	0	0	0	1	12	0	0
655	0	0	0	0	0	0	0	0	0	0	0	0	0	0	0	0	0	0
656	0	0	0	0	0	0	0	0	0	0	0	0	0	0	1	44	0	0
657	0	0	0	0	0	0	0	0	0	0	0	0	0	0	0	0	0	0
658	0	0	0	0	0	0	0	0	0	0	0	0	0	0	0	0	0	0
659	0	0	0	0	0	0	0	0	0	0	0	0	0	0	1	20	0	0
660	0	0	0	0	0	0	0	0	0	0	0	0	0	0	1	14	0	0
661	0	0	0	0	0	0	0	0	0	0	0	0	0	0	2	39	0	0
662	0	0	0	0	0	0	0	0	0	0	0	0	0	0	0	0	0	0
663	0	0	0	0	0	0	0	0	0	0	0	0	0	0	0	0	0	0
664	0	0	0	0	0	0	0	0	0	0	0	0	0	0	0	0	0	0
665	0	0	0	0	0	0	0	0	0	0	0	0	0	0	0	0	0	0
666	0	0	0	0	0	0	0	0	0	0	0	0	0	0	2	42	0	0
667	0	0	0	0	0	0	0	0	0	0	0	0	0	0	0	0	0	0
668	0	0	0	0	0	0	0	0	0	0	0	0	0	0	0	0	0	0
669	0	0	0	0	0	0	0	0	0	0	0	0	0	0	0	0	0	0
670	0	0	0	0	0	0	0	0	0	0	0	0	0	0	0	0	0	0
671	0	0	0	0	0	0	0	0	0	0	0	0	0	0	0	0	0	0
672	0	0	0	0	0	0	0	0	0	0	0	0	0	0	0	0	0	0
673	0	0	0	0	0	0	0	0	0	0	0	0	0	0	1	12	0	0
674	0	0	0	0	0	0	0	0	0	0	0	0	0	0	1	14	0	0
675	0	0	0	0	0	0	0	0	0	0	0	0	0	0	0	0	0	0
676	0	0	0	0	0	0	0	0	0	0	0	0	0	0	0	0	0	0
678	0	0	0	0	0	0	0	0	0	0	0	0	0	0	0	0	0	0
679	1	41	1	2	0	0	0	0	0	0	0	0	0	0	2	57	0	0
680	0	0	0	0	0	0	0	0	0	0	0	0	0	0	0	0	0	0
681	0	0	0	0	0	0	0	0	0	0	0	0	0	0	1	24	0	0

TABLE V-9: DEDICATED SPECIAL CARE UNITS AND BEDS BY HSA, 1997 (CONTINUED)

HSA	Rehabilitation Units	Rehabilitation Beds	Hospice Units	Hospice Beds	AIDS Units	AIDS Beds	Head Trauma Units	Head Trauma Beds	Disabled Children & Young Adults Units	Disabled Children & Young Adults Beds	Respiratory Units	Respiratory Beds	Dialysis Units	Dialysis Beds	Alzheimer's Units	Alzheimer's Beds	Huntington's Disease Units	Huntington's Disease Beds
682	0	0	0	0	0	0	0	0	0	0	0	0	0	0	0	0	0	0
683	0	0	0	0	0	0	0	0	0	0	0	0	0	0	1	37	0	0
684	0	0	0	0	0	0	0	0	0	0	0	0	0	0	0	0	0	0
685	0	0	0	0	0	0	0	0	0	0	0	0	0	0	0	0	0	0
686	0	0	0	0	0	0	0	0	0	0	0	0	0	0	1	16	0	0
687	0	0	0	0	0	0	0	0	0	0	0	0	0	0	1	15	0	0
688	7	168	2	16	1	10	1	10	0	0	0	0	1	20	23	770	1	10
689	2	27	4	26	1	12	1	12	2	70	3	39	1	12	14	423	0	0
690	1	17	0	0	0	0	0	0	0	0	0	0	0	0	3	117	0	0
691	0	0	0	0	0	0	0	0	0	0	0	0	0	0	5	93	0	0
692	1	14	0	0	0	0	0	0	0	0	0	0	0	0	3	55	0	0
693	0	0	0	0	0	0	0	0	0	0	0	0	0	0	2	78	0	0
694	0	0	1	2	0	0	0	0	0	0	0	0	0	0	2	38	0	0
695	1	29	0	0	0	0	0	0	0	0	0	0	0	0	2	48	0	0
696	1	24	0	0	0	0	0	0	0	0	1	4	0	0	1	30	0	0
697	2	54	0	0	0	0	0	0	0	0	0	0	0	0	3	89	0	0
698	2	35	0	0	0	0	0	0	0	0	0	0	0	0	8	218	0	0
699	5	175	2	6	1	31	0	0	1	5	5	87	0	0	31	1,053	0	0
700	4	88	3	78	1	126	1	126	1	126	2	66	1	60	17	644	1	126
701	0	0	0	0	0	0	0	0	1	7	0	0	0	0	5	164	0	0
702	0	0	0	0	0	0	0	0	0	0	0	0	0	0	2	61	0	0
703	1	28	1	6	0	0	0	0	0	0	0	0	0	0	3	45	0	0
704	2	46	1	8	0	0	0	0	0	0	1	6	0	0	6	154	0	0
705	1	15	0	0	0	0	0	0	0	0	0	0	0	0	4	167	0	0
707	1	24	1	2	0	0	0	0	0	0	2	145	0	0	5	162	0	0
708	4	93	0	0	0	0	0	0	0	0	0	0	0	0	9	313	0	0
709	3	100	0	0	0	0	0	0	0	0	1	34	0	0	5	342	0	0
710	1	99	0	0	0	0	0	0	0	0	0	0	0	0	1	20	0	0

TABLE V-9: DEDICATED SPECIAL CARE UNITS AND BEDS BY HSA, 1997 (CONTINUED)

HSA	Rehabilitation Units	Rehabilitation Beds	Hospice Units	Hospice Beds	AIDS Units	AIDS Beds	Head Trauma Units	Head Trauma Beds	Disabled Children & Young Adults Units	Disabled Children & Young Adults Beds	Respiratory Units	Respiratory Beds	Dialysis Units	Dialysis Beds	Alzheimer's Units	Alzheimer's Beds	Huntington's Disease Units	Huntington's Disease Beds
711	0	0	2	5	0	0	0	0	0	0	0	0	0	0	4	142	0	0
712	0	0	0	0	0	0	0	0	0	0	0	0	0	0	1	14	0	0
713	0	0	0	0	0	0	0	0	0	0	0	0	0	0	2	77	0	0
714	0	0	0	0	0	0	0	0	0	0	0	0	0	0	1	21	0	0
715	0	0	0	0	0	0	0	0	0	0	0	0	0	0	2	60	0	0
716	3	43	0	0	0	0	0	0	1	42	0	0	0	0	8	173	0	0
717	0	0	1	1	0	0	0	0	0	0	0	0	0	0	3	76	0	0
718	2	145	0	0	0	0	0	0	0	0	2	52	0	0	3	200	0	0
719	0	0	0	0	0	0	0	0	0	0	0	0	0	0	1	17	0	0
720	0	0	0	0	0	0	0	0	0	0	0	0	0	0	0	0	0	0
721	1	12	0	0	0	0	0	0	0	0	0	0	0	0	1	10	0	0
722	0	0	1	12	0	0	0	0	0	0	0	0	0	0	3	63	0	0
723	15	611	7	298	5	153	2	21	0	0	19	477	2	51	34	1,986	1	1
724	0	0	0	0	0	0	0	0	0	0	0	0	0	0	1	22	0	0
725	0	0	0	0	0	0	0	0	0	0	0	0	0	0	1	20	0	0
726	0	0	0	0	0	0	0	0	0	0	0	0	0	0	3	88	0	0
727	0	0	0	0	0	0	0	0	0	0	0	0	0	0	1	24	0	0
728	0	0	0	0	0	0	0	0	0	0	0	0	0	0	2	76	0	0
729	0	0	0	0	0	0	0	0	0	0	0	0	0	0	1	19	0	0
730	0	0	0	0	0	0	0	0	0	0	0	0	0	0	0	0	0	0
731	0	0	1	1	0	0	0	0	0	0	0	0	0	0	2	34	0	0
732	0	0	0	0	0	0	0	0	0	0	0	0	0	0	2	43	0	0
733	0	0	0	0	0	0	0	0	0	0	0	0	0	0	0	0	0	0
734	1	23	0	0	0	0	0	0	0	0	1	8	0	0	5	105	0	0
735	0	0	0	0	0	0	0	0	0	0	0	0	0	0	1	14	0	0
736	10	259	6	81	1	35	2	145	0	0	2	22	0	0	35	1,033	0	0
737	3	114	0	0	0	0	0	0	0	0	1	20	0	0	1	25	0	0
738	1	10	1	71	0	0	0	0	0	0	0	0	0	0	0	0	0	0

Table V-9: Dedicated Special Care Units and Beds by HSA, 1997 (Continued)

HSA	Rehabilitation Units	Rehabilitation Beds	Hospice Units	Hospice Beds	AIDS Units	AIDS Beds	Head Trauma Units	Head Trauma Beds	Disabled Children & Young Adults Units	Disabled Children & Young Adults Beds	Respiratory Units	Respiratory Beds	Dialysis Units	Dialysis Beds	Alzheimer's Units	Alzheimer's Beds	Huntington's Disease Units	Huntington's Disease Beds
739	0	0	0	0	0	0	0	0	1	120	0	0	0	0	2	46	0	0
740	0	0	0	0	0	0	0	0	0	0	0	0	0	0	3	54	0	0
741	1	29	0	0	0	0	0	0	0	0	0	0	0	0	2	31	0	0
742	0	0	0	0	0	0	0	0	0	0	0	0	0	0	1	32	0	0
743	0	0	0	0	0	0	0	0	0	0	0	0	0	0	1	20	0	0
744	1	7	1	2	0	0	0	0	1	1	0	0	0	0	4	98	0	0
745	0	0	0	0	0	0	0	0	0	0	0	0	0	0	3	56	0	0
746	1	59	0	0	0	0	0	0	0	0	1	28	0	0	1	23	0	0
747	0	0	0	0	0	0	0	0	0	0	0	0	0	0	4	174	0	0
748	0	0	1	1	0	0	0	0	0	0	0	0	0	0	3	57	0	0
749	0	0	0	0	0	0	0	0	0	0	0	0	0	0	3	74	0	0
750	2	32	0	0	0	0	0	0	0	0	2	59	0	0	3	123	0	0
751	7	414	2	31	0	0	0	0	2	53	3	58	1	1	10	432	1	1
752	1	20	0	0	0	0	0	0	0	0	1	4	0	0	4	105	0	0
753	0	0	0	0	0	0	0	0	0	0	0	0	0	0	0	0	0	0
754	1	25	2	48	0	0	0	0	0	0	2	36	0	0	5	167	0	0
755	0	0	0	0	0	0	0	0	0	0	0	0	0	0	0	0	0	0
756	0	0	0	0	0	0	0	0	0	0	0	0	0	0	1	24	0	0
757	4	291	2	40	4	82	1	2	0	0	6	113	1	4	5	227	0	0
758	1	20	1	152	1	40	0	0	0	0	0	0	1	1	7	168	0	0
759	0	0	0	0	0	0	0	0	0	0	0	0	0	0	1	47	0	0
760	3	60	0	0	0	0	0	0	0	0	1	14	0	0	7	226	0	0
761	1	16	0	0	0	0	0	0	0	0	0	0	0	0	3	60	0	0
763	0	0	0	0	0	0	0	0	0	0	0	0	0	0	0	0	0	0
764	2	101	0	0	0	0	0	0	0	0	0	0	0	0	2	86	0	0
765	0	0	0	0	0	0	0	0	0	0	0	0	0	0	0	0	0	0
766	6	291	0	0	0	0	0	0	0	0	3	54	0	0	5	157	0	0
767	0	0	0	0	0	0	0	0	0	0	0	0	0	0	2	30	0	0

TABLE V-9: DEDICATED SPECIAL CARE UNITS AND BEDS BY HSA, 1997 (CONTINUED)

HSA	Rehabilitation Units	Rehabilitation Beds	Hospice Units	Hospice Beds	AIDS Units	AIDS Beds	Head Trauma Units	Head Trauma Beds	Disabled Children & Young Adults Units	Disabled Children & Young Adults Beds	Respiratory Units	Respiratory Beds	Dialysis Units	Dialysis Beds	Alzheimer's Units	Alzheimer's Beds	Huntington's Disease Units	Huntington's Disease Beds
768	3	266	4	49	0	0	0	0	1	59	5	125	0	0	10	366	0	0
769	0	0	0	0	0	0	0	0	0	0	0	0	0	0	2	43	0	0
770	0	0	0	0	0	0	0	0	0	0	0	0	0	0	2	46	0	0
771	0	0	1	1	0	0	0	0	0	0	0	0	0	0	1	18	0	0
772	0	0	0	0	0	0	0	0	0	0	0	0	0	0	1	7	0	0
773	0	0	1	1	0	0	1	19	0	0	0	0	0	0	0	0	0	0
774	5	299	0	0	0	0	0	0	1	59	5	181	0	0	12	559	0	0
775	0	0	0	0	0	0	0	0	0	0	0	0	0	0	0	0	0	0
777	0	0	0	0	0	0	0	0	0	0	0	0	0	0	3	49	0	0
778	0	0	0	0	0	0	0	0	0	0	0	0	0	0	0	0	0	0
779	0	0	0	0	0	0	0	0	0	0	0	0	0	0	0	0	0	0
780	0	0	0	0	0	0	0	0	0	0	0	0	0	0	0	0	0	0
781	1	12	0	0	0	0	0	0	0	0	0	0	0	0	0	0	0	0
782	1	15	1	2	0	0	0	0	1	10	1	1	0	0	4	86	0	0
783	0	0	0	0	0	0	0	0	0	0	0	0	0	0	1	21	0	0
784	1	16	0	0	0	0	0	0	0	0	0	0	0	0	4	46	0	0
785	0	0	0	0	0	0	0	0	0	0	0	0	0	0	0	0	0	0
786	0	0	0	0	0	0	0	0	0	0	0	0	0	0	1	12	0	0
787	0	0	0	0	0	0	0	0	0	0	0	0	0	0	2	76	0	0
788	0	0	0	0	0	0	0	0	0	0	0	0	0	0	0	0	0	0
789	0	0	0	0	0	0	0	0	0	0	0	0	0	0	0	0	0	0
790	1	23	0	0	0	0	0	0	0	0	1	36	0	0	0	0	0	0
792	0	0	0	0	0	0	0	0	0	0	0	0	0	0	0	0	0	0
793	0	0	0	0	0	0	0	0	0	0	0	0	0	0	0	0	0	0
794	1	33	1	23	0	0	0	0	0	0	2	22	0	0	5	126	0	0
795	0	0	0	0	0	0	0	0	0	0	0	0	0	0	5	123	0	0
796	0	0	0	0	0	0	0	0	0	0	0	0	1	2	4	95	0	0
797	0	0	0	0	0	0	0	0	0	0	0	0	0	0	0	0	0	0

TABLE V-9: DEDICATED SPECIAL CARE UNITS AND BEDS BY HSA, 1997 (CONTINUED)

HSA	Rehabilitation Units	Rehabilitation Beds	Hospice Units	Hospice Beds	AIDS Units	AIDS Beds	Head Trauma Units	Head Trauma Beds	Disabled Children & Young Adults Units	Disabled Children & Young Adults Beds	Respiratory Units	Respiratory Beds	Dialysis Units	Dialysis Beds	Alzheimer's Units	Alzheimer's Beds	Huntington's Disease Units	Huntington's Disease Beds
799	0	0	0	0	0	0	0	0	0	0	0	0	0	0	1	12	0	0
800	1	85	0	0	0	0	0	0	0	0	0	0	0	0	0	0	0	0
801	0	0	0	0	0	0	0	0	0	0	0	0	0	0	0	0	0	0
802	1	99	0	0	0	0	0	0	0	0	0	0	0	0	0	0	0	0
803	0	0	0	0	0	0	0	0	0	0	0	0	0	0	0	0	0	0
804	0	0	0	0	0	0	0	0	0	0	0	0	0	0	0	0	0	0
805	0	0	0	0	0	0	0	0	0	0	0	0	0	0	0	0	0	0
806	0	0	0	0	0	0	0	0	0	0	0	0	0	0	0	0	0	0
807	1	18	1	2	0	0	0	0	0	0	1	45	0	0	0	0	0	0
808	0	0	0	0	0	0	0	0	0	0	0	0	0	0	0	0	0	0
809	0	0	0	0	0	0	0	0	0	0	0	0	0	0	1	23	0	0
810	1	9	0	0	0	0	0	0	0	0	0	0	0	0	0	0	0	0
811	1	8	0	0	0	0	0	0	0	0	0	0	0	0	0	0	0	0
812	0	0	0	0	0	0	0	0	0	0	0	0	0	0	4	66	0	0
813	0	0	0	0	0	0	0	0	0	0	0	0	0	0	0	0	0	0
814	0	0	0	0	0	0	0	0	0	0	0	0	0	0	0	0	0	0
815	0	0	0	0	0	0	0	0	0	0	0	0	0	0	6	135	0	0
816	0	0	0	0	0	0	0	0	0	0	0	0	0	0	0	0	0	0
817	0	0	0	0	0	0	0	0	0	0	0	0	0	0	0	0	0	0
818	0	0	0	0	0	0	0	0	0	0	0	0	0	0	0	0	0	0
819	0	0	0	0	0	0	0	0	0	0	0	0	0	0	0	0	0	0
820	0	0	0	0	0	0	0	0	0	0	0	0	0	0	0	0	0	0
821	1	12	0	0	0	0	0	0	0	0	0	0	0	0	0	0	0	0
822	0	0	1	6	0	0	0	0	0	0	0	0	0	0	0	0	0	0
823	1	10	1	82	0	0	0	0	0	0	0	0	0	0	2	88	0	0

Section VI

Staffing Information

TABLE VI-1

PHYSICAL THERAPIST STAFFING BY STATE, 1997

	% None	% On Staff Only	% Contract Only	% Both Contract and Staff
UNITED STATES	12.33%	24.98%	59.79%	2.90%
Alabama	16.07%	25.00%	57.14%	1.79%
Alaska	12.50%	62.50%	25.00%	0.00%
Arizona	7.27%	33.94%	52.73%	6.06%
Arkansas	17.63%	22.61%	57.47%	2.30%
California	10.29%	25.58%	59.27%	4.86%
Colorado	0.44%	41.33%	54.67%	3.56%
Connecticut	4.23%	26.92%	60.39%	8.46%
Delaware	9.30%	44.19%	46.51%	0.00%
District of Columbia	0.00%	19.05%	76.19%	4.76%
Florida	4.88%	37.45%	53.23%	4.45%
Georgia	4.24%	19.49%	73.16%	3.11%
Hawaii	23.26%	44.19%	30.23%	2.33%
Idaho	4.65%	44.19%	51.16%	0.00%
Illinois	17.09%	16.74%	63.63%	2.54%
Indiana	14.39%	22.01%	61.53%	2.08%
Iowa	18.98%	14.07%	66.53%	0.43%
Kansas	11.82%	17.97%	68.79%	1.42%
Kentucky	18.10%	27.30%	53.02%	1.59%
Louisiana	28.61%	15.34%	54.57%	1.47%
Maine	16.30%	23.70%	58.52%	1.48%
Maryland	10.48%	27.42%	59.68%	2.42%
Massachusetts	5.51%	32.33%	59.50%	2.66%
Michigan	9.46%	16.89%	71.85%	1.80%
Minnesota	10.91%	17.37%	70.82%	0.89%
Mississippi	7.39%	29.06%	61.58%	1.97%
Missouri	9.47%	22.28%	66.67%	1.58%
Montana	8.74%	43.69%	44.66%	2.91%
Nebraska	13.92%	22.36%	62.87%	0.84%
Nevada	13.33%	31.11%	51.11%	4.44%
New Hampshire	11.11%	37.04%	46.91%	4.94%
New Jersey	4.23%	15.11%	76.13%	4.53%
New Mexico	10.59%	32.94%	55.29%	1.18%
New York	3.38%	43.00%	45.73%	7.89%
North Carolina	2.49%	25.12%	68.91%	3.48%
North Dakota	14.77%	22.73%	62.50%	0.00%
Ohio	15.29%	18.15%	65.09%	1.48%
Oklahoma	44.31%	14.29%	40.92%	0.48%
Oregon	19.63%	26.99%	51.53%	1.84%
Pennsylvania	4.67%	29.29%	63.13%	2.90%

TABLE VI-1: PHYSICAL THERAPIST STAFFING BY STATE, 1997 (CONTINUED)

	% None	% On Staff Only	% Contract Only	% Both Contract and Staff
Rhode Island	22.00%	12.00%	63.00%	3.00%
South Carolina	9.66%	18.18%	69.89%	2.27%
South Dakota	15.79%	21.93%	61.40%	0.88%
Tennessee	7.76%	29.31%	59.77%	3.16%
Texas	21.15%	24.31%	51.77%	2.77%
Utah	11.46%	21.88%	64.58%	2.08%
Vermont	15.91%	38.64%	40.91%	4.55%
Virginia	8.12%	20.66%	68.64%	2.58%
Washington	3.16%	40.35%	49.47%	7.02%
West Virginia	17.65%	29.41%	51.47%	1.47%
Wisconsin	13.95%	26.48%	56.97%	2.60%
Wyoming	13.16%	31.58%	50.00%	5.26%

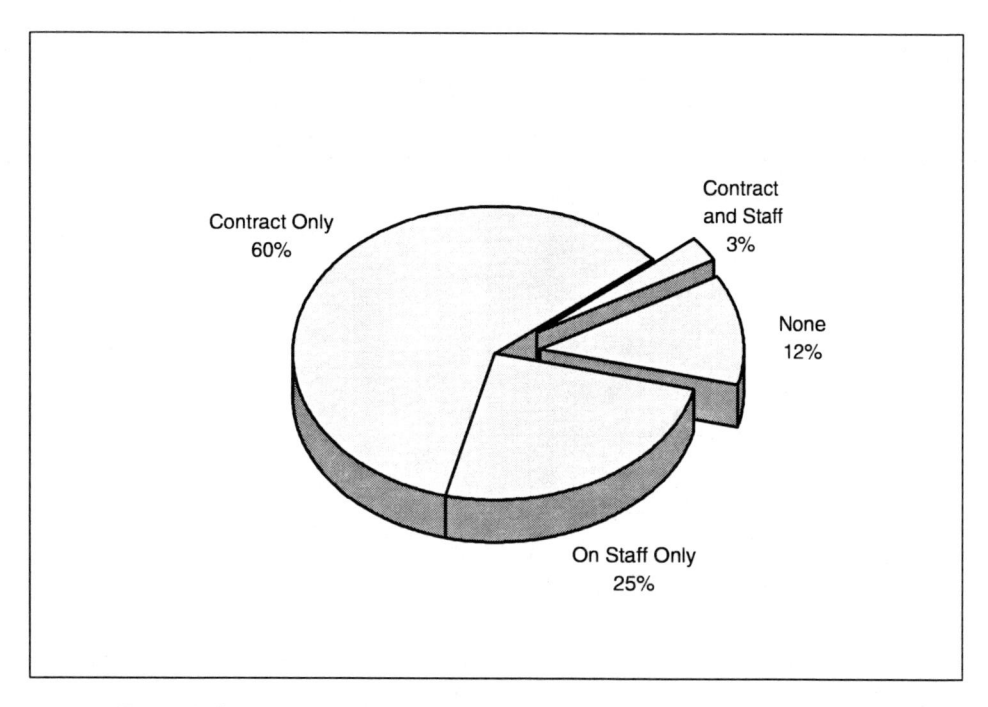

FIG. VI-A: PHYSICAL THERAPIST STAFFING, UNITED STATES, 1997

TABLE VI-2

OCCUPATIONAL THERAPIST STAFFING BY STATE, 1997

	% None	% On Staff Only	% Contract Only	% Both Contract and Staff
UNITED STATES	20.23%	19.82%	57.77%	2.17%
Alabama	24.55%	15.18%	58.93%	1.34%
Alaska	31.25%	37.50%	31.25%	0.00%
Arizona	9.70%	35.76%	49.70%	4.85%
Arkansas	30.27%	15.33%	51.34%	3.07%
California	14.45%	21.07%	60.61%	3.88%
Colorado	0.44%	37.78%	58.22%	3.56%
Connecticut	8.85%	17.69%	70.00%	3.46%
Delaware	20.93%	20.93%	55.81%	2.33%
District of Columbia	0.00%	14.29%	85.71%	0.00%
Florida	6.46%	32.71%	57.10%	3.73%
Georgia	9.89%	15.54%	72.88%	1.69%
Hawaii	34.88%	41.86%	20.93%	2.33%
Idaho	13.95%	37.21%	47.67%	1.16%
Illinois	30.25%	14.20%	54.04%	1.50%
Indiana	19.76%	19.58%	58.58%	2.08%
Iowa	34.97%	11.94%	52.88%	0.21%
Kansas	27.42%	14.42%	56.97%	1.18%
Kentucky	29.21%	20.32%	49.84%	0.63%
Louisiana	36.28%	13.86%	48.67%	1.18%
Maine	25.93%	18.52%	54.07%	1.48%
Maryland	13.71%	19.76%	63.31%	3.23%
Massachusetts	9.06%	24.33%	65.19%	1.42%
Michigan	13.51%	11.71%	73.42%	1.35%
Minnesota	17.37%	13.59%	68.82%	0.22%
Mississippi	16.75%	22.17%	59.61%	1.48%
Missouri	16.32%	19.47%	62.46%	1.75%
Montana	34.95%	31.07%	32.04%	1.94%
Nebraska	28.69%	18.57%	51.90%	0.84%
Nevada	17.78%	26.67%	48.89%	6.67%
New Hampshire	19.75%	23.46%	53.09%	3.70%
New Jersey	9.97%	13.60%	73.11%	3.32%
New Mexico	18.82%	27.06%	54.12%	0.00%
New York	12.56%	31.56%	50.08%	5.80%
North Carolina	6.22%	22.64%	69.15%	1.99%
North Dakota	47.73%	11.36%	40.91%	0.00%
Ohio	23.67%	14.79%	59.86%	1.68%
Oklahoma	59.56%	9.69%	30.51%	0.24%
Oregon	23.93%	21.47%	52.76%	1.84%
Pennsylvania	7.32%	23.61%	66.54%	2.53%

TABLE VI-2: OCCUPATIONAL THERAPIST STAFFING BY STATE, 1997 (CONTINUED)

	% None	% On Staff Only	% Contract Only	% Both Contract and Staff
Rhode Island	38.00%	5.00%	55.00%	2.00%
South Carolina	14.21%	10.80%	73.86%	1.14%
South Dakota	47.37%	14.91%	36.84%	0.88%
Tennessee	20.40%	19.83%	57.76%	2.01%
Texas	27.77%	18.77%	51.62%	1.85%
Utah	21.88%	19.79%	57.29%	1.04%
Vermont	31.82%	15.91%	52.27%	0.00%
Virginia	15.87%	15.87%	66.42%	1.85%
Washington	6.67%	31.58%	57.90%	3.86%
West Virginia	52.94%	9.56%	36.03%	1.47%
Wisconsin	17.73%	27.19%	52.72%	2.36%
Wyoming	26.32%	28.95%	44.74%	0.00%

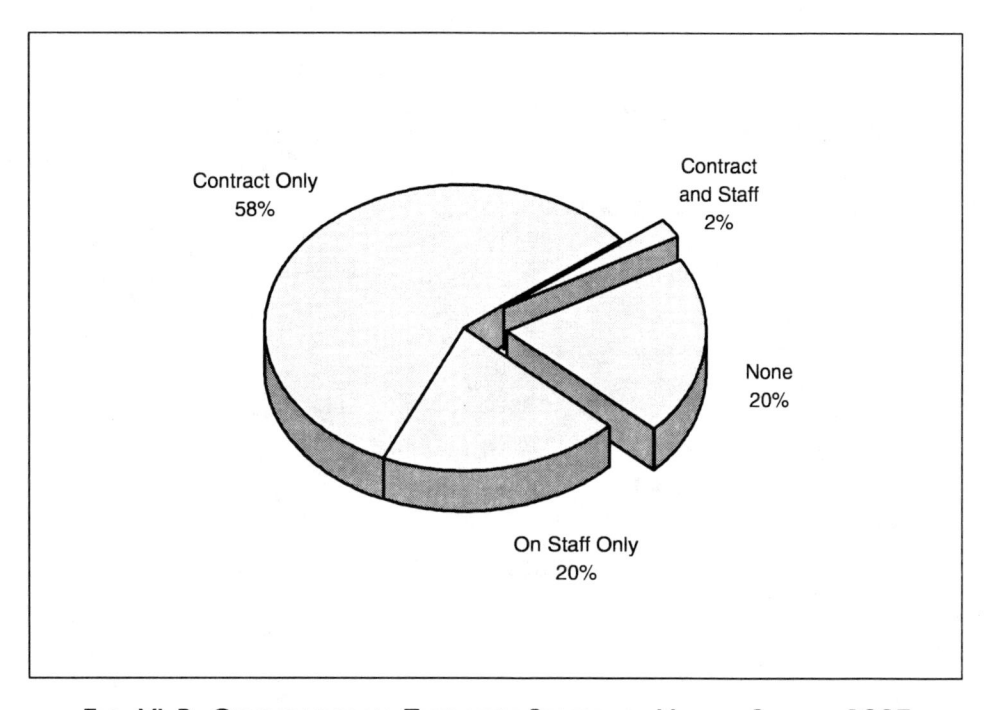

FIG. VI-B: OCCUPATIONAL THERAPIST STAFFING, UNITED STATES, 1997

TABLE VI-3

SPEECH AND LANGUAGE PATHOLOGIST STAFFING BY STATE, 1997

	% None	% On Staff Only	% Contract Only	% Both Contract and Staff
UNITED STATES	26.30%	16.79%	55.89%	1.02%
Alabama	22.77%	16.52%	59.38%	1.34%
Alaska	50.00%	6.25%	43.75%	0.00%
Arizona	15.15%	32.12%	50.91%	1.82%
Arkansas	34.87%	16.09%	48.28%	0.77%
California	21.28%	16.91%	59.48%	2.33%
Colorado	0.00%	32.89%	64.44%	2.67%
Connecticut	11.15%	11.92%	76.54%	0.38%
Delaware	27.91%	16.28%	53.49%	2.33%
District of Columbia	4.76%	9.52%	85.71%	0.00%
Florida	10.76%	30.70%	55.52%	3.01%
Georgia	11.30%	14.97%	71.19%	2.54%
Hawaii	53.49%	13.95%	27.91%	4.65%
Idaho	20.93%	31.40%	47.67%	0.00%
Illinois	36.95%	12.82%	50.00%	0.23%
Indiana	27.56%	17.68%	54.42%	0.35%
Iowa	41.58%	9.17%	49.04%	0.21%
Kansas	35.70%	12.77%	51.30%	0.24%
Kentucky	32.06%	20.00%	47.94%	0.00%
Louisiana	40.12%	13.57%	46.31%	0.00%
Maine	42.22%	11.11%	45.19%	1.48%
Maryland	18.55%	18.55%	61.29%	1.61%
Massachusetts	19.54%	17.41%	61.81%	1.24%
Michigan	20.05%	9.01%	70.50%	0.45%
Minnesota	34.74%	7.13%	58.13%	0.00%
Mississippi	15.76%	18.23%	66.01%	0.00%
Missouri	21.93%	17.72%	59.83%	0.53%
Montana	43.69%	16.51%	39.81%	0.00%
Nebraska	38.82%	18.14%	43.04%	0.00%
Nevada	20.00%	31.11%	48.89%	0.00%
New Hampshire	34.57%	13.58%	50.62%	1.23%
New Jersey	16.31%	12.39%	70.70%	0.60%
New Mexico	25.88%	18.82%	55.29%	0.00%
New York	27.86%	14.33%	56.52%	1.29%
North Carolina	6.97%	21.89%	70.40%	0.75%
North Dakota	52.27%	2.27%	45.46%	0.00%
Ohio	28.99%	14.79%	55.23%	0.99%
Oklahoma	58.84%	9.44%	31.48%	0.24%
Oregon	29.45%	16.56%	52.15%	1.84%
Pennsylvania	11.11%	20.08%	67.55%	1.26%

TABLE VI-3: SPEECH AND LANGUAGE PATHOLOGIST STAFFING BY STATE, 1997 (CONTINUED)

	% None	% On Staff Only	% Contract Only	% Both Contract and Staff
Rhode Island	46.00%	6.00%	48.00%	0.00%
South Carolina	18.18%	9.66%	69.89%	2.27%
South Dakota	52.63%	14.04%	32.46%	0.88%
Tennessee	22.13%	22.70%	54.02%	1.15%
Texas	33.85%	16.69%	48.39%	1.08%
Utah	25.00%	18.75%	56.25%	0.00%
Vermont	45.46%	22.73%	31.82%	0.00%
Virginia	19.93%	17.34%	62.73%	0.00%
Washington	14.74%	27.02%	56.14%	2.11%
West Virginia	46.32%	13.24%	40.44%	0.00%
Wisconsin	25.77%	20.57%	53.19%	0.47%
Wyoming	36.84%	31.58%	31.58%	0.00%

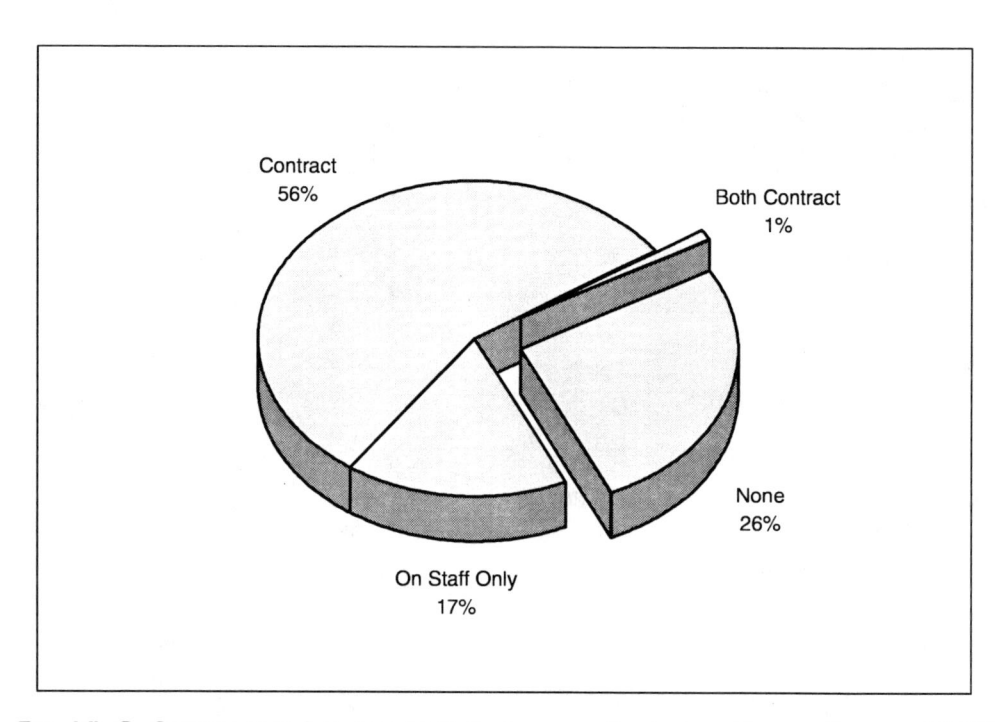

FIG. VI-C: SPEECH AND LANGUAGE PATHOLOGIST STAFFING, UNITED STATES, 1997

- Contract 56%
- Both Contract 1%
- None 26%
- On Staff Only 17%

TABLE VI-4

CONTRACT LABOR USAGE FOR NURSING SERVICES BY STATE, 1997

	Percentage of Facilities Using Contract Nursing Services For:		
	RNs	LPNs	Aides
UNITED STATES	**4.96%**	**6.66%**	**8.68%**
Alabama	1.34%	3.57%	4.91%
Alaska	6.25%	6.25%	0.00%
Arizona	16.36%	17.58%	21.82%
Arkansas	2.30%	4.98%	2.68%
California	4.30%	4.51%	6.48%
Colorado	8.89%	10.22%	14.67%
Connecticut	18.85%	16.92%	13.46%
Delaware	6.98%	13.95%	11.63%
District of Columbia	0.00%	14.29%	14.29%
Florida	4.88%	9.47%	11.76%
Georgia	0.57%	2.83%	5.37%
Hawaii	6.98%	4.65%	4.65%
Idaho	0.00%	1.16%	0.00%
Illinois	4.04%	3.23%	6.93%
Indiana	2.43%	5.20%	7.80%
Iowa	2.56%	2.13%	5.97%
Kansas	4.26%	4.73%	8.98%
Kentucky	1.91%	5.71%	8.57%
Louisiana	2.66%	1.77%	0.89%
Maine	2.96%	2.96%	8.15%
Maryland	12.10%	15.32%	14.11%
Massachusetts	13.32%	15.45%	15.81%
Michigan	8.11%	12.16%	16.89%
Minnesota	3.79%	6.90%	10.47%
Mississippi	3.45%	3.94%	2.96%
Missouri	1.93%	2.28%	5.26%
Montana	2.91%	2.91%	4.85%
Nebraska	1.69%	2.11%	8.02%
Nevada	8.89%	8.89%	11.11%
New Hampshire	11.11%	9.88%	12.35%
New Jersey	7.55%	11.78%	11.18%
New Mexico	5.88%	5.88%	10.59%
New York	8.53%	16.26%	16.26%
North Carolina	3.98%	7.71%	10.45%
North Dakota	1.14%	1.14%	0.00%
Ohio	5.52%	9.17%	12.53%
Oklahoma	4.36%	2.91%	2.42%
Oregon	3.68%	5.52%	16.56%
Pennsylvania	4.42%	6.44%	8.21%

TABLE VI-4: CONTRACT LABOR USAGE FOR NURSING SERVICES BY STATE, 1997 (CONTINUED)

	Percentage of Facilities Using Contract Nursing Services For:		
	RNs	LPNs	Aides
Rhode Island	14.00%	11.00%	21.00%
South Carolina	5.11%	9.09%	11.36%
South Dakota	2.63%	1.75%	0.88%
Tennessee	2.59%	6.03%	7.18%
Texas	3.85%	4.00%	3.38%
Utah	3.12%	3.12%	2.08%
Vermont	0.00%	0.00%	2.27%
Virginia	1.85%	4.80%	3.69%
Washington	3.51%	4.56%	7.37%
West Virginia	0.74%	0.74%	2.94%
Wisconsin	6.38%	6.62%	14.18%
Wyoming	2.63%	2.63%	2.63%

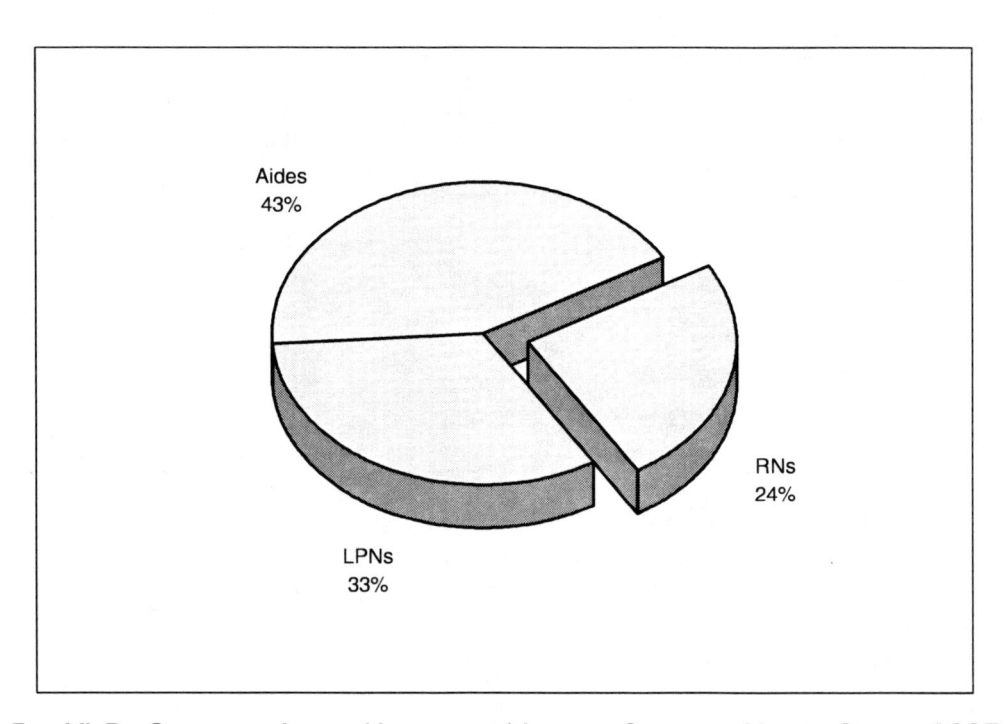

FIG. VI-D: CONTRACT LABOR USAGE FOR NURSING SERVICES, UNITED STATES, 1997

Table VI-5

Nurse Staffing Hours Per Patient Day, 1997

	RN Director of Nurses	Nurses with Administrative Duties	Other Registered Nurses	Licensed Practical Nurses
UNITED STATES	**0.093**	**0.117**	**0.476**	**0.703**
Alabama	0.073	0.107	0.282	0.939
Alaska	0.217	0.132	0.958	0.778
Arizona	0.107	0.109	0.675	0.798
Arkansas	0.085	0.069	0.281	0.758
California	0.107	0.109	0.549	0.695
Colorado	0.103	0.107	0.607	0.695
Connecticut	0.062	0.164	0.548	0.508
Delaware	0.085	0.155	0.750	0.652
District of Columbia	0.085	0.149	0.633	0.805
Florida	0.087	0.154	0.529	0.861
Georgia	0.071	0.078	0.209	0.827
Hawaii	0.115	0.132	0.757	0.683
Idaho	0.123	0.144	0.541	0.821
Illinois	0.088	0.109	0.571	0.581
Indiana	0.106	0.106	0.421	0.828
Iowa	0.104	0.084	0.408	0.506
Kansas	0.121	0.085	0.393	0.582
Kentucky	0.098	0.114	0.486	0.904
Louisiana	0.084	0.078	0.355	0.838
Maine	0.116	0.142	0.594	0.478
Maryland	0.080	0.108	0.556	0.603
Massachusetts	0.087	0.175	0.580	0.597
Michigan	0.074	0.146	0.395	0.624
Minnesota	0.079	0.119	0.361	0.668
Mississippi	0.103	0.096	0.402	0.887
Missouri	0.100	0.086	0.438	0.732
Montana	0.128	0.111	0.511	0.597
Nebraska	0.113	0.120	0.440	0.665
Nevada	0.116	0.133	0.811	0.852
New Hampshire	0.097	0.130	0.656	0.527
New Jersey	0.063	0.104	0.548	0.548
New Mexico	0.104	0.106	0.527	0.590
New York	0.048	0.150	0.386	0.671
North Carolina	0.077	0.146	0.464	0.755
North Dakota	0.097	0.118	0.419	0.586
Ohio	0.103	0.155	0.530	0.792
Oklahoma	0.102	0.055	0.264	0.647
Oregon	0.104	0.165	0.560	0.425
Pennsylvania	0.091	0.137	0.665	0.756

TABLE VI-5: NURSE STAFFING HOURS PER PATIENT DAY, 1997 (CONTINUED)

	RN Director of Nurses	Nurses with Administrative Duties	Other Registered Nurses	Licensed Practical Nurses
Rhode Island	0.081	0.081	0.610	0.402
South Carolina	0.084	0.116	0.379	0.907
South Dakota	0.097	0.095	0.516	0.338
Tennessee	0.086	0.092	0.354	0.798
Texas	0.109	0.106	0.372	0.816
Utah	0.103	0.090	0.477	0.618
Vermont	0.087	0.090	0.489	0.664
Virginia	0.080	0.113	0.420	0.785
Washington	0.090	0.184	0.657	0.600
West Virginia	0.088	0.114	0.427	0.839
Wisconsin	0.075	0.090	0.542	0.446
Wyoming	0.091	0.094	0.482	0.561

TABLE VI-6

NURSE AIDE STAFFING HOURS PER PATIENT DAY, 1997

	Certified Nurse Aides	Nurse Aides in Training	Medication Aides/ Technicians
UNITED STATES	**2.041**	**0.083**	**0.034**
Alabama	2.355	0.165	0.002
Alaska	3.351	0.000	0.000
Arizona	2.061	0.143	0.002
Arkansas	1.888	0.101	0.002
California	2.258	0.055	0.002
Colorado	1.963	0.112	0.002
Connecticut	2.188	0.023	0.000
Delaware	2.268	0.059	0.002
District of Columbia	2.579	0.148	0.000
Florida	2.143	0.030	0.002
Georgia	2.074	0.060	0.000
Hawaii	2.515	0.007	0.003
Idaho	2.499	0.174	0.003
Illinois	1.878	0.046	0.001
Indiana	1.601	0.081	0.084
Iowa	1.718	0.071	0.052
Kansas	1.668	0.055	0.141
Kentucky	2.186	0.182	0.118
Louisiana	1.989	0.056	0.003
Maine	2.576	0.019	0.135
Maryland	2.058	0.076	0.139
Massachusetts	2.240	0.033	0.001
Michigan	2.276	0.089	0.004
Minnesota	1.896	0.028	0.055
Mississippi	2.051	0.151	0.000
Missouri	1.815	0.303	0.163
Montana	2.218	0.040	0.000
Nebraska	1.798	0.030	0.083
Nevada	2.064	0.201	0.000
New Hampshire	2.389	0.041	0.000
New Jersey	2.056	0.089	0.001
New Mexico	2.146	0.216	0.000
New York	2.098	0.035	0.002
North Carolina	2.281	0.030	0.004
North Dakota	2.206	0.088	0.019
Ohio	2.097	0.090	0.001
Oklahoma	1.608	0.206	0.180
Oregon	2.131	0.101	0.134
Pennsylvania	2.096	0.048	0.000

TABLE VI-6: NURSE AIDE STAFFING HOURS PER PATIENT DAY, 1997 (CONTINUED)

	Certified Nurse Aides	Nurse Aides in Training	Medication Aides/ Technicians
Rhode Island	2.258	0.011	0.060
South Carolina	2.293	0.046	0.001
South Dakota	1.882	0.153	0.025
Tennessee	1.912	0.078	0.001
Texas	1.883	0.105	0.123
Utah	1.893	0.255	0.005
Vermont	2.269	0.062	0.000
Virginia	2.064	0.028	0.002
Washington	2.399	0.157	0.002
West Virginia	2.133	0.054	0.002
Wisconsin	2.152	0.026	0.016
Wyoming	1.923	0.153	0.000

Table VI-7

Occupational Therapist Hours Per Patient Day, 1997

	Occupational Therapists	Occupational Therapy Assistants	Occupational Therapy Aides
UNITED STATES	**0.054**	**0.027**	**0.005**
Alabama	0.037	0.029	0.003
Alaska	0.045	0.011	0.005
Arizona	0.086	0.054	0.005
Arkansas	0.045	0.006	0.007
California	0.069	0.026	0.007
Colorado	0.095	0.039	0.006
Connecticut	0.047	0.027	0.003
Delaware	0.055	0.041	0.008
District of Columbia	0.061	0.019	0.004
Florida	0.113	0.046	0.016
Georgia	0.046	0.018	0.005
Hawaii	0.033	0.023	0.001
Idaho	0.090	0.036	0.005
Illinois	0.042	0.034	0.013
Indiana	0.061	0.021	0.006
Iowa	0.021	0.015	0.002
Kansas	0.038	0.016	0.001
Kentucky	0.058	0.016	0.005
Louisiana	0.039	0.011	0.004
Maine	0.056	0.014	0.001
Maryland	0.055	0.028	0.006
Massachusetts	0.059	0.043	0.005
Michigan	0.059	0.025	0.005
Minnesota	0.039	0.024	0.003
Mississippi	0.064	0.016	0.005
Missouri	0.060	0.030	0.006
Montana	0.048	0.014	0.004
Nebraska	0.042	0.008	0.002
Nevada	0.088	0.041	0.015
New Hampshire	0.056	0.022	0.004
New Jersey	0.046	0.016	0.006
New Mexico	0.060	0.027	0.003
New York	0.021	0.020	0.006
North Carolina	0.058	0.032	0.004
North Dakota	0.018	0.017	0.001
Ohio	0.040	0.035	0.003
Oklahoma	0.023	0.013	0.001
Oregon	0.058	0.024	0.002
Pennsylvania	0.067	0.049	0.005

TABLE VI-7: OCCUPATIONAL THERAPIST HOURS PER PATIENT DAY, 1997 (CONTINUED)

	Occupational Therapists	Occupational Therapy Assistants	Occupational Therapy Aides
Rhode Island	0.015	0.012	0.001
South Carolina	0.065	0.035	0.005
South Dakota	0.027	0.005	0.000
Tennessee	0.052	0.035	0.007
Texas	0.058	0.023	0.004
Utah	0.095	0.036	0.010
Vermont	0.022	0.009	0.003
Virginia	0.050	0.026	0.006
Washington	0.085	0.036	0.006
West Virginia	0.026	0.020	0.003
Wisconsin	0.056	0.039	0.008
Wyoming	0.053	0.021	0.007

Table VI-8

Physical and Speech Therapist Hours Per Patient Day, 1997

	Physical Therapists	Physical Therapy Assistants	Physical Therapy Aides	Speech Language Pathologists
UNITED STATES	**0.064**	**0.035**	**0.040**	**0.030**
Alabama	0.035	0.044	0.031	0.038
Alaska	0.073	0.006	0.054	0.011
Arizona	0.124	0.036	0.049	0.045
Arkansas	0.050	0.022	0.035	0.027
California	0.081	0.033	0.032	0.034
Colorado	0.104	0.056	0.045	0.047
Connecticut	0.076	0.022	0.042	0.023
Delaware	0.076	0.049	0.051	0.028
District of Columbia	0.076	0.004	0.057	0.029
Florida	0.140	0.060	0.067	0.063
Georgia	0.051	0.026	0.037	0.035
Hawaii	0.076	0.019	0.026	0.015
Idaho	0.127	0.038	0.082	0.042
Illinois	0.051	0.034	0.054	0.022
Indiana	0.075	0.029	0.030	0.032
Iowa	0.027	0.021	0.043	0.011
Kansas	0.039	0.044	0.051	0.022
Kentucky	0.065	0.044	0.033	0.034
Louisiana	0.056	0.015	0.018	0.022
Maine	0.058	0.024	0.020	0.019
Maryland	0.068	0.026	0.047	0.030
Massachusetts	0.063	0.052	0.035	0.029
Michigan	0.066	0.033	0.041	0.030
Minnesota	0.043	0.035	0.036	0.016
Mississippi	0.071	0.033	0.034	0.045
Missouri	0.061	0.043	0.051	0.035
Montana	0.065	0.010	0.066	0.014
Nebraska	0.051	0.019	0.039	0.019
Nevada	0.114	0.040	0.057	0.043
New Hampshire	0.059	0.026	0.039	0.019
New Jersey	0.057	0.021	0.034	0.024
New Mexico	0.064	0.022	0.041	0.033
New York	0.038	0.022	0.035	0.008
North Carolina	0.064	0.061	0.041	0.040
North Dakota	0.032	0.023	0.084	0.005
Ohio	0.043	0.038	0.030	0.024
Oklahoma	0.035	0.017	0.027	0.018
Oregon	0.071	0.037	0.038	0.033
Pennsylvania	0.081	0.037	0.047	0.038

TABLE VI-8: PHYSICAL AND SPEECH THERAPIST HOURS PER PATIENT DAY, 1997 (CONTINUED)

	Physical Therapists	Physical Therapy Assistants	Physical Therapy Aides	Speech Language Pathologists
Rhode Island	0.029	0.025	0.012	0.014
South Carolina	0.068	0.046	0.038	0.040
South Dakota	0.038	0.016	0.061	0.016
Tennessee	0.076	0.047	0.036	0.040
Texas	0.065	0.028	0.028	0.034
Utah	0.118	0.041	0.075	0.045
Vermont	0.043	0.016	0.038	0.013
Virginia	0.057	0.042	0.040	0.033
Washington	0.097	0.042	0.049	0.040
West Virginia	0.048	0.025	0.047	0.025
Wisconsin	0.060	0.040	0.046	0.032
Wyoming	0.083	0.036	0.055	0.029

APPENDIX A

HEALTH SERVICE AREA MAPS

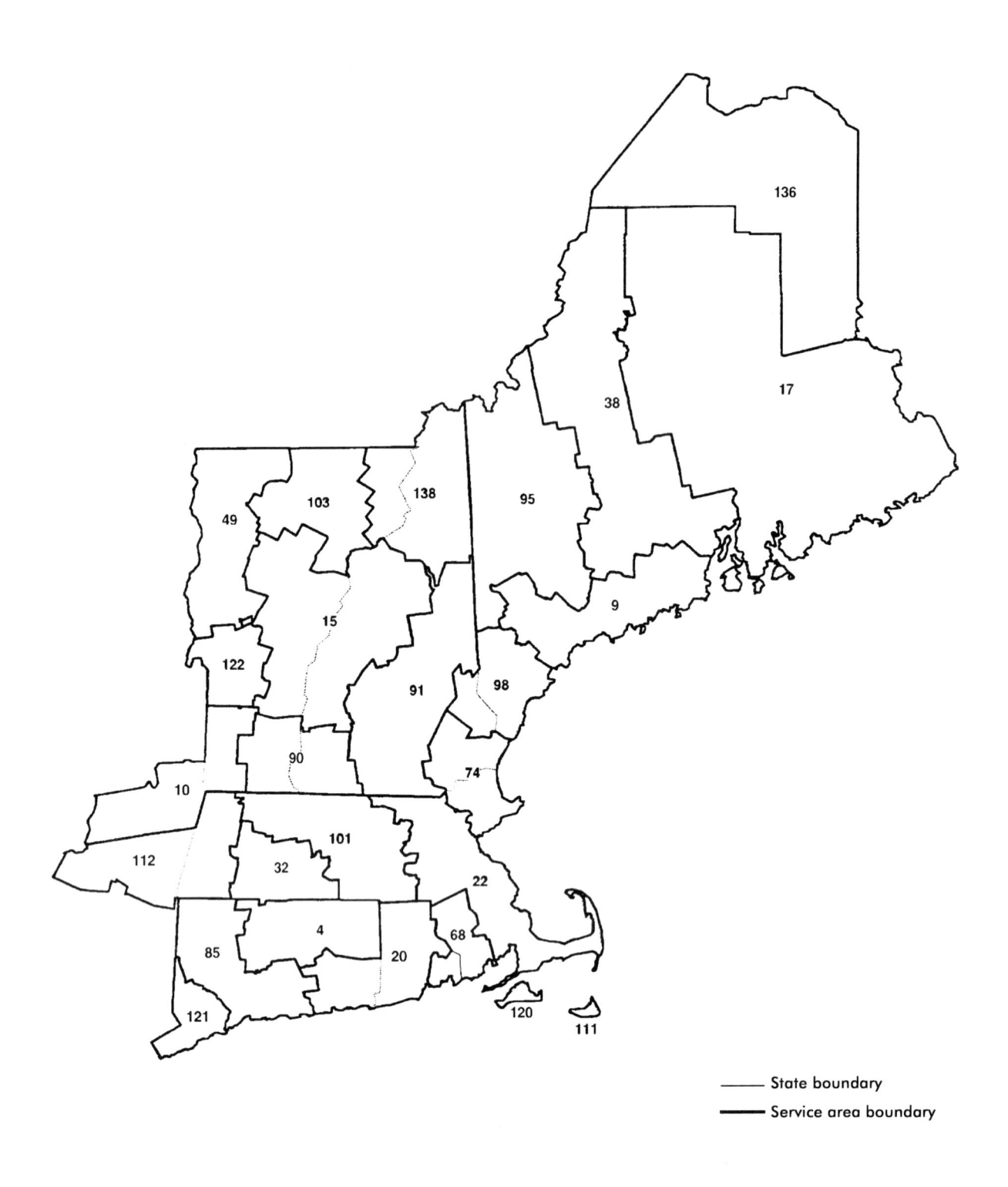

MAP A-1: HEALTH SERVICE AREAS IN MAINE, NEW HAMPSHIRE, VERMONT, MASSACHUSETTS, RHODE ISLAND, AND CONNECTICUT

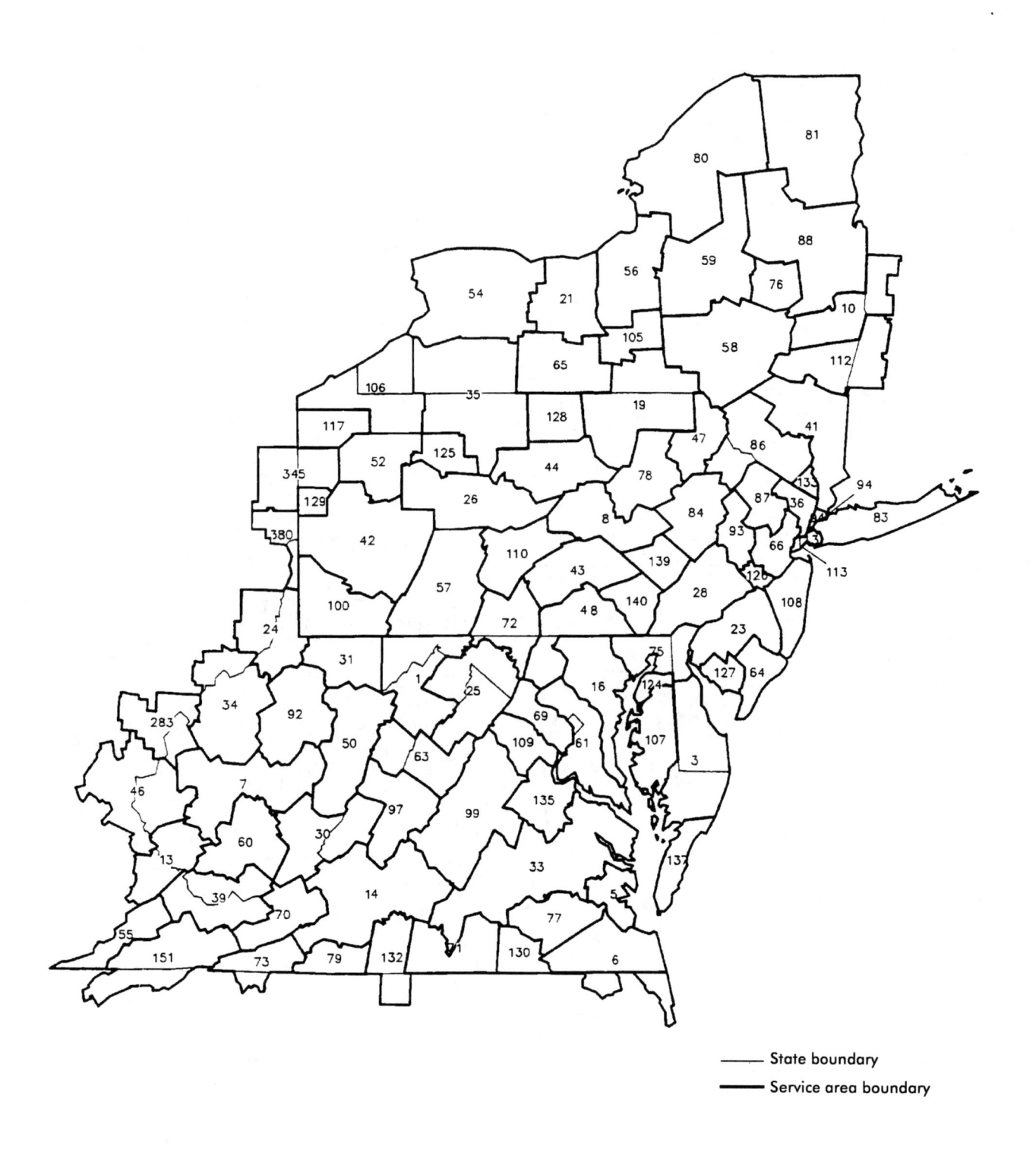

MAP A-2: HEALTH SERVICE AREAS IN NEW YORK, NEW JERSEY, PENNSYLVANIA, DELAWARE, MARYLAND, WASHINGTON, D.C., VIRGINIA, AND WEST VIRGINIA

APPENDIX A: HEALTH SERVICE AREA MAPS **227**

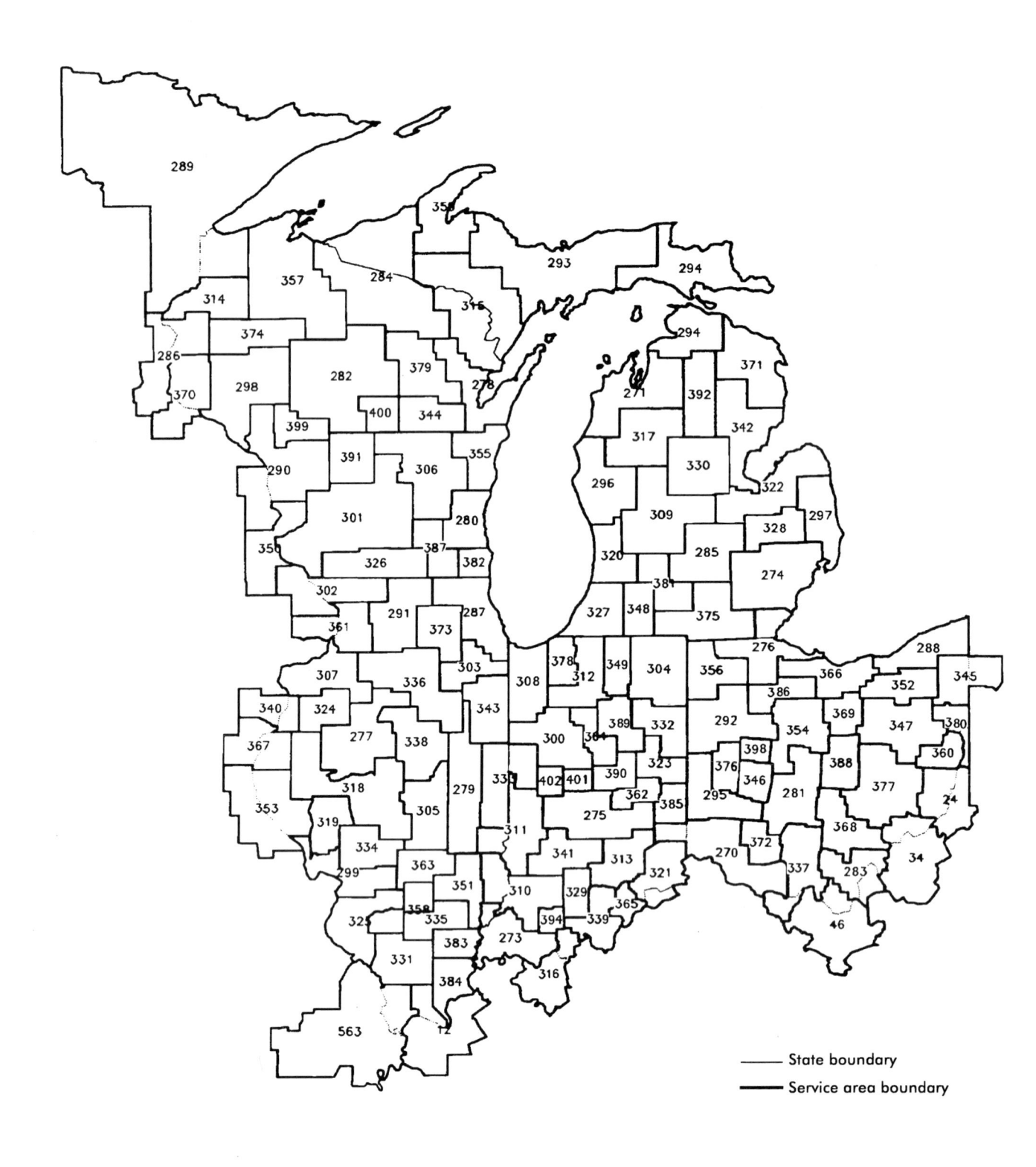

MAP A-3: HEALTH SERVICE AREAS IN OHIO, INDIANA, ILLINOIS, MICHIGAN, AND WISCONSIN

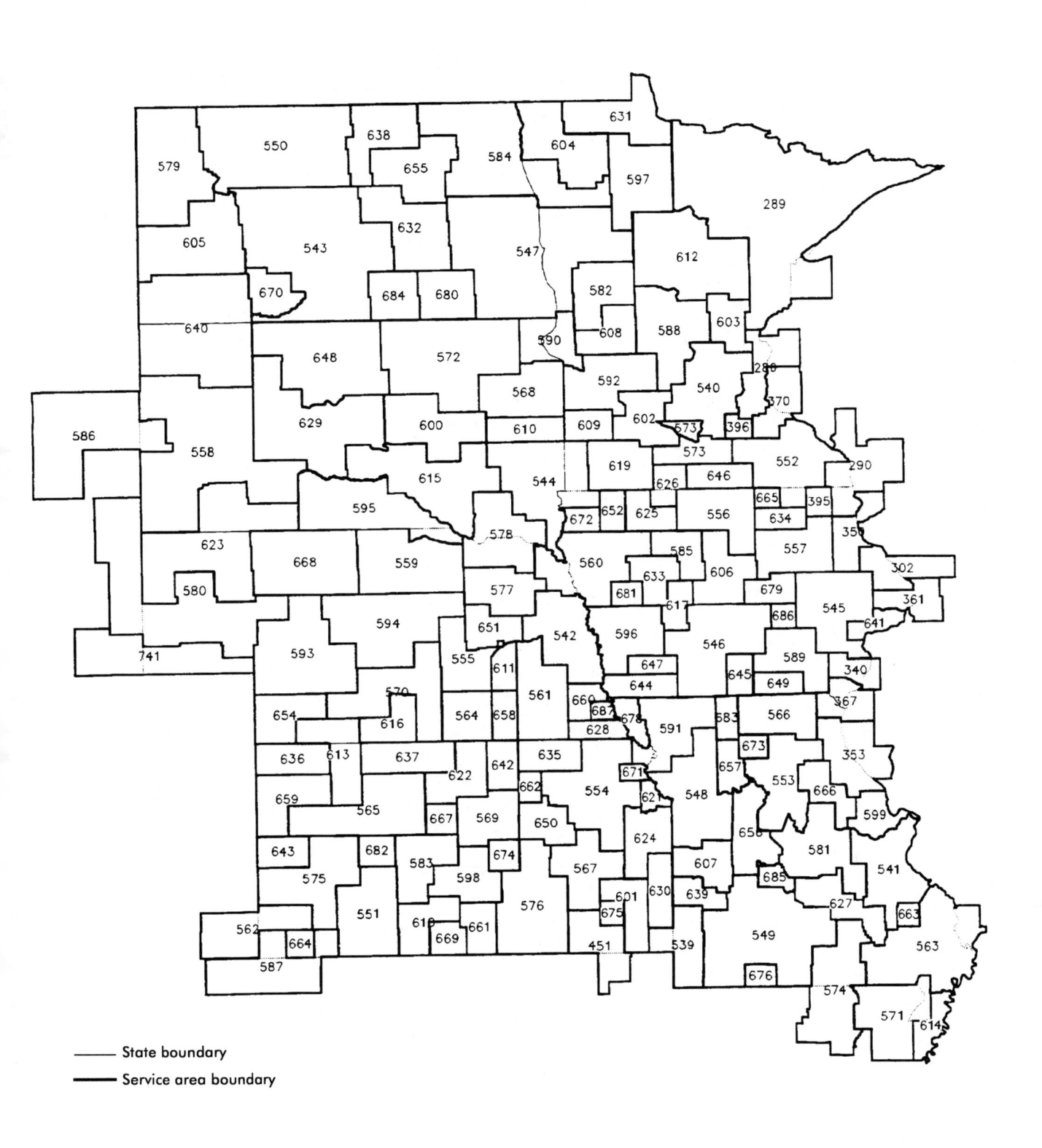

MAP A-4: HEALTH SERVICE AREAS IN MINNESOTA, IOWA, MISSOURI, NORTH DAKOTA, SOUTH DAKOTA, NEBRASKA, AND KANSAS

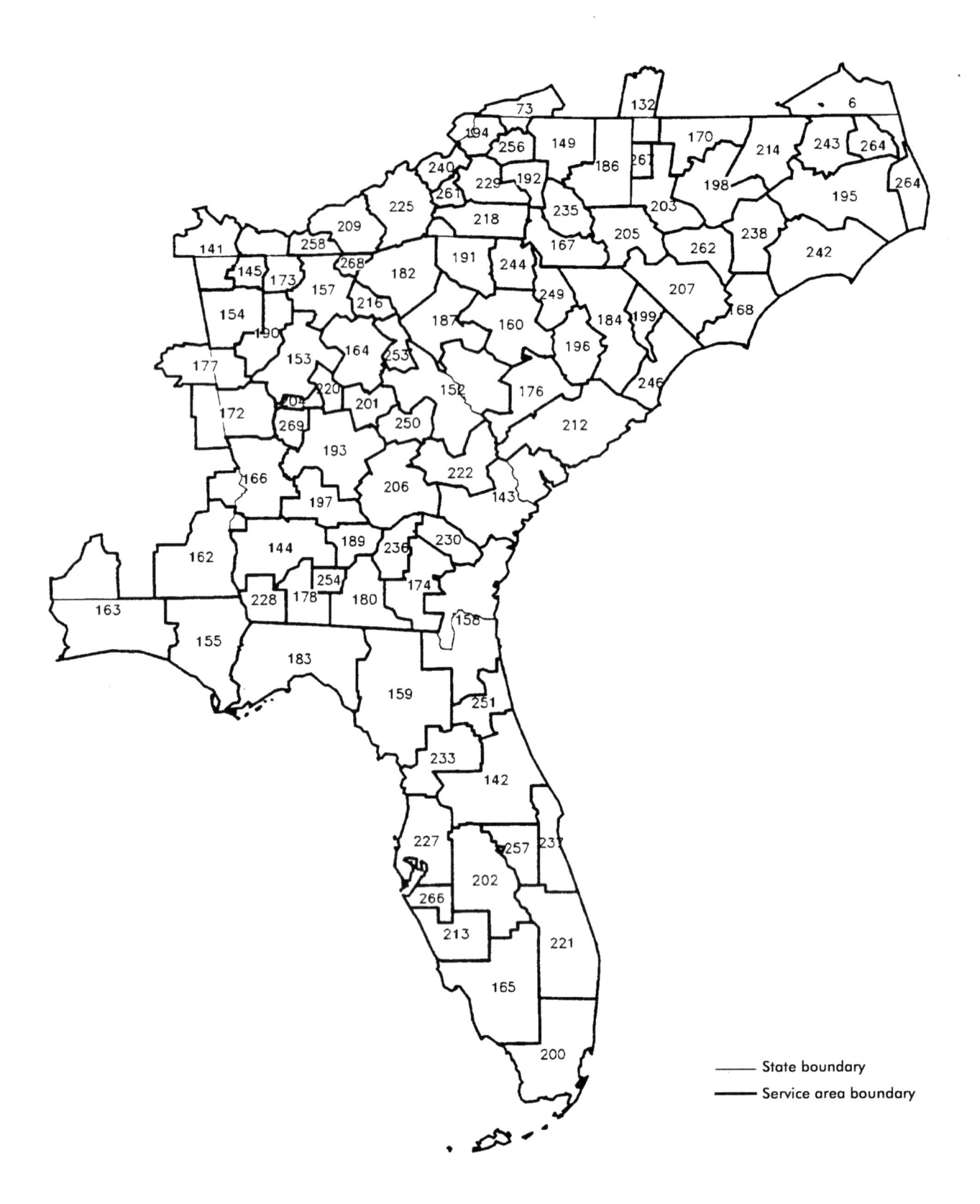

MAP A-5: HEALTH SERVICE AREAS IN NORTH CAROLINA, SOUTH CAROLINA, GEORGIA, AND FLORIDA

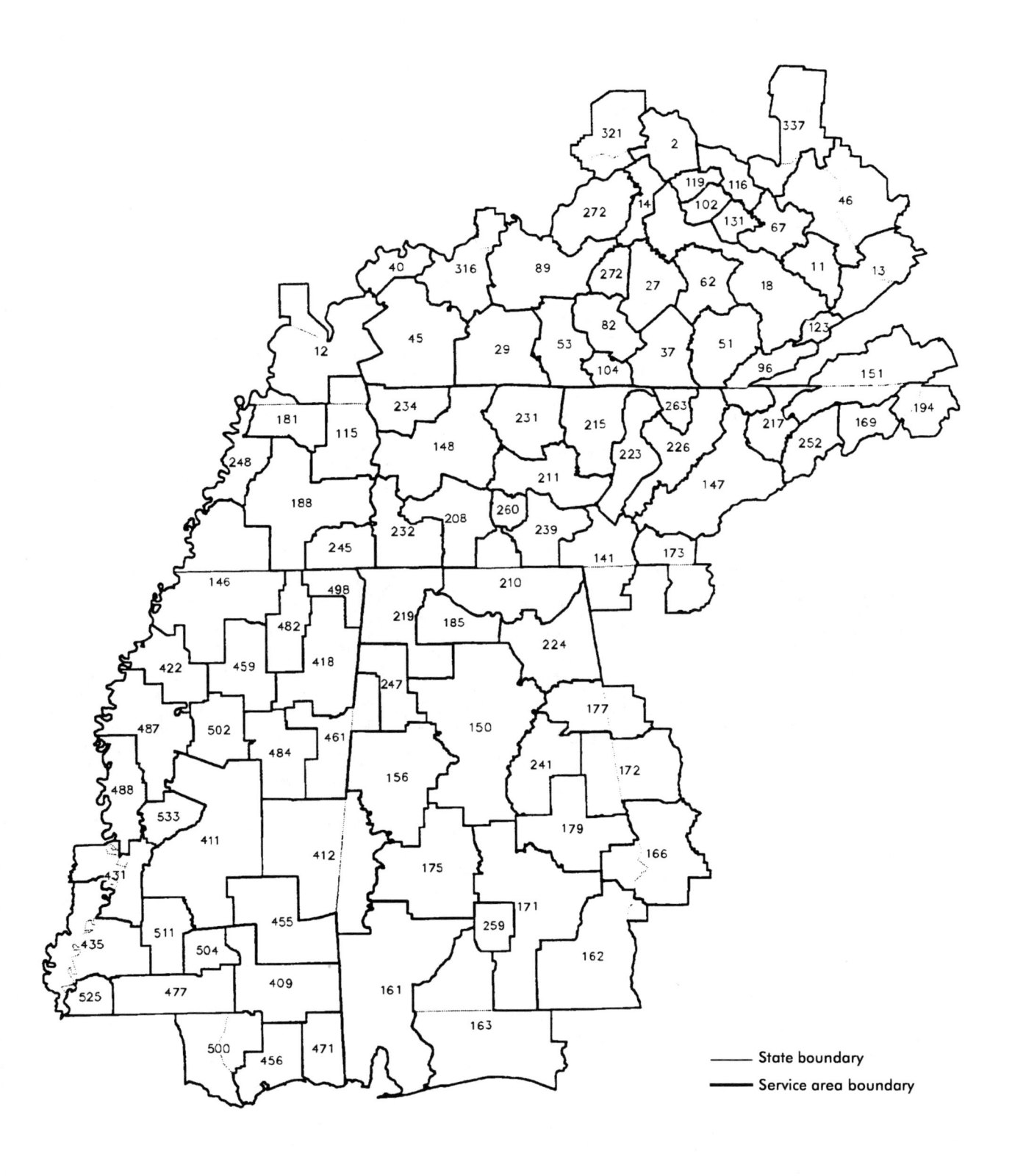

MAP A-6: HEALTH SERVICE AREAS IN KENTUCKY, TENNESSEE, ALABAMA, AND MISSISSIPPI

APPENDIX A: HEALTH SERVICE AREA MAPS **231**

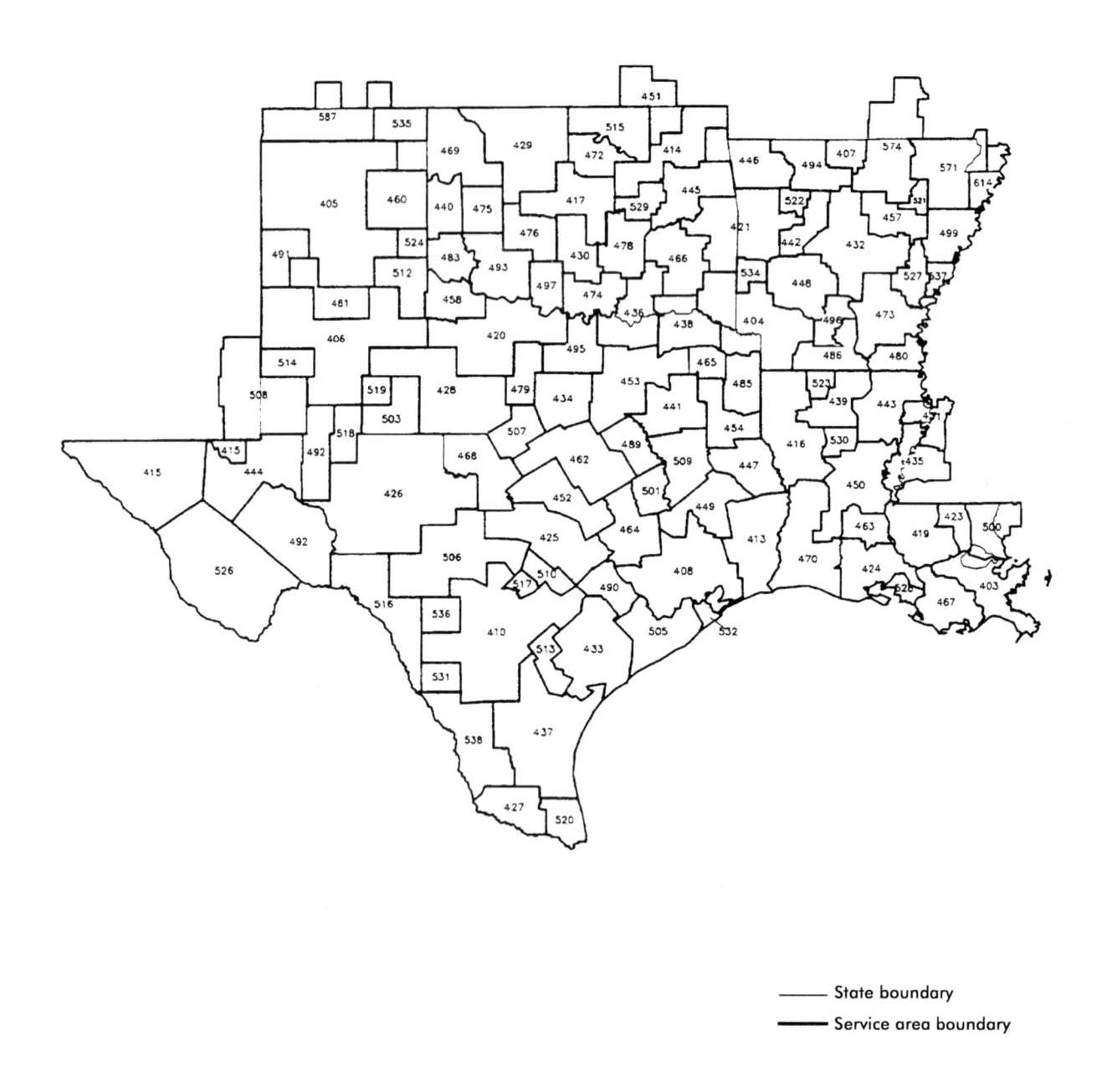

MAP A-7: HEALTH SERVICE AREAS IN ARKANSAS, LOUISIANA, OKLAHOMA, AND TEXAS

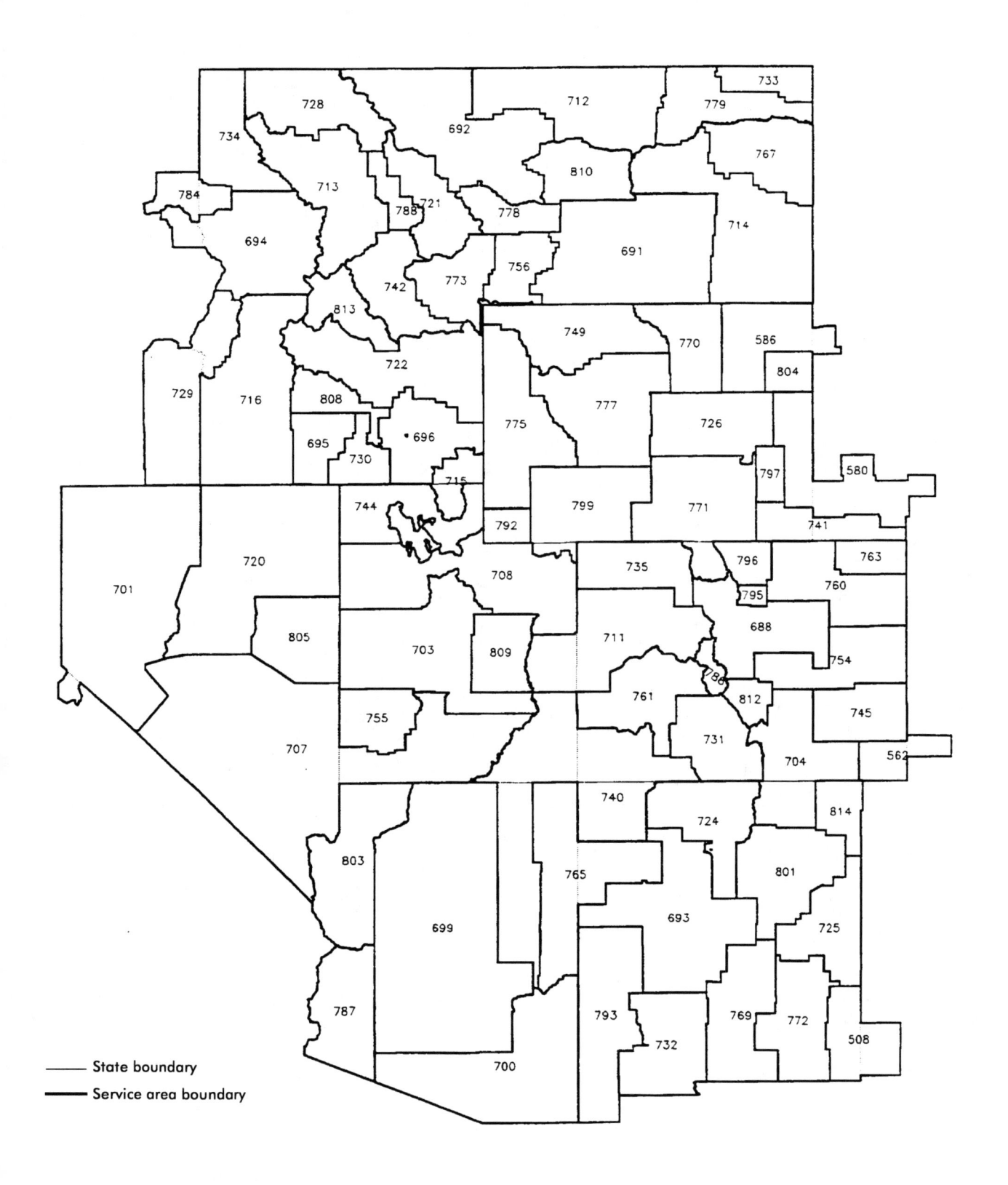

MAP A-8: HEALTH SERVICE AREAS IN MONTANA, IDAHO, WYOMING, COLORADO, NEW MEXICO, ARIZONA, UTAH, AND NEVADA

APPENDIX A: HEALTH SERVICE AREA MAPS **233**

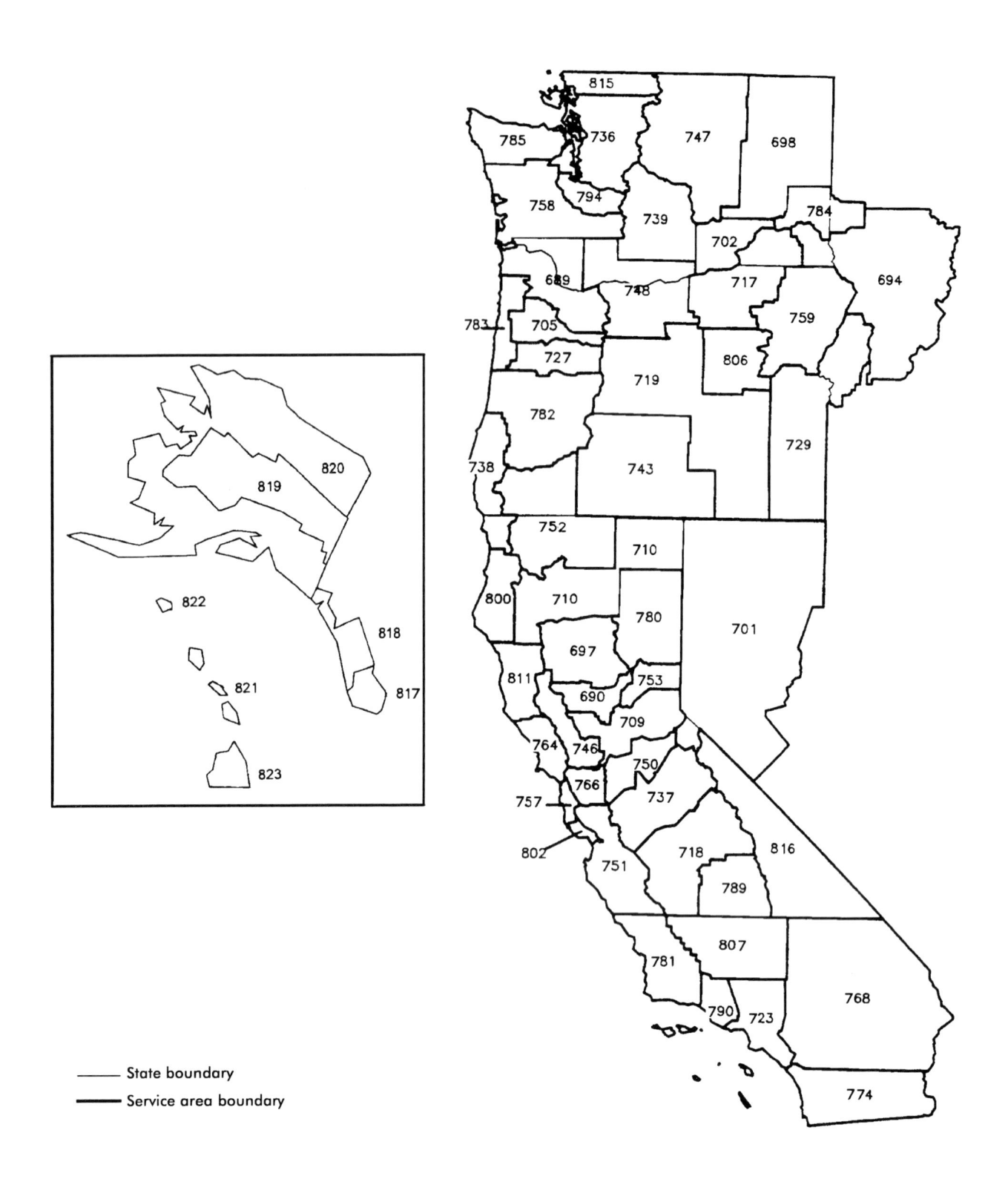

MAP A-9: HEALTH SERVICE AREAS IN WASHINGTON, OREGON, CALIFORNIA, ALASKA, AND HAWAII

APPENDIX B

HEALTH SERVICE AREA DEFINITIONS

TABLE B-1

HEALTH SERVICE AREAS BY STATE AND COUNTY

AL

County	Code
Autauga	171
Baldwin	161
Barbour	162
Bibb	150
Blount	150
Bullock	171
Butler	259
Calhoun	177
Chambers	172
Cherokee	224
Chilton	150
Choctaw	412
Clarke	161
Clay	241
Cleburne	177
Coffee	162
Colbert	219
Conecuh	163
Coosa	241
Covington	171
Crenshaw	171
Cullman	150
Dale	162
Dallas	175
De Kalb	224
Elmore	179
Escambia	163
Etowah	224
Fayette	247
Franklin	219
Geneva	162
Greene	156
Hale	156
Henry	162
Houston	162
Jackson	210
Jefferson	150
Lamar	461
Lauderdale	219
Lawrence	185
Lee	179
Limestone	210
Lowndes	171
Macon	179
Madison	210
Marengo	175
Marion	247
Marshall	224
Mobile	161
Monroe	161
Montgomery	171
Morgan	185
Perry	175
Pickens	156
Pike	171
Randolph	172
Russell	166
St. Clair	150
Shelby	150
Sumter	412
Talladega	241
Tallapoosa	179
Tuscaloosa	156
Walker	150
Washington	161
Wilcox	175
Winston	219

AK

County	Code
Aleutian Islands	820
Anchorage	820
Angoon	818
Barrow-North Slope	820
Bethel	820
Bristol Bay	820
Bristol Bay Borough	820
Fairbanks North Star	819
Kenai-Cook Inlet	820
Haines	818
Juneau	818
Ketchikan Gateway	817
Kodiak Island	820
Matanuska-Susitna	820
Nome	820
Outer Ketchikan	817
Prince of Wales	817
Sitka	818
Skagway-Yakutat	818
Southeast Fairbanks	819
Upper Yukon	819
Valdez-Chitina-Whittier	820
Wade Hampton	820
Wrangell-Petersburg	817
Yukon-Koyukuk	819

AR

County	Code
Arkansas	527
Ashley	480
Baxter	407
Benton	446
Boone	494
Bradley	473
Calhoun	486
Carroll	494
Chicot	480
Clark	448
Clay	571
Cleburne	457
Cleveland	473
Columbia	486
Conway	432
Craighead	571
Crawford	421
Crittenden	499
Cross	499
Dallas	496
Desha	473
Drew	473
Faulkner	432
Franklin	421
Fulton	574
Garland	448
Grant	432
Greene	571
Hempstead	404
Hot Spring	448
Howard	404
Independence	574
Izard	574
Jackson	521
Jefferson	473
Johnson	522
Lafayette	404
Lawrence	571
Lee	499
Lincoln	473
Little River	404
Logan	421
Lonoke	432
Madison	446
Marion	407
Miller	404
Mississippi	614
Monroe	527
Montgomery	448
Nevada	404
Newton	494
Ouachita	496
Perry	432
Phillips	537
Pike	448
Poinsett	571
Polk	534
Pope	442
Prairie	432
Pulaski	432
Randolph	571
St. Francis	499
Saline	432
Scott	421
Searcy	494
Sebastian	421
Sevier	404
Sharp	574
Stone	574
Union	486
Van Buren	432
Washington	446
White	457
Woodruff	457
Yell	442

AZ

County	Code
Apache	765
Cochise	700
Coconino	699
Gila	699
Graham	700
Greenlee	700
Maricopa	699
Mohave	803
Navajo	740
Pima	700
Pinal	699
Santa Cruz	700
Yavapai	699
Yuma	787

CA

County	Code
Alameda	766
Alpine	701
Amador	750
Butte	697
Calaveras	750
Colusa	690
Contra Costa	766
Del Norte	738
Eldorado	709
Fresno	718
Glenn	697
Humboldt	800
Imperial	774
Inyo	816
Kern	807
Kings	718
Lake	746
Lassen	780
Los Angeles	723
Madera	718
Marin	764
Mariposa	737
Mendocino	811
Merced	737
Modoc	710
Mono	816
Monterey	751
Napa	746
Nevada	753
Orange	723
Placer	709
Plumas	780
Riverside	768
Sacramento	709
San Benito	751
San Bernardino	768
San Diego	774
San Francisco	757
San Joaquin	750
San Luis Obispo	781

Table B-1: Health Service Areas by State and County

San Mateo	757	Otero	745	Gadsden	183	Bryan	143
Santa Barbara	781	Ouray	761	Gilchrist	159	Bulloch	222
Santa Clara	751	Park	688	Glades	165	Burke	152
Santa Cruz	802	Phillips	763	Gulf	155	Butts	204
Shasta	710	Pitkin	711	Hamilton	159	Calhoun	144
Sierra	753	Prowers	745	Hardee	202	Camden	158
Siskiyou	752	Pueblo	704	Hendry	165	Candler	222
Solano	746	Rio Blanco	711	Hernando	227	Carroll	177
Sonoma	764	Rio Grande	731	Highlands	202	Catoosa	141
Stanislaus	737	Routt	735	Hillsborough	227	Charlton	158
Sutter	690	Saguache	731	Holmes	155	Chatham	143
Tehama	697	San Juan	740	Indian River	237	Chattahoochee	166
Trinity	710	San Miguel	761	Jackson	155	Chattooga	154
Tulare	789	Sedgwick	763	Jefferson	183	Cherokee	190
Tuolumne	737	Summit	688	Lafayette	159	Clarke	164
Ventura	790	Teller	754	Lake	142	Clay	144
Yolo	709	Washington	760	Lee	165	Clayton	153
Yuba	690	Weld	760	Leon	183	Clinch	174
		Yuma	760	Levy	159	Cobb	190
				Liberty	183	Coffee	236
				Madison	183	Colquitt	254
				Manatee	266	Columbia	152

CO

				Marion	233	Cook	180
Adams	688			Martin	221	Coweta	172
Alamosa	731	Fairfield	121	Monroe	200	Crawford	193
Arapahoe	688	Hartford	4	Nassau	158	Crisp	197
Archuleta	740	Litchfield	85	Okaloosa	163	Dade	141
Baca	562	Middlesex	85	Okeechobee	221	Dawson	157
Bent	745	New Haven	85	Orange	142	Decatur	228
Boulder	795	New London	20	Osceola	257	De Kalb	153
Chaffee	786	Tolland	4	Palm Beach	221	Dodge	206
Cheyenne	754	Windham	4	Pasco	227	Dooly	197
Clear Creek	688			Pinellas	227	Dougherty	144
Conejos	731			Polk	202	Douglas	190
Costilla	731			Putnam	251	Early	144

CT

DC

District of Columbia 61

DE

Kent	3
New Castle	75
Sussex	3

FL

Alachua	159		
Baker	158		
Bay	155		
Bradford	159		
Brevard	237		
Broward	200		
Calhoun	155		
Charlotte	213		
Citrus	233		
Clay	158		
Collier	165		
Columbia	159		
Dade	200		
De Soto	213		
Dixie	159		
Duval	158		
Escambia	163		
Flagler	142		
Franklin	183		

St. Johns	251	Echols	180
St. Lucie	221	Effingham	143
Santa Rosa	163	Elbert	253
Sarasota	213	Emanuel	222
Seminole	142	Evans	143
Sumter	142	Fannin	173
Suwannee	159	Fayette	153
Taylor	183	Floyd	154
Union	159	Forsyth	153
Volusia	142	Franklin	216
Wakulla	183	Fulton	153
Walton	163	Gilmer	173
Washington	155	Glascock	152
		Glynn	158
		Gordon	154

GA

		Grady	178
		Greene	164
Appling	230	Gwinnett	153
Atkinson	236	Habersham	157
Bacon	174	Hall	157
Baker	144	Hancock	201
Baldwin	201	Haralson	177
Banks	157	Harris	166
Barrow	164	Hart	216
Bartow	154	Heard	172
Ben Hill	189	Henry	153
Berrien	180	Houston	193
Bibb	193	Irwin	189
Bleckley	193	Jackson	164
Brantley	158	Jasper	220
Brooks	180	Jeff Davis	236

CO colorado counties list:
Dolores 740
Douglas 688
Eagle 711
Elbert 688
El Paso 754
Fremont 812
Garfield 711
Gilpin 688
Grand 688
Gunnison 761
Hinsdale 761
Huerfano 704
Jackson 771
Jefferson 688
Kiowa 745
Kit Carson 754
Lake 786
La Plata 740
Larimer 796
Las Animas 704
Lincoln 754
Logan 763
Mesa 711
Mineral 731
Moffat 735
Montezuma 740
Montrose 761
Morgan 760
Custer 812
Delta 761
Denver 688

Appendix B: Health Service Area Definitions — **237**

TABLE B-1: HEALTH SERVICE AREAS BY STATE AND COUNTY

County	#	County	#	County	#	County	#
Jefferson	250	Walton	153	Hancock	556	Bear Lake	715
Jenkins	152	Ware	174	Hardin	606	Benewah	734
Johnson	206	Warren	152	Harrison	596	Bingham	696
Jones	193	Washington	250	Henry	340	Blaine	808
Lamar	269	Wayne	230	Howard	552	Boise	716
Lanier	180	Webster	166	Humboldt	585	Bonner	734
Laurens	206	Wheeler	206	Ida	560	Bonneville	722
Lee	144	White	157	Iowa	545	Boundary	734
Liberty	143	Whitfield	145	Jackson	302	Butte	722
Lincoln	152	Wilcox	197	Jasper	546	Camas	808
Long	143	Wilkes	253	Jefferson	589	Canyon	716
Lowndes	180	Wilkinson	193	Johnson	545	Caribou	696
Lumpkin	157	Worth	144	Jones	545	Cassia	730
McDuffie	152			Keokuk	589	Clark	722
McIntosh	158			Kossuth	556	Clearwater	694
Macon	197		**HI**	Lee	367	Custer	722
Madison	164			Linn	545	Elmore	716
Marion	166	Hawaii	823	Louisa	545	Franklin	715
Meriwether	172	Honolulu	821	Lucas	645	Fremont	722
Miller	228	Kauai	822	Lyon	544	Gem	716
Mitchell	178	Maui	821	Madison	546	Gooding	695
Monroe	193	Kalawao	821	Mahaska	589	Idaho	694
Montgomery	206			Marion	546	Jefferson	722
Morgan	164			Marshall	679	Jerome	695
Murray	145		**IA**	Mills	596	Kootenai	734
Muscogee	166			Mitchell	665	Latah	784
Newton	220	Adair	546	Monona	560	Lemhi	813
Oconee	164	Adams	647	Monroe	589	Lewis	694
Oglethorpe	164	Allamakee	290	Montgomery	647	Lincoln	695
Paulding	190	Appanoose	649	Muscatine	641	Madison	722
Peach	193	Audubon	596	Obrien	652	Minidoka	730
Pickens	190	Benton	545	Osceola	652	Nez Perce	694
Pierce	174	Black Hawk	557	Page	644	Oneida	696
Pike	269	Boone	606	Palo Alto	625	Owyhee	716
Polk	154	Bremer	557	Plymouth	560	Payette	729
Pulaski	193	Buchanan	557	Pocahontas	585	Power	696
Putnam	201	Buena Vista	560	Polk	546	Shoshone	734
Quitman	162	Butler	557	Pottawattamie	596	Teton	722
Rabun	268	Calhoun	633	Poweshiek	686	Twin Falls	695
Randolph	144	Carroll	633	Ringgold	546	Valley	716
Richmond	152	Cass	596	Sac	633	Washington	729
Rockdale	153	Cedar	545	Scott	641		
Schley	166	Cerro Gordo	556	Shelby	596		**IL**
Screven	222	Cherokee	560	Sioux	672		
Seminole	228	Chickasaw	634	Story	606	Adams	353
Spalding	204	Clarke	546	Tama	679	Alexander	563
Stephens	216	Clay	625	Taylor	644	Bond	299
Stewart	166	Clayton	350	Union	546	Boone	291
Sumter	197	Clinton	361	Van Buren	589	Brown	318
Talbot	166	Crawford	681	Wapello	589	Bureau	336
Taliaferro	152	Dallas	546	Warren	546	Calhoun	299
Tattnall	143	Davis	649	Washington	545	Carroll	361
Taylor	193	Decatur	546	Wayne	645	Cass	318
Telfair	206	Delaware	350	Webster	585	Champaign	279
Terrell	144	Des Moines	340	Winnebago	556	Christian	318
Thomas	178	Dickinson	625	Winneshiek	395	Clark	311
Tift	189	Dubuque	302	Woodbury	560	Clay	351
Toombs	206	Emmet	626	Worth	556	Clinton	325
Towns	157	Fayette	557	Wright	606	Coles	279
Treutlen	206	Floyd	634			Cook	287
Troup	172	Franklin	556			Crawford	310
Turner	189	Fremont	644		**ID**	Cumberland	279
Twiggs	193	Greene	617			DeKalb	373
Union	157	Grundy	557	Ada	716	DeWitt	338
Upson	269	Guthrie	617	Adams	729	Douglas	279
Walker	141	Hamilton	606	Bannock	696		

TABLE B-1: HEALTH SERVICE AREAS BY STATE AND COUNTY

County	#	County	#	County	#	County	#
DuPage	287	Stark	307	Madison	390	Cowley	576
Edgar	333	Stephenson	302	Marion	275	Crawford	630
Edwards	351	Tazewell	277	Marshall	312	Decatur	613
Effingham	363	Union	563	Martin	310	Dickinson	650
Fayette	363	Vermilion	333	Miami	389	Doniphan	591
Ford	279	Wabash	273	Monroe	341	Douglas	624
Franklin	331	Warren	324	Montgomery	402	Edwards	583
Fulton	277	Washington	358	Morgan	275	Elk	451
Gallatin	384	Wayne	335	Newton	308	Ellis	565
Greene	319	White	383	Noble	304	Ellsworth	569
Grundy	303	Whiteside	361	Ohio	321	Finney	575
Hamilton	383	Will	303	Orange	329	Ford	551
Hancock	367	Williamson	331	Owen	341	Franklin	624
Hardin	384	Winnebago	291	Parke	311	Geary	650
Henderson	340	Woodford	338	Perry	316	Gove	565
Henry	307			Pike	310	Graham	565
Iroquois	343			Porter	308	Grant	562
Jackson	331		**IN**	Posey	273	Gray	551
Jasper	351			Pulaski	312	Greeley	643
Jefferson	335	Adams	332	Putnam	275	Greenwood	567
Jersey	299	Allen	304	Randolph	323	Hamilton	575
Jo Daviess	302	Bartholomew	313	Ripley	321	Harper	661
Johnson	12	Benton	300	Rush	275	Harvey	576
Kane	373	Blackford	323	St. Joseph	312	Haskell	575
Kankakee	343	Boone	401	Scott	365	Hodgeman	551
Kendall	373	Brown	341	Shelby	275	Jackson	554
Knox	324	Carroll	300	Spencer	273	Jefferson	554
Lake	287	Cass	364	Starke	378	Jewell	622
LaSalle	336	Clark	365	Steuben	304	Johnson	624
Lawrence	310	Clay	311	Sullivan	311	Kearny	575
Lee	291	Clinton	300	Switzerland	321	Kingman	661
Livingston	336	Crawford	339	Tippecanoe	300	Kiowa	618
Logan	318	Daviess	310	Tipton	364	Labette	601
McDonough	318	Dearborn	321	Union	385	Lane	575
McHenry	287	Decatur	313	Vanderburgh	273	Leavenworth	621
McLean	338	DeKalb	304	Vermillion	311	Lincoln	569
Macon	305	Delaware	323	Vigo	311	Linn	630
Macoupin	334	Dubois	394	Wabash	389	Logan	565
Madison	299	Elkhart	349	Warren	333	Lyon	567
Marion	358	Fayette	385	Warrick	273	Mcpherson	674
Marshall	277	Floyd	339	Washington	339	Marion	576
Mason	277	Fountain	333	Wayne	385	Marshall	635
Massac	12	Franklin	270	Wells	332	Meade	551
Menard	318	Fulton	312	White	300	Miami	624
Mercer	307	Gibson	273	Whitley	304	Mitchell	622
Monroe	325	Grant	389			Montgomery	451
Montgomery	334	Greene	341			Morris	650
Morgan	319	Hamilton	390		**KS**	Morton	587
Moultrie	305	Hancock	362			Nemaha	554
Ogle	291	Harrison	339	Allen	601	Neosho	601
Peoria	277	Hendricks	275	Anderson	624	Ness	682
Perry	331	Henry	362	Atchison	671	Norton	637
Piatt	305	Howard	364	Barber	669	Osage	554
Pike	353	Huntington	332	Barton	583	Osborne	622
Pope	384	Jackson	313	Bourbon	630	Ottawa	569
Pulaski	563	Jasper	308	Brown	554	Pawnee	583
Putnam	336	Jay	332	Butler	576	Phillips	637
Randolph	325	Jefferson	321	Chase	567	Pottawatomie	554
Richland	351	Jennings	313	Chautauqua	451	Pratt	618
Rock Island	307	Johnson	275	Cherokee	539	Rawlins	636
St. Clair	325	Knox	310	Cheyenne	636	Reno	598
Saline	384	Kosciusko	349	Clark	551	Republic	642
Sangamon	318	Lagrange	304	Clay	662	Rice	598
Schuyler	318	Lake	308	Cloud	642	Riley	554
Scott	319	LaPorte	378	Coffey	567	Rooks	565
Shelby	305	Lawrence	329	Comanche	618	Rush	583

APPENDIX B: HEALTH SERVICE AREA DEFINITIONS

TABLE B-1: HEALTH SERVICE AREAS BY STATE AND COUNTY

County	#	County	#	County	#	County	#
Russell	667	Grant	2	Simpson	29	St. Landry	463
Saline	569	Graves	12	Spencer	272	St. Martin	424
Scott	575	Grayson	89	Taylor	82	St. Mary	528
Sedgwick	576	Green	82	Todd	45	St. Tammany	500
Seward	587	Greenup	46	Trigg	45	Tangipahoa	423
Shawnee	554	Hancock	316	Trimble	321	Tensas	435
Sheridan	613	Hardin	89	Union	40	Terrebonne	467
Sherman	659	Harlan	96	Warren	29	Union	439
Smith	637	Harrison	119	Washington	272	Vermilion	424
Stafford	598	Hart	53	Wayne	37	Vernon	470
Stanton	562	Henderson	40	Webster	45	Washington	500
Stevens	664	Henry	272	Whitley	51	Webster	416
Sumner	576	Hickman	12	Wolfe	18	West Baton Rouge	419
Thomas	659	Hopkins	45	Woodford	18	West Carroll	443
Trego	565	Jackson	62			West Feliciana	419
Wabaunsee	554	Jefferson	272			Winn	530
Wallace	659	Jessamine	18	——— LA			
Washington	635	Johnson	11			——— MA	
Wichita	643	Kenton	2	Acadia	424		
Wilson	675	Knott	18	Allen	450	Barnstable	22
Woodson	601	Knox	51	Ascension	419	Berkshire	112
Wyandotte	621	Larue	89	Assumption	467	Bristol	68
		Laurel	51	Avoyelles	450	Dukes	120
——— KY		Lawrence	46	Beauregard	470	Essex	74
		Lee	18	Bienville	439	Franklin	101
Adair	82	Leslie	18	Bossier	416	Hampden	32
Allen	29	Letcher	123	Caddo	416	Hampshire	32
Anderson	114	Lewis	337	Calcasieu	470	Middlesex	22
Ballard	12	Lincoln	27	Caldwell	443	Nantucket	111
Barren	53	Livingston	12	Cameron	470	Norfolk	22
Bath	131	Logan	29	Catahoula	450	Plymouth	22
Bell	96	Lyon	12	Claiborne	523	Suffolk	22
Boone	2	McCracken	12	Concordia	435	Worcester	101
Bourbon	102	McCreary	37	De Soto	416		
Boyd	46	McLean	316	East Baton Rouge	419	——— MD	
Boyle	27	Madison	62	East Carroll	443		
Bracken	116	Magoffin	11	East Feliciana	419	Allegany	1
Breathitt	18	Marion	272	Evangeline	463	Anne Arundel	16
Breckinridge	89	Marshall	12	Franklin	443	Baltimore	16
Bullitt	272	Martin	46	Grant	450	Baltimore City	16
Butler	29	Mason	116	Iberia	424	Calvert	16
Caldwell	45	Meade	89	Iberville	419	Caroline	107
Calloway	115	Menifee	67	Jackson	439	Carroll	16
Campbell	2	Mercer	27	Jefferson	403	Cecil	75
Carlisle	12	Metcalfe	53	Jefferson Davis	470	Charles	61
Carroll	321	Monroe	53	Lafayette	424	Dorchester	107
Carter	46	Montgomery	131	Lafourche	467	Frederick	48
Casey	27	Morgan	67	LaSalle	450	Garrett	1
Christian	45	Muhlenberg	45	Lincoln	439	Harford	75
Clark	18	Nelson	272	Livingston	419	Howard	16
Clay	51	Nicholas	102	Madison	431	Kent	124
Clinton	104	Ohio	316	Morehouse	443	Montgomery	61
Crittenden	12	Oldham	272	Natchitoches	416	Prince George's	61
Cumberland	104	Owen	114	Orleans	403	Queen Anne's	107
Daviess	316	Owsley	18	Ouachita	443	St. Mary's	61
Edmonson	29	Pendleton	2	Plaquemines	403	Somerset	3
Elliott	67	Perry	18	Pointe Coupee	419	Talbot	107
Estill	62	Pike	13	Rapides	450	Washington	72
Fayette	18	Powell	18	Red River	416	Wicomico	3
Fleming	116	Pulaski	37	Richland	443	Worcester	3
Floyd	11	Robertson	119	Sabine	416		
Franklin	114	Rockcastle	62	St. Bernard	403		
Fulton	181	Rowan	67	St. Charles	403		
Gallatin	2	Russell	82	St. Helena	423		
Garrard	27	Scott	18	St. James	403		
		Shelby	272	St. John the Baptist	403		

Table B-1: Health Service Areas by State and County

ME

County	
Androscoggin	95
Aroostook	136
Cumberland	9
Franklin	95
Hancock	17
Kennebec	38
Knox	9
Lincoln	9
Oxford	95
Penobscot	17
Piscataquis	17
Sagadahoc	9
Somerset	38
Waldo	38
Washington	17
York	98

MI

County	
Alcona	371
Alger	293
Allegan	320
Alpena	371
Antrim	271
Arenac	342
Baraga	359
Barry	381
Bay	342
Benzie	271
Berrien	327
Branch	375
Calhoun	381
Cass	327
Charlevoix	294
Cheboygan	294
Chippewa	294
Clare	330
Clinton	285
Crawford	392
Delta	293
Dickinson	315
Eaton	285
Emmet	294
Genesee	328
Gladwin	330
Gogebic	284
Grand Traverse	271
Gratiot	309
Hillsdale	375
Houghton	359
Huron	322
Ingham	285
Ionia	309
Iosco	342
Iron	315
Isabella	330
Jackson	375
Kalamazoo	348
Kalkaska	271
Kent	309
Keweenaw	359
Lake	317
Lapeer	328
Leelanau	271
Lenawee	375
Livingston	274
Luce	293
Mackinac	294
Macomb	274
Manistee	271
Marquette	293
Mason	296
Mecosta	309
Menominee	315
Midland	330
Missaukee	317
Monroe	276
Montcalm	309
Montmorency	371
Muskegon	296
Newaygo	296
Oakland	274
Oceana	296
Ogemaw	342
Ontonagon	284
Osceola	317
Oscoda	342
Otsego	392
Ottawa	320
Presque Isle	371
Roscommon	392
Saginaw	322
St. Clair	297
St. Joseph	348
Sanilac	297
Schoolcraft	293
Shiawassee	285
Tuscola	322
Van Buren	327
Washtenaw	274
Wayne	274
Wexford	317

MN

County	
Aitkin	612
Anoka	540
Becker	547
Beltrami	597
Benton	588
Big Stone	590
Blue Earth	573
Brown	602
Carlton	289
Carver	540
Cass	612
Chippewa	592
Chisago	286
Clay	547
Clearwater	597
Cook	289
Cottonwood	619
Crow Wing	612
Dakota	286
Dodge	552
Douglas	608
Faribault	646
Fillmore	552
Freeborn	646
Goodhue	370
Grant	582
Hennepin	540
Houston	290
Hubbard	612
Isanti	603
Itasca	289
Jackson	619
Kanabec	603
Kandiyohi	592
Kittson	604
Koochiching	289
Lac Qui Parle	592
Lake	289
Lake of the Woods	631
Le Sueur	540
Lincoln	609
Lyon	609
McLeod	540
Mahnomen	547
Marshall	604
Martin	626
Meeker	588
Mille Lacs	603
Morrison	580
Mower	552
Murray	619
Nicollet	573
Nobles	619
Norman	547
Olmsted	552
Otter Tail	582
Pennington	604
Pine	289
Pipestone	544
Polk	584
Pope	608
Ramsey	286
Red Lake	604
Redwood	602
Renville	602
Rice	396
Rock	544
Roseau	631
St. Louis	289
Scott	540
Sherburne	540
Sibley	540
Stearns	588
Steele	552
Stevens	608
Swift	592
Todd	580
Traverse	590
Wabasha	552
Wadena	612
Waseca	573
Washington	286
Watonwan	573
Wilkin	547
Winona	552
Wright	540
Yellow Medicine	592

MO

County	
Adair	566
Andrew	591
Atchison	678
Audrain	666
Barry	549
Barton	539
Bates	607
Benton	656
Bollinger	563
Boone	553
Buchanan	591
Butler	563
Caldwell	548
Callaway	581
Camden	685
Cape Girardeau	563
Carroll	657
Carter	563
Cass	548
Cedar	639
Chariton	553
Christian	549
Clark	367
Clay	548
Clinton	548
Cole	581
Cooper	553
Crawford	581
Dade	549
Dallas	549
Daviess	548
DeKalb	591
Dent	627
Douglas	549
Dunklin	571
Franklin	541
Gasconade	581
Gentry	591
Greene	549
Grundy	683
Harrison	591
Henry	607
Hickory	549
Holt	678
Howard	553
Howell	574
Iron	541
Jackson	548
Jasper	539
Jefferson	541
Johnson	548
Knox	566
Laclede	549
Lafayette	548
Lawrence	549
Lewis	353
Lincoln	599
Linn	673
Livingston	657
McDonald	539
Macon	553
Madison	663
Maries	581
Marion	353

Appendix B: Health Service Area Definitions

TABLE B-1: HEALTH SERVICE AREAS BY STATE AND COUNTY

County	#	County	#	County	#	County	#
Mercer	683	Clarke	412	Webster	484		**NC**
Miller	581	Clay	461	Wilkinson	525		
Mississippi	563	Coahoma	422	Winston	484	Alamance	267
Moniteau	581	Copiah	511	Yalobusha	459	Alexander	192
Monroe	666	Covington	409	Yazoo	533	Alleghany	73
Montgomery	666	De Soto	146			Anson	167
Morgan	656	Forrest	409			Ashe	194
New Madrid	563	Franklin	435		**MT**	Avery	240
Newton	539	George	471			Beaufort	195
Nodaway	591	Greene	409	Beaverhead	742	Bertie	243
Oregon	574	Grenada	502	Big Horn	691	Bladen	207
Osage	581	Hancock	456	Blaine	712	Brunswick	168
Ozark	549	Harrison	456	Broadwater	721	Buncombe	225
Pemiscot	614	Hinds	411	Carbon	691	Burke	229
Perry	563	Holmes	411	Carter	714	Cabarrus	235
Pettis	656	Humphreys	487	Cascade	692	Caldwell	229
Phelps	627	Issaquena	488	Chouteau	692	Camden	264
Pike	353	Itawamba	418	Custer	714	Carteret	242
Platte	548	Jackson	471	Daniels	733	Caswell	132
Polk	549	Jasper	455	Dawson	767	Catawba	229
Pulaski	627	Jefferson	435	Deer Lodge	742	Chatham	203
Putnam	566	Jefferson Davis	504	Fallon	714	Cherokee	258
Ralls	353	Jones	455	Fergus	810	Chowan	243
Randolph	553	Kemper	412	Flathead	728	Clay	258
Ray	548	Lafayette	459	Gallatin	773	Cleveland	218
Reynolds	627	Lamar	409	Garfield	714	Columbus	207
Ripley	563	Lauderdale	412	Glacier	692	Craven	242
St. Charles	599	Lawrence	504	Golden Valley	691	Cumberland	262
St. Clair	607	Leake	411	Granite	713	Currituck	6
St. Genevieve	541	Lee	418	Hill	712	Dare	264
St. Francois	541	Leflore	487	Jefferson	721	Davidson	186
St. Louis	541	Lincoln	511	Judith Basin	692	Davie	149
St. Louis City	541	Lowndes	461	Lake	713	Duplin	238
Saline	656	Madison	411	Lewis and Clark	721	Durham	170
Schuyler	566	Marion	477	Liberty	712	Edgecombe	214
Scotland	566	Marshall	146	Lincoln	728	Forsyth	149
Scott	563	Monroe	418	McCone	767	Franklin	198
Shannon	574	Montgomery	502	Madison	773	Gaston	218
Shelby	553	Neshoba	412	Meagher	778	Gates	243
Stoddard	563	Newton	412	Mineral	713	Graham	209
Stone	549	Noxubee	461	Missoula	713	Granville	170
Sullivan	566	Oktibbeha	484	Musselshell	691	Greene	238
Taney	676	Panola	146	Park	756	Guilford	186
Texas	549	Pearl River	500	Petroleum	810	Halifax	214
Vernon	639	Perry	409	Phillips	712	Harnett	203
Warren	599	Pike	477	Pondera	692	Haywood	225
Washington	541	Pontotoc	482	Powder River	714	Henderson	225
Wayne	563	Prentiss	418	Powell	788	Hertford	243
Webster	549	Quitman	422	Prairie	714	Hoke	205
Worth	591	Rankin	411	Ravalli	713	Hyde	195
Wright	549	Scott	411	Richland	767	Iredell	192
		Sharkey	488	Roosevelt	779	Jackson	209
		Simpson	411	Rosebud	691	Johnston	198
	MS	Smith	455	Sanders	713	Jones	242
		Stone	456	Sheridan	733	Lee	203
Adams	435	Sunflower	487	Silver Bow	742	Lenoir	238
Alcorn	498	Tallahatchie	422	Stillwater	691	Lincoln	218
Amite	477	Tate	146	Sweet Grass	756	McDowell	261
Attala	411	Tippah	482	Teton	692	Macon	209
Benton	146	Tishomingo	498	Toole	692	Madison	225
Bolivar	487	Tunica	146	Treasure	691	Martin	195
Calhoun	459	Union	482	Valley	779	Mecklenburg	167
Carroll	502	Walthall	477	Wheatland	778	Mitchell	240
Chickasaw	418	Warren	431	Wibaux	767	Montgomery	205
Choctaw	484	Washington	488	Yellowstone	691	Moore	205
Claiborne	431	Wayne	455	Yellowstone Park	691	Nash	214

Table B-1: Health Service Areas by State and County

County	HSA	County	HSA	County	HSA	County	HSA
New Hanover	168	McKenzie	579	Garfield	594	Grafton	15
Northampton	214	McLean	543	Gosper	570	Hillsborough	91
Onslow	242	Mercer	543	Grant	580	Merrimack	91
Orange	203	Morton	543	Greeley	555	Rockingham	74
Pamlico	242	Mountrail	550	Hall	555	Strafford	98
Pasquotank	264	Nelson	584	Hamilton	555	Sullivan	15
Pender	168	Oliver	543	Harlan	616		
Perquimans	264	Pembina	584	Hayes	654	**NJ**	
Person	170	Pierce	638	Hitchcock	613		
Pitt	195	Ramsey	655	Holt	559	Atlantic	64
Polk	191	Ransom	547	Hooker	593	Bergen	36
Randolph	186	Renville	550	Howard	555	Burlington	23
Richmond	205	Richland	547	Jefferson	561	Camden	23
Robeson	207	Rolette	638	Johnson	660	Cape May	64
Rockingham	186	Sargent	547	Kearney	570	Cumberland	127
Rowan	235	Sheridan	543	Keith	593	Essex	66
Rutherford	218	Sioux	543	Keya Paha	559	Gloucester	23
Sampson	262	Slope	640	Kimball	741	Hudson	36
Scotland	207	Stark	605	Knox	578	Hunterdon	93
Stanly	235	Steele	547	Lancaster	561	Mercer	126
Stokes	149	Stutsman	632	Lincoln	593	Middlesex	66
Surry	149	Towner	638	Logan	594	Monmouth	108
Swain	209	Traill	547	Loup	594	Morris	87
Transylvania	225	Walsh	584	McPherson	593	Ocean	108
Tyrrell	195	Ward	550	Madison	577	Passaic	36
Union	167	Wells	632	Merrick	555	Salem	23
Vance	170	Williams	579	Morrill	580	Somerset	66
Wake	198			Nance	651	Sussex	87
Warren	170			Nemaha	687	Union	66
Washington	195	**NE**		Nuckolls	564	Warren	93
Watauga	194			Otoe	660		
Wayne	238	Adams	564	Pawnee	628		
Wilkes	256	Antelope	577	Perkins	593	**NM**	
Wilson	198	Arthur	593	Phelps	616		
Yadkin	149	Banner	580	Pierce	577	Bernalillo	693
Yancey	240	Blaine	594	Platte	651	Catron	793
		Boone	651	Polk	611	Chaves	772
		Box Butte	580	Red Willow	613	Colfax	704
ND		Boyd	595	Richardson	628	Curry	725
		Brown	559	Rock	559	De Baca	725
Adams	640	Buffalo	570	Saline	561	Dona Ana	732
Barnes	547	Burt	542	Sarpy	542	Eddy	772
Benson	655	Butler	561	Saunders	542	Grant	793
Billings	605	Cass	542	Scotts Bluff	580	Guadalupe	801
Bottineau	550	Cedar	578	Seward	561	Cibola	801
Bowman	640	Chase	654	Sheridan	623	Harding	801
Burke	550	Cherry	668	Sherman	570	Hidalgo	793
Burleigh	543	Cheyenne	741	Sioux	623	Lea	508
Cass	547	Clay	564	Stanton	577	Lincoln	769
Cavalier	584	Colfax	542	Thayer	658	Los Alamos	724
Dickey	680	Cuming	542	Thomas	594	Luna	732
Divide	579	Custer	594	Thurston	560	McKinley	765
Dunn	605	Dakota	560	Valley	594	Mora	801
Eddy	655	Dawes	623	Washington	542	Otero	769
Emmons	543	Dawson	570	Wayne	577	Quay	725
Foster	632	Deuel	741	Webster	564	Rio Arriba	724
Golden Valley	605	Dixon	560	Wheeler	594	Roosevelt	725
Grand Forks	584	Dodge	542	York	611	Sandoval	693
Grant	670	Douglas	542			San Juan	740
Griggs	547	Dundy	654			San Miguel	801
Hettinger	640	Fillmore	658	**NH**		Santa Fe	724
Kidder	543	Franklin	570			Sierra	732
LaMoure	680	Frontier	570	Belknap	91	Socorro	693
Logan	684	Furnas	616	Carroll	91	Taos	724
McHenry	550	Gage	561	Cheshire	90	Torrance	693
McIntosh	684	Garden	580	Coos	138		

APPENDIX B: HEALTH SERVICE AREA DEFINITIONS

Table B-1: Health Service Areas by State and County

County	Code	County	Code	County	Code	County	Code
Union	814	Otsego	58	Huron	366	Cimarron	587
Valencia	693	Putnam	41	Jackson	283	Cleveland	430
		Queens	83	Jefferson	360	Coal	478
		Rensselaer	10	Knox	388	Comanche	493
NV		Richmond	113	Lake	288	Cotton	493
		Rockland	133	Lawrence	46	Craig	414
Carson City	701	St. Lawrence	80	Licking	388	Creek	414
Churchill	701	Saratoga	88	Logan	398	Custer	475
Clark	707	Schenectady	88	Lorain	366	Delaware	446
Douglas	701	Schoharie	58	Lucas	276	Dewey	469
Elko	720	Schuyler	65	Madison	281	Ellis	469
Esmeralda	707	Seneca	21	Mahoning	345	Garfield	429
Eureka	720	Steuben	65	Marion	354	Garvin	430
Humboldt	701	Suffolk	83	Medina	352	Grady	476
Lander	720	Sullivan	86	Meigs	283	Grant	429
Lincoln	707	Tioga	19	Mercer	292	Greer	483
Lyon	701	Tompkins	105	Miami	376	Harmon	483
Mineral	701	Ulster	41	Monroe	24	Harper	469
Nye	707	Warren	88	Montgomery	295	Haskell	421
Ormsby	701	Washington	88	Morgan	377	Hughes	478
Pershing	701	Wayne	21	Morrow	354	Jackson	483
Storey	701	Westchester	41	Muskingum	377	Jefferson	497
Washoe	701	Wyoming	54	Noble	377	Johnston	474
White Pine	805	Yates	21	Ottawa	276	Kay	515
				Paulding	356	Kingfisher	429
				Perry	377	Kiowa	493
NY		**OH**		Pickaway	281	Latimer	466
				Pike	337	Le Flore	421
Albany	10	Adams	270	Portage	352	Lincoln	417
Allegany	35	Allen	292	Preble	295	Logan	417
Bronx	94	Ashland	369	Putnam	292	Love	474
Broome	19	Ashtabula	288	Richland	369	McClain	430
Cattaraugus	35	Athens	368	Ross	337	McCurtain	404
Cayuga	56	Auglaize	292	Sandusky	366	McIntosh	445
Chautauqua	106	Belmont	24	Scioto	337	Major	429
Chemung	65	Brown	270	Seneca	386	Marshall	474
Chenango	58	Butler	270	Shelby	376	Mayes	414
Clinton	81	Carroll	347	Stark	347	Murray	430
Columbia	112	Champaign	346	Summit	352	Muskogee	445
Cortland	105	Clark	346	Trumbull	345	Noble	472
Delaware	58	Clermont	270	Tuscarawas	347	Nowata	451
Dutchess	41	Clinton	372	Union	354	Okfuskee	529
Erie	54	Columbiana	380	Van Wert	292	Oklahoma	417
Essex	81	Coshocton	377	Vinton	368	Okmulgee	529
Franklin	81	Crawford	354	Warren	270	Osage	515
Fulton	76	Cuyahoga	288	Washington	34	Ottawa	414
Genesee	54	Darke	295	Wayne	347	Pawnee	472
Greene	112	Defiance	356	Williams	356	Payne	472
Hamilton	88	Delaware	281	Wood	276	Pittsburg	466
Herkimer	59	Erie	366	Wyandot	354	Pontotoc	478
Jefferson	80	Fairfield	368			Pottawatomie	417
Kings	113	Fayette	281			Pushmataha	466
Lewis	80	Franklin	281	**OK**		Roger Mills	440
Livingston	54	Fulton	276			Rogers	414
Madison	59	Gallia	283	Adair	445	Seminole	478
Monroe	54	Geauga	288	Alfalfa	429	Sequoyah	421
Montgomery	76	Greene	295	Atoka	436	Stephens	497
Nassau	83	Guernsey	377	Beaver	535	Texas	587
New York	94	Hamilton	270	Beckham	440	Tillman	493
Niagara	54	Hancock	386	Blaine	429	Tulsa	414
Oneida	59	Hardin	292	Bryan	436	Wagoner	445
Onondaga	56	Harrison	360	Caddo	476	Washington	451
Ontario	21	Henry	356	Canadian	417	Washita	475
Orange	86	Highland	372	Carter	474	Woods	429
Orleans	54	Hocking	368	Cherokee	445	Woodward	469
Oswego	56	Holmes	347	Choctaw	438		

TABLE B-1: HEALTH SERVICE AREAS BY STATE AND COUNTY

OR

County	
Baker	759
Benton	727
Clackamas	689
Clatsop	689
Columbia	689
Coos	738
Crook	719
Curry	738
Deschutes	719
Douglas	782
Gilliam	748
Grant	806
Harney	719
Hood River	748
Jackson	752
Jefferson	719
Josephine	752
Klamath	743
Lake	743
Lane	782
Lincoln	783
Linn	727
Malheur	729
Marion	705
Morrow	717
Multnomah	689
Polk	705
Sherman	748
Tillamook	783
Umatilla	717
Union	759
Wallowa	759
Wasco	748
Washington	689
Wheeler	719
Yamhill	705

PA

County	
Adams	48
Allegheny	42
Armstrong	42
Beaver	42
Bedford	57
Berks	139
Blair	57
Bradford	19
Bucks	28
Butler	42
Cambria	57
Cameron	35
Carbon	84
Centre	26
Chester	28
Clarion	52
Clearfield	26
Clinton	44
Columbia	78
Crawford	117
Cumberland	43
Dauphin	43
Delaware	28
Elk	125
Erie	106
Fayette	100
Forest	52
Franklin	72
Fulton	72
Greene	100
Huntingdon	110
Indiana	42
Jefferson	26
Juniata	110
Lackawanna	47
Lancaster	140
Lawrence	129
Lebanon	43
Lehigh	84
Luzerne	78
Lycoming	44
McKean	35
Mercer	345
Mifflin	110
Monroe	84
Montgomery	28
Montour	8
Northampton	84
Northumberland	8
Perry	43
Philadelphia	28
Pike	86
Potter	35
Schuylkill	8
Snyder	8
Somerset	57
Sullivan	19
Susquehanna	19
Tioga	128
Union	8
Venango	52
Warren	106
Washington	100
Wayne	47
Westmoreland	42
Wyoming	78
York	48

RI

County	
Bristol	20
Kent	20
Newport	68
Providence	20
Washington	20

SC

County	
Abbeville	187
Aiken	152
Allendale	176
Anderson	182
Bamberg	176
Barnwell	152
Beaufort	143
Berkeley	212
Calhoun	176
Charleston	212
Cherokee	191
Chester	244
Chesterfield	184
Clarendon	196
Colleton	212
Darlington	184
Dillon	199
Dorchester	212
Edgefield	152
Fairfield	160
Florence	184
Georgetown	246
Greenville	182
Greenwood	187
Hampton	212
Horry	246
Jasper	143
Kershaw	249
Lancaster	249
Laurens	187
Lee	196
Lexington	160
McCormick	187
Marion	199
Marlboro	184
Newberry	160
Oconee	182
Orangeburg	176
Pickens	182
Richland	160
Saluda	187
Spartanburg	191
Sumter	196
Union	191
Williamsburg	184
York	244

SD

County	
Aurora	615
Beadle	600
Bennett	623
Bon Homme	578
Brookings	610
Brown	572
Brule	615
Buffalo	615
Butte	558
Campbell	648
Charles Mix	615
Clark	568
Clay	578
Codington	568
Corson	648
Custer	558
Davison	615
Day	572
Deuel	568
Dewey	648
Douglas	615
Edmunds	572
Fall River	558
Faulk	572
Grant	568
Gregory	595
Haakon	629
Hamlin	568
Hand	600
Hanson	615
Harding	640
Hughes	629
Hutchinson	578
Hyde	600
Jackson	558
Jerauld	600
Jones	629
Kingsbury	610
Lake	544
Lawrence	586
Lincoln	544
Lyman	615
McCook	544
McPherson	572
Marshall	572
Meade	558
Mellette	595
Miner	544
Minnehaha	544
Moody	544
Pennington	558
Perkins	640
Potter	648
Roberts	590
Sanborn	615
Shannon	623
Spink	572
Stanley	629
Sully	629
Todd	595
Tripp	595
Turner	544
Union	544
Walworth	648
Yankton	578
Ziebach	629

TN

County	
Anderson	226
Bedford	260
Benton	115
Bledsoe	223
Blount	147
Bradley	173
Campbell	226
Cannon	211
Carroll	115
Carter	169
Cheatham	148
Chester	188
Claiborne	96
Clay	215
Cocke	252
Coffee	239
Crockett	188
Cumberland	223
Davidson	148
Decatur	188
De Kalb	211

APPENDIX B: HEALTH SERVICE AREA DEFINITIONS

TABLE B-1: HEALTH SERVICE AREAS BY STATE AND COUNTY

County	HSA	County	HSA	County	HSA	County	HSA
Dickson	148	Van Buren	211	Culberson	415	Jasper	413
Dyer	248	Warren	211	Dallam	405	Jeff Davis	526
Fayette	146	Washington	169	Dallas	453	Jefferson	413
Fentress	223	Wayne	232	Dawson	406	Jim Hogg	538
Franklin	239	Weakley	181	Deaf Smith	491	Jim Wells	437
Gibson	188	White	215	Delta	438	Johnson	434
Giles	208	Williamson	148	Denton	495	Jones	428
Grainger	217	Wilson	231	De Witt	433	Karnes	513
Greene	252			Dickens	406	Kaufman	453
Grundy	239			Dimmit	531	Kendall	410
Hamblen	217		TX	Donley	405	Kenedy	437
Hamilton	141			Duval	437	Kent	428
Hancock	217	Anderson	509	Eastland	428	Kerr	506
Hardeman	188	Andrews	508	Ector	444	Kimble	506
Hardin	245	Angelina	449	Edwards	506	King	406
Hawkins	151	Aransas	437	Ellis	453	Kinney	516
Haywood	188	Archer	420	El Paso	415	Kleberg	437
Henderson	188	Armstrong	405	Erath	507	Knox	420
Henry	115	Atascosa	410	Falls	462	Lamar	438
Hickman	148	Austin	408	Fannin	436	Lamb	406
Houston	234	Bailey	406	Fayette	490	Lampasas	452
Humphreys	148	Bandera	410	Fisher	503	LaSalle	410
Jackson	215	Bastrop	425	Floyd	481	Lavaca	433
Jefferson	217	Baylor	420	Foard	458	Lee	425
Johnson	194	Bee	513	Fort Bend	408	Leon	501
Knox	147	Bell	452	Franklin	465	Liberty	408
Lake	248	Bexar	410	Freestone	489	Limestone	462
Lauderdale	248	Blanco	506	Frio	410	Lipscomb	469
Lawrence	232	Borden	406	Gaines	508	Live Oak	437
Lewis	208	Bosque	462	Galveston	532	Llano	425
Lincoln	210	Bowie	404	Garza	406	Loving	415
Loudon	147	Brazoria	505	Gillespie	506	Lubbock	406
McMinn	147	Brazos	464	Glasscock	518	Lynn	406
McNairy	245	Brewster	526	Goliad	433	McCulloch	426
Macon	231	Briscoe	405	Gonzales	410	McLennan	462
Madison	188	Brooks	437	Gray	460	McMullen	410
Marion	141	Brown	468	Grayson	436	Madison	501
Marshall	208	Burleson	464	Gregg	454	Marion	485
Maury	208	Burnet	425	Grimes	464	Martin	492
Meigs	147	Caldwell	510	Guadalupe	410	Mason	506
Monroe	147	Calhoun	433	Hale	481	Matagorda	505
Montgomery	234	Callahan	428	Hall	512	Maverick	516
Moore	239	Cameron	520	Hamilton	462	Medina	410
Morgan	226	Camp	465	Hansford	405	Menard	426
Obion	181	Carson	405	Hardeman	458	Midland	492
Overton	215	Cass	485	Hardin	413	Milam	452
Perry	232	Castro	481	Harris	408	Mills	468
Pickett	215	Chambers	408	Harrison	485	Mitchell	503
Polk	173	Cherokee	509	Hartley	405	Montague	420
Putnam	215	Childress	512	Haskell	428	Montgomery	408
Rhea	226	Clay	420	Hays	510	Moore	405
Roane	226	Cochran	406	Hemphill	460	Morris	465
Robertson	148	Coke	426	Henderson	441	Motley	406
Rutherford	211	Coleman	468	Hidalgo	427	Nacogdoches	447
Scott	263	Collin	453	Hill	462	Navarro	489
Sequatchie	141	Collingsworth	524	Hockley	406	Newton	413
Sevier	147	Colorado	490	Hood	434	Nolan	503
Shelby	146	Comal	517	Hopkins	453	Nueces	437
Smith	231	Comanche	507	Houston	509	Ochiltree	405
Stewart	234	Concho	426	Howard	518	Oldham	405
Sullivan	151	Cooke	495	Hudspeth	415	Orange	413
Sumner	231	Coryell	452	Hunt	453	Palo Pinto	479
Tipton	146	Cottle	512	Hutchinson	405	Panola	454
Trousdale	231	Crane	444	Irion	426	Parker	434
Unicoi	169	Crockett	426	Jack	479	Parmer	491
Union	147	Crosby	406	Jackson	433	Pecos	492

TABLE B-1: HEALTH SERVICE AREAS BY STATE AND COUNTY

County	HSA	County	HSA	County	HSA	County	HSA
Polk	449	Zapata	538	Chesterfield	33	Patrick	79
Potter	405	Zavala	410	Clarke	25	Petersburg City	77
Presidio	526			Clifton Forge City	30	Pittsylvania	132
Rains	453			Colonial Heights City	33	Poquoson	5
Randall	405		**UT**	Craig	14	Portsmouth City	6
Reagan	426			Culpeper	99	Powhatan	33
Real	506	Beaver	755	Cumberland	33	Prince Edward	33
Red River	438	Box Elder	744	Danville City	132	Prince George	77
Reeves	444	Cache	715	Dickenson	55	Prince William	109
Refugio	433	Carbon	809	Dinwiddie	77	Pulaski	70
Roberts	460	Daggett	799	Emporia City	130	Radford City	70
Robertson	464	Davis	744	Essex	33	Rappahannock	99
Rockwall	453	Duchesne	708	Fairfax	69	Richmond	33
Runnels	426	Emery	809	Fairfax City	69	Richmond City	33
Rusk	454	Garfield	707	Fauquier	109	Roanoke	14
Sabine	447	Grand	711	Floyd	14	Roanoke City	14
San Augustine	447	Iron	755	Fluvanna	99	Rockbridge	97
San Jacinto	408	Juab	703	Franklin	14	Rockingham	63
San Patricio	437	Kane	707	Franklin City	6	Russell	151
San Saba	468	Millard	703	Frederick	25	Salem City	14
Schleicher	426	Morgan	744	Fredericksburg City	135	Scott	151
Scurry	519	Piute	707	Galax City	73	Shenandoah	25
Shackelford	428	Rich	744	Giles	70	Smyth	151
Shelby	447	Salt Lake	708	Gloucester	5	South Boston City	71
Sherman	405	San Juan	740	Goochland	33	Southampton	6
Smith	441	Sanpete	703	Grayson	73	Spotsylvania	135
Somervell	434	Sevier	703	Greene	99	Stafford	135
Starr	427	Summit	708	Greensville	130	Staunton City	97
Stephens	428	Tooele	708	Halifax	71	Suffolk City	6
Sterling	426	Uintah	708	Hanover	33	Surry	77
Stonewall	428	Utah	703	Harrisonburg City	63	Sussex	77
Sutton	426	Wasatch	708	Henrico	33	Tazewell	39
Swisher	405	Washington	707	Henry	79	Warren	25
Tarrant	434	Wayne	703	Highland	97	Washington	151
Taylor	428	Weber	744	Hopewell City	33	Westmoreland	33
Terrell	492			Isle of Wight	6	Wise	55
Terry	514			James City	5	Wythe	70
Throckmorton	420		**VA**	King and Queen	33	York	5
Titus	465			King George	135	Alexandria City	69
Tom Green	426	Accomack	137	King William	33	Chesapeake City	6
Travis	425	Albermarle	99	Lancaster	33	Hampton City	5
Trinity	449	Alleghany	30	Lee	55	Newport News	5
Tyler	413	Amelia	33	Lexington City	97	Virginia Beach City	6
Upshur	454	Amherst	14	Loudoun	69	Waynesboro City	99
Upton	492	Appomattox	14	Louisa	99	Williamsburg City	5
Uvalde	536	Arlington	69	Lunenburg	71	Winchester City	25
Val Verde	516	Alexandria	69	Lynchburg City	14		
Van Zandt	441	Alexandria City	69	Madison	99		**VT**
Victoria	433	Augusta	97	Manassas	69		
Walker	449	Bath	30	Martinsville City	79	Addison	49
Waller	408	Bedford	14	Mathews	5	Bennington	10
Ward	444	Bedford City	14	Mecklenburg	71	Caledonia	103
Washington	464	Buena Vista City	14	Middlesex	33	Chittenden	49
Webb	538	Bland	39	Montgomery	70	Essex	138
Wharton	505	Botetourt	14	Nansemond	6	Franklin	49
Wheeler	460	Bristol City	151	Nelson	99	Grand Isle	49
Wichita	420	Brunswick	130	New Kent	33	Lamoille	103
Wilbarger	458	Buchanan	39	Newport News City	5	Orange	15
Willacy	520	Buckingham	99	Norfolk/Ports	6	Orleans	103
Williamson	425	Campbell	14	Norfolk City	6	Rutland	122
Wilson	410	Caroline	135	Northampton	137	Washington	15
Winkler	444	Carroll	73	Northumberland	33	Windham	90
Wise	495	Charles City	33	Norton City	55	Windsor	15
Wood	441	Charlotte	33	Nottoway	33		
Yoakum	514	Charlottesville City	99	Orange	99		
Young	420	Chesapeake City	6	Page	63		

APPENDIX B: HEALTH SERVICE AREA DEFINITIONS **247**

Table B-1: Health Service Areas by State and County

WA

County	Code
Adams	698
Asotin	694
Benton	702
Chelan	747
Clallam	785
Clark	689
Columbia	717
Cowlitz	689
Douglas	747
Ferry	698
Franklin	702
Garfield	694
Grant	747
Grays Harbor	758
Island	736
Jefferson	785
King	736
Kitsap	736
Kittitas	739
Klickitat	748
Lewis	758
Lincoln	698
Mason	758
Okanogan	747
Pacific	758
Pend Oreille	698
Pierce	794
San Juan	736
Skagit	736
Skamania	748
Snohomish	736
Spokane	698
Stevens	698
Thurston	758
Wahkiakum	689
Walla Walla	717
Whatcom	815
Whitman	784
Yakima	739

WI

County	Code
Adams	391
Ashland	357
Barron	374
Bayfield	357
Brown	278
Buffalo	298
Burnett	314
Calumet	355
Chippewa	298
Clark	282
Columbia	301
Crawford	350
Dane	301
Dodge	306
Door	278
Douglas	289
Dunn	298
Eau Claire	298
Florence	315
Fond Du Lac	306
Forest	284
Grant	301
Green	326
Green Lake	306
Iowa	301
Iron	284
Jackson	399
Jefferson	387
Juneau	391
Kenosha	382
Kewaunee	278
LaCrosse	290
Lafayette	326
Langlade	379
Lincoln	282
Manitowoc	355
Marathon	282
Marinette	315
Marquette	301
Menominee	379
Milwaukee	280
Monroe	290
Oconto	278
Oneida	284
Outagamie	344
Ozaukee	280
Pepin	298
Pierce	370
Polk	286
Portage	400
Price	357
Racine	382
Richland	301
Rock	326
Rusk	374
St. Croix	370
Sauk	301
Sawyer	357
Shawano	379
Sheboygan	355
Taylor	282
Trempealeau	290
Vernon	290
Vilas	284
Walworth	387
Washburn	314
Washington	280
Waukesha	280
Waupaca	344
Waushara	306
Winnebago	306
Wood	282

WV

County	Code
Barbour	50
Berkeley	25
Boone	7
Braxton	92
Brooke	380
Cabell	46
Calhoun	34
Clay	7
Doddridge	92
Fayette	60
Gilmer	92
Grant	1
Greenbrier	30
Hampshire	25
Hancock	380
Hardy	1
Harrison	92
Jackson	34
Jefferson	25
Kanawha	7
Lewis	92
Lincoln	46
Logan	13
McDowell	39
Marion	31
Marshall	24
Mason	283
Mercer	39
Mineral	1
Mingo	13
Monongalia	31
Monroe	30
Morgan	25
Nicholas	7
Ohio	24
Pendleton	63
Pleasants	34
Pocahontas	50
Preston	31
Putnam	7
Raleigh	60
Randolph	50
Ritchie	34
Roane	34
Summers	60
Taylor	31
Tucker	50
Tyler	24
Upshur	92
Wayne	46
Webster	7
Wetzel	24
Wirt	34
Wood	34
Wyoming	60

WY

County	Code
Albany	771
Big Horn	749
Campbell	586
Carbon	771
Converse	726
Crook	586
Fremont	777
Goshen	580
Hot Springs	777
Johnson	770
Laramie	741
Lincoln	775
Natrona	726
Niobrara	580
Park	749
Platte	797
Sheridan	770
Sublette	775
Sweetwater	799
Teton	775
Uinta	792
Washakie	777
Weston	804

Table B-2

Numeric List of Health Service Areas

HSA	County, State
1	Allegany, MD
1	Garrett, MD
1	Grant, WV
1	Hardy, WV
1	Mineral, WV
2	Boone, KY
2	Campbell, KY
2	Gallatin, KY
2	Grant, KY
2	Kenton, KY
2	Pendleton, KY
3	Kent, DE
3	Sussex, DE
3	Somerset, MD
3	Wicomico, MD
3	Worcester, MD
4	Hartford, CT
4	Tolland, CT
4	Windham, CT
5	Gloucester, VA
5	Hampton City, VA
5	James City, VA
5	Mathews, VA
5	Newport News, VA
5	Newport News City, VA
5	Poquoson, VA
5	Williamsburg City, VA
5	York, VA
6	Currituck, NC
6	Chesapeake City, VA
6	Franklin City, VA
6	Isle of Wight, VA
6	Nansemond, VA
6	Norfolk City, VA
6	Norfolk/Ports, VA
6	Portsmouth City, VA
6	Southampton, VA
6	Suffolk City, VA
6	Virginia Beach City, VA
7	Boone, WV
7	Clay, WV
7	Kanawha, WV
7	Nicholas, WV
7	Putnam, WV
7	Webster, WV
8	Montour, PA
8	Northumberland, PA
8	Schuylkill, PA
8	Snyder, PA
8	Union, PA
9	Cumberland, ME
9	Knox, ME
9	Lincoln, ME
9	Sagadahoc, ME
10	Albany, NY
10	Rensselaer, NY
10	Bennington, VT
11	Floyd, KY
11	Johnson, KY
11	Magoffin, KY
12	Johnson, IL
12	Massac, IL
12	Ballard, KY
12	Carlisle, KY
12	Crittenden, KY
12	Graves, KY
12	Hickman, KY
12	Livingston, KY
12	Lyon, KY
12	Marshall, KY
12	McCracken, KY
13	Pike, KY
13	Logan, WV
13	Mingo, WV
14	Amherst, VA
14	Appomattox, VA
14	Bedford, VA
14	Bedford City, VA
14	Botetourt, VA
14	Buena Vista City, VA
14	Campbell, VA
14	Craig, VA
14	Floyd, VA
14	Franklin, VA
14	Lynchburg City, VA
14	Roanoke, VA
14	Roanoke City, VA
14	Salem City, VA
15	Grafton, NH
15	Sullivan, NH
15	Orange, VT
15	Washington, VT
15	Windsor, VT
16	Anne Arundel, MD
16	Baltimore, MD
16	Baltimore City, MD
16	Calvert, MD
16	Carroll, MD
16	Howard, MD
17	Hancock, ME
17	Penobscot, ME
17	Piscataquis, ME
17	Washington, ME
18	Breathitt, KY
18	Clark, KY
18	Fayette, KY
18	Jessamine, KY
18	Knott, KY
18	Lee, KY
18	Leslie, KY
18	Owsley, KY
18	Perry, KY
18	Powell, KY
18	Scott, KY
18	Wolfe, KY
18	Woodford, KY
19	Broome, NY
19	Tioga, NY
19	Bradford, PA
19	Sullivan, PA
19	Susquehanna, PA
20	New London, CT
20	Bristol, RI
20	Kent, RI
20	Providence, RI
20	Washington, RI
21	Ontario, NY
21	Seneca, NY
21	Wayne, NY
21	Yates, NY
22	Barnstable, MA
22	Middlesex, MA
22	Norfolk, MA
22	Plymouth, MA
22	Suffolk, MA
23	Burlington, NJ
23	Camden, NJ
23	Gloucester, NJ
23	Salem, NJ
24	Belmont, OH
24	Monroe, OH
24	Marshall, WV
24	Ohio, WV
24	Tyler, WV
24	Wetzel, WV
25	Clarke, VA
25	Frederick, VA
25	Shenandoah, VA
25	Warren, VA
25	Winchester City, VA
25	Berkeley, WV
25	Hampshire, WV
25	Jefferson, WV
25	Morgan, WV
26	Centre, PA
26	Clearfield, PA
26	Jefferson, PA
27	Boyle, KY
27	Casey, KY
27	Garrard, KY
27	Lincoln, KY
27	Mercer, KY
28	Bucks, PA
28	Chester, PA
28	Delaware, PA
28	Montgomery, PA
28	Philadelphia, PA
29	Allen, KY
29	Butler, KY
29	Edmonson, KY
29	Logan, KY
29	Simpson, KY
29	Warren, KY
30	Alleghany, VA
30	Bath, VA
30	Clifton Forge City, VA
30	Greenbrier, WV
30	Monroe, WV
31	Marion, WV
31	Monongalia, WV
31	Preston, WV
31	Taylor, WV
32	Hampden, MA
32	Hampshire, MA
33	Amelia, VA
33	Charles City, VA
33	Charlotte, VA
33	Chesterfield, VA
33	Colonial Heights City, VA
33	Cumberland, VA
33	Essex, VA
33	Goochland, VA
33	Hanover, VA
33	Henrico, VA
33	Hopewell City, VA
33	King and Queen, VA
33	King William, VA
33	Lancaster, VA
33	Middlesex, VA
33	New Kent, VA
33	Northumberland, VA
33	Nottoway, VA
33	Powhatan, VA
33	Prince Edward, VA
33	Richmond, VA
33	Richmond City, VA
33	Westmoreland, VA
34	Washington, OH
34	Calhoun, WV
34	Jackson, WV
34	Pleasants, WV
34	Ritchie, WV
34	Roane, WV
34	Wirt, WV
34	Wood, WV
35	Allegany, NY
35	Cattaraugus, NY
35	Cameron, PA
35	McKean, PA
35	Potter, PA
36	Bergen, NJ
36	Hudson, NJ
36	Passaic, NJ
37	McCreary, KY
37	Pulaski, KY
37	Wayne, KY
38	Kennebec, ME
38	Somerset, ME
38	Waldo, ME
39	Bland, VA
39	Buchanan, VA
39	Tazewell, VA
39	McDowell, WV
39	Mercer, WV
40	Henderson, KY
40	Union, KY
41	Dutchess, NY
41	Putnam, NY
41	Ulster, NY

Appendix B: Health Service Area Definitions

Table B-2: Numeric List of Health Service Areas

41	Westchester, NY	56	Oswego, NY	73	Grayson, VA	93	Hunterdon, NJ
42	Allegheny, PA	57	Bedford, PA	74	Essex, MA	93	Warren, NJ
42	Armstrong, PA	57	Blair, PA	74	Rockingham, NH	94	Bronx, NY
42	Beaver, PA	57	Cambria, PA	75	New Castle, DE	94	New York, NY
42	Butler, PA	57	Somerset, PA	75	Cecil, MD	95	Androscoggin, ME
42	Indiana, PA	58	Chenango, NY	75	Harford, MD	95	Franklin, ME
42	Westmoreland, PA	58	Delaware, NY	76	Fulton, NY	95	Oxford, ME
43	Cumberland, PA	58	Otsego, NY	76	Montgomery, NY	96	Bell, KY
43	Dauphin, PA	58	Schoharie, NY	77	Dinwiddie, VA	96	Harlan, KY
43	Lebanon, PA	59	Herkimer, NY	77	Petersburg City, VA	96	Claiborne, TN
43	Perry, PA	59	Madison, NY	77	Prince George, VA	97	Augusta, VA
44	Clinton, PA	59	Oneida, NY	77	Surry, VA	97	Highland, VA
44	Lycoming, PA	60	Fayette, WV	77	Sussex, VA	97	Lexington City, VA
45	Caldwell, KY	60	Raleigh, WV	78	Columbia, PA	97	Rockbridge, VA
45	Christian, KY	60	Summers, WV	78	Luzerne, PA	97	Staunton City, VA
45	Hopkins, KY	60	Wyoming, WV	78	Wyoming, PA	98	York, ME
45	Muhlenberg, KY	61	District of Columbia, DC	79	Henry, VA	98	Strafford, NH
45	Todd, KY	61	Charles, MD	79	Martinsville City, VA	99	Albermarle, VA
45	Trigg, KY	61	Montgomery, MD	79	Patrick, VA	99	Buckingham, VA
45	Webster, KY	61	Prince George's, MD	80	Jefferson, NY	99	Charlottesville City, VA
46	Boyd, KY	61	St. Mary's, MD	80	Lewis, NY	99	Culpeper, VA
46	Carter, KY	62	Estill, KY	80	St. Lawrence, NY	99	Fluvanna, VA
46	Greenup, KY	62	Jackson, KY	81	Clinton, NY	99	Greene, VA
46	Lawrence, KY	62	Madison, KY	81	Essex, NY	99	Louisa, VA
46	Martin, KY	62	Rockcastle, KY	81	Franklin, NY	99	Madison, VA
46	Lawrence, OH	63	Harrisonburg City, VA	82	Adair, KY	99	Nelson, VA
46	Cabell, WV	63	Page, VA	82	Green, KY	99	Orange, VA
46	Lincoln, WV	63	Rockingham, VA	82	Russell, KY	99	Rappahannock, VA
46	Wayne, WV	63	Pendleton, WV	82	Taylor, KY	99	Waynesboro City, VA
47	Lackawanna, PA	64	Atlantic, NJ	83	Nassau, NY	100	Fayette, PA
47	Wayne, PA	64	Cape May, NJ	83	Queens, NY	100	Greene, PA
48	Frederick, MD	65	Chemung, NY	83	Suffolk, NY	100	Washington, PA
48	Adams, PA	65	Schuyler, NY	84	Carbon, PA	101	Franklin, MA
48	York, PA	65	Steuben, NY	84	Lehigh, PA	101	Worcester, MA
49	Addison, VT	66	Essex, NJ	84	Monroe, PA	102	Bourbon, KY
49	Chittenden, VT	66	Middlesex, NJ	84	Northampton, PA	102	Nicholas, KY
49	Franklin, VT	66	Somerset, NJ	85	Litchfield, CT	103	Caledonia, VT
49	Grand Isle, VT	66	Union, NJ	85	Middlesex, CT	103	Lamoille, VT
50	Barbour, WV	67	Elliott, KY	85	New Haven, CT	103	Orleans, VT
50	Pocahontas, WV	67	Menifee, KY	86	Orange, NY	104	Clinton, KY
50	Randolph, WV	67	Morgan, KY	86	Sullivan, NY	104	Cumberland, KY
50	Tucker, WV	67	Rowan, KY	86	Pike, PA	105	Cortland, NY
51	Clay, KY	68	Bristol, MA	87	Morris, NJ	105	Tompkins, NY
51	Knox, KY	68	Newport, RI	87	Sussex, NJ	106	Chautauqua, NY
51	Laurel, KY	69	Alexandria, VA	88	Hamilton, NY	106	Erie, PA
51	Whitley, KY	69	Alexandria City, VA	88	Saratoga, NY	106	Warren, PA
52	Clarion, PA	69	Arlington, VA	88	Schenectady, NY	107	Caroline, MD
52	Forest, PA	69	Fairfax, VA	88	Warren, NY	107	Dorchester, MD
52	Venango, PA	69	Fairfax City, VA	88	Washington, NY	107	Queen Anne's, MD
53	Barren, KY	69	Loudoun, VA	89	Breckinridge, KY	107	Talbot, MD
53	Hart, KY	69	Manassas, VA	89	Grayson, KY	108	Monmouth, NJ
53	Metcalfe, KY	70	Giles, VA	89	Hardin, KY	108	Ocean, NJ
53	Monroe, KY	70	Montgomery, VA	89	Larue, KY	109	Fauquier, VA
54	Erie, NY	70	Pulaski, VA	89	Meade, KY	109	Prince William, VA
54	Genesee, NY	70	Radford City, VA	90	Cheshire, NH	110	Huntingdon, PA
54	Livingston, NY	70	Wythe, VA	90	Windham, VT	110	Juniata, PA
54	Monroe, NY	71	Halifax, VA	91	Belknap, NH	110	Mifflin, PA
54	Niagara, NY	71	Lunenburg, VA	91	Carroll, NH	111	Nantucket, MA
54	Orleans, NY	71	Mecklenburg, VA	91	Hillsborough, NH	112	Berkshire, MA
54	Wyoming, NY	71	South Boston City, VA	91	Merrimack, NH	112	Columbia, NY
55	Dickenson, VA	72	Washington, MD	92	Braxton, WV	112	Greene, NY
55	Lee, VA	72	Franklin, PA	92	Doddridge, WV	113	Kings, NY
55	Norton City, VA	72	Fulton, PA	92	Gilmer, WV	113	Richmond, NY
55	Wise, VA	73	Alleghany, NC	92	Harrison, WV	114	Anderson, KY
56	Cayuga, NY	73	Carroll, VA	92	Lewis, WV	114	Franklin, KY
56	Onondaga, NY	73	Galax City, VA	92	Upshur, WV	114	Owen, KY

Table B-2: Numeric List of Health Service Areas

115	Calloway, KY	144	Early, GA	153	Forsyth, GA	163	Escambia, FL
115	Benton, TN	144	Lee, GA	153	Fulton, GA	163	Okaloosa, FL
115	Carroll, TN	144	Randolph, GA	153	Gwinnett, GA	163	Santa Rosa, FL
115	Henry, TN	144	Terrell, GA	153	Henry, GA	163	Walton, FL
116	Bracken, KY	144	Worth, GA	153	Rockdale, GA	164	Barrow, GA
116	Fleming, KY	145	Murray, GA	153	Walton, GA	164	Clarke, GA
116	Mason, KY	145	Whitfield, GA	154	Bartow, GA	164	Greene, GA
117	Crawford, PA	146	Benton, MS	154	Chattooga, GA	164	Jackson, GA
119	Harrison, KY	146	De Soto, MS	154	Floyd, GA	164	Madison, GA
119	Robertson, KY	146	Marshall, MS	154	Gordon, GA	164	Morgan, GA
120	Dukes, MA	146	Panola, MS	154	Polk, GA	164	Oconee, GA
121	Fairfield, CT	146	Tate, MS	155	Bay, FL	164	Oglethorpe, GA
122	Rutland, VT	146	Tunica, MS	155	Calhoun, FL	165	Collier, FL
123	Letcher, KY	146	Fayette, TN	155	Gulf, FL	165	Glades, FL
124	Kent, MD	146	Shelby, TN	155	Holmes, FL	165	Hendry, FL
125	Elk, PA	146	Tipton, TN	155	Jackson, FL	165	Lee, FL
126	Mercer, NJ	147	Blount, TN	155	Washington, FL	166	Russell, AL
127	Cumberland, NJ	147	Knox, TN	156	Greene, AL	166	Chattahoochee, GA
128	Tioga, PA	147	Loudon, TN	156	Hale, AL	166	Harris, GA
129	Lawrence, PA	147	McMinn, TN	156	Pickens, AL	166	Marion, GA
130	Brunswick, VA	147	Meigs, TN	156	Tuscaloosa, AL	166	Muscogee, GA
130	Emporia City, VA	147	Monroe, TN	157	Banks, GA	166	Schley, GA
130	Greensville, VA	147	Sevier, TN	157	Dawson, GA	166	Stewart, GA
131	Bath, KY	147	Union, TN	157	Habersham, GA	166	Talbot, GA
131	Montgomery, KY	148	Cheatham, TN	157	Hall, GA	166	Webster, GA
132	Caswell, NC	148	Davidson, TN	157	Lumpkin, GA	167	Anson, NC
132	Danville City, VA	148	Dickson, TN	157	Towns, GA	167	Mecklenburg, NC
132	Pittsylvania, VA	148	Hickman, TN	157	Union, GA	167	Union, NC
133	Rockland, NY	148	Humphreys, TN	157	White, GA	168	Brunswick, NC
135	Caroline, VA	148	Robertson, TN	158	Baker, FL	168	New Hanover, NC
135	Fredericksburg City, VA	148	Williamson, TN	158	Clay, FL	168	Pender, NC
135	King George, VA	149	Davie, NC	158	Duval, FL	169	Carter, TN
135	Spotsylvania, VA	149	Forsyth, NC	158	Nassau, FL	169	Unicoi, TN
135	Stafford, VA	149	Stokes, NC	158	Brantley, GA	169	Washington, TN
136	Aroostook, ME	149	Surry, NC	158	Camden, GA	170	Durham, NC
137	Accomack, VA	149	Yadkin, NC	158	Charlton, GA	170	Granville, NC
137	Northampton, VA	150	Bibb, AL	158	Glynn, GA	170	Person, NC
138	Coos, NH	150	Blount, AL	158	McIntosh, GA	170	Vance, NC
138	Essex, VT	150	Chilton, AL	159	Alachua, FL	170	Warren, NC
139	Berks, PA	150	Cullman, AL	159	Bradford, FL	171	Autauga, AL
140	Lancaster, PA	150	Jefferson, AL	159	Columbia, FL	171	Bullock, AL
141	Catoosa, GA	150	Shelby, AL	159	Dixie, FL	171	Covington, AL
141	Dade, GA	150	St. Clair, AL	159	Gilchrist, FL	171	Crenshaw, AL
141	Walker, GA	150	Walker, AL	159	Hamilton, FL	171	Lowndes, AL
141	Hamilton, TN	151	Hawkins, TN	159	Lafayette, FL	171	Montgomery, AL
141	Marion, TN	151	Sullivan, TN	159	Levy, FL	171	Pike, AL
141	Sequatchie, TN	151	Bristol City, VA	159	Suwannee, FL	172	Chambers, AL
142	Flagler, FL	151	Russell, VA	159	Union, FL	172	Randolph, AL
142	Lake, FL	151	Scott, VA	160	Fairfield, SC	172	Coweta, GA
142	Orange, FL	151	Smyth, VA	160	Lexington, SC	172	Heard, GA
142	Seminole, FL	151	Washington, VA	160	Newberry, SC	172	Meriwether, GA
142	Sumter, FL	152	Burke, GA	160	Richland, SC	172	Troup, GA
142	Volusia, FL	152	Columbia, GA	161	Baldwin, AL	173	Fannin, GA
143	Bryan, GA	152	Glascock, GA	161	Clarke, AL	173	Gilmer, GA
143	Chatham, GA	152	Jenkins, GA	161	Mobile, AL	173	Bradley, TN
143	Effingham, GA	152	Lincoln, GA	161	Monroe, AL	173	Polk, TN
143	Evans, GA	152	McDuffie, GA	161	Washington, AL	174	Bacon, GA
143	Liberty, GA	152	Richmond, GA	162	Barbour, AL	174	Clinch, GA
143	Long, GA	152	Taliaferro, GA	162	Coffee, AL	174	Pierce, GA
143	Tattnall, GA	152	Warren, GA	162	Dale, AL	174	Ware, GA
143	Beaufort, SC	152	Aiken, SC	162	Geneva, AL	175	Dallas, AL
143	Jasper, SC	152	Barnwell, SC	162	Henry, AL	175	Marengo, AL
144	Baker, GA	152	Edgefield, SC	162	Houston, AL	175	Perry, AL
144	Calhoun, GA	153	Clayton, GA	162	Quitman, GA	175	Wilcox, AL
144	Clay, GA	153	De Kalb, GA	163	Conecuh, AL	176	Allendale, SC
144	Dougherty, GA	153	Fayette, GA	163	Escambia, AL	176	Bamberg, SC

Appendix B: Health Service Area Definitions

Table B-2: Numeric List of Health Service Areas

176 Calhoun, SC	190 Pickens, GA	206 Treutlen, GA	223 Bledsoe, TN
176 Orangeburg, SC	191 Polk, NC	206 Wheeler, GA	223 Cumberland, TN
177 Calhoun, AL	191 Cherokee, SC	207 Bladen, NC	223 Fentress, TN
177 Cleburne, AL	191 Spartanburg, SC	207 Columbus, NC	224 Cherokee, AL
177 Carroll, GA	191 Union, SC	207 Robeson, NC	224 DeKalb, AL
177 Haralson, GA	192 Alexander, NC	207 Scotland, NC	224 Etowah, AL
178 Grady, GA	192 Iredell, NC	208 Giles, TN	224 Marshall, AL
178 Mitchell, GA	193 Bibb, GA	208 Lewis, TN	225 Buncombe, NC
178 Thomas, GA	193 Bleckley, GA	208 Marshall, TN	225 Haywood, NC
179 Elmore, AL	193 Crawford, GA	208 Maury, TN	225 Henderson, NC
179 Lee, AL	193 Houston, GA	209 Graham, NC	225 Madison, NC
179 Macon, AL	193 Jones, GA	209 Jackson, NC	225 Transylvania, NC
179 Tallapoosa, AL	193 Monroe, GA	209 Macon, NC	226 Anderson, TN
180 Berrien, GA	193 Peach, GA	209 Swain, NC	226 Campbell, TN
180 Brooks, GA	193 Pulaski, GA	210 Jackson, AL	226 Morgan, TN
180 Cook, GA	193 Taylor, GA	210 Limestone, AL	226 Rhea, TN
180 Echols, GA	193 Twiggs, GA	210 Madison, AL	226 Roane, TN
180 Lanier, GA	193 Wilkinson, GA	210 Lincoln, TN	227 Hernando, FL
180 Lowndes, GA	194 Ashe, NC	211 Cannon, TN	227 Hillsborough, FL
181 Fulton, KY	194 Watauga, NC	211 De Kalb, TN	227 Pasco, FL
181 Obion, TN	194 Johnson, TN	211 Rutherford, TN	227 Pinellas, FL
181 Weakley, TN	195 Beaufort, NC	211 Van Buren, TN	228 Decatur, GA
182 Anderson, SC	195 Hyde, NC	211 Warren, TN	228 Miller, GA
182 Greenville, SC	195 Martin, NC	212 Berkeley, SC	228 Seminole, GA
182 Oconee, SC	195 Pitt, NC	212 Charleston, SC	229 Burke, NC
182 Pickens, SC	195 Tyrrell, NC	212 Colleton, SC	229 Caldwell, NC
183 Franklin, FL	195 Washington, NC	212 Dorchester, SC	229 Catawba, NC
183 Gadsden, FL	196 Clarendon, SC	212 Hampton, SC	230 Appling, GA
183 Jefferson, FL	196 Lee, SC	213 Charlotte, FL	230 Wayne, GA
183 Leon, FL	196 Sumter, SC	213 De Soto, FL	231 Macon, TN
183 Liberty, FL	197 Crisp, GA	213 Sarasota, FL	231 Smith, TN
183 Madison, FL	197 Dooly, GA	214 Edgecombe, NC	231 Sumner, TN
183 Taylor, FL	197 Macon, GA	214 Halifax, NC	231 Trousdale, TN
183 Wakulla, FL	197 Sumter, GA	214 Nash, NC	231 Wilson, TN
184 Chesterfield, SC	197 Wilcox, GA	214 Northampton, NC	232 Lawrence, TN
184 Darlington, SC	198 Franklin, NC	215 Clay, TN	232 Perry, TN
184 Florence, SC	198 Johnston, NC	215 Jackson, TN	232 Wayne, TN
184 Marlboro, SC	198 Wake, NC	215 Overton, TN	233 Citrus, FL
184 Williamsburg, SC	198 Wilson, NC	215 Pickett, TN	233 Marion, FL
185 Lawrence, AL	199 Dillon, SC	215 Putnam, TN	234 Houston, TN
185 Morgan, AL	199 Marion, SC	215 White, TN	234 Montgomery, TN
186 Davidson, NC	200 Broward, FL	216 Franklin, GA	234 Stewart, TN
186 Guilford, NC	200 Dade, FL	216 Hart, GA	235 Cabarrus, NC
186 Randolph, NC	200 Monroe, FL	216 Stephens, GA	235 Rowan, NC
186 Rockingham, NC	201 Baldwin, GA	217 Grainger, TN	235 Stanly, NC
187 Abbeville, SC	201 Hancock, GA	217 Hamblen, TN	236 Atkinson, GA
187 Greenwood, SC	201 Putnam, GA	217 Hancock, TN	236 Coffee, GA
187 Laurens, SC	202 Hardee, FL	217 Jefferson, TN	236 Jeff Davis, GA
187 McCormick, SC	202 Highlands, FL	218 Cleveland, NC	237 Brevard, FL
187 Saluda, SC	202 Polk, FL	218 Gaston, NC	237 Indian River, FL
188 Chester, TN	203 Chatham, NC	218 Lincoln, NC	238 Duplin, NC
188 Crockett, TN	203 Harnett, NC	218 Rutherford, NC	238 Greene, NC
188 Decatur, TN	203 Lee, NC	219 Colbert, AL	238 Lenoir, NC
188 Gibson, TN	203 Orange, NC	219 Franklin, AL	238 Wayne, NC
188 Hardeman, TN	204 Butts, GA	219 Lauderdale, AL	239 Coffee, TN
188 Haywood, TN	204 Spalding, GA	219 Winston, AL	239 Franklin, TN
188 Henderson, TN	205 Hoke, NC	220 Jasper, GA	239 Grundy, TN
188 Madison, TN	205 Montgomery, NC	220 Newton, GA	239 Moore, TN
189 Ben Hill, GA	205 Moore, NC	221 Martin, FL	240 Avery, NC
189 Irwin, GA	205 Richmond, NC	221 Okeechobee, FL	240 Mitchell, NC
189 Tift, GA	206 Dodge, GA	221 Palm Beach, FL	240 Yancey, NC
189 Turner, GA	206 Johnson, GA	221 St. Lucie, FL	241 Clay, AL
190 Cherokee, GA	206 Laurens, GA	222 Bulloch, GA	241 Coosa, AL
190 Cobb, GA	206 Montgomery, GA	222 Candler, GA	241 Talladega, AL
190 Douglas, GA	206 Telfair, GA	222 Emanuel, GA	242 Carteret, NC
190 Paulding, GA	206 Toombs, GA	222 Screven, GA	242 Craven, NC

Table B-2: Numeric List of Health Service Areas

242	Jones, NC	272	Nelson, KY	285	Clinton, MI	299	Bond, IL
242	Onslow, NC	272	Oldham, KY	285	Eaton, MI	299	Calhoun, IL
242	Pamlico, NC	272	Shelby, KY	285	Ingham, MI	299	Jersey, IL
243	Bertie, NC	272	Spencer, KY	285	Shiawassee, MI	299	Madison, IL
243	Chowan, NC	272	Washington, KY	286	Chisago, MN	300	Benton, IN
243	Gates, NC	273	Wabash, IL	286	Dakota, MN	300	Carroll, IN
243	Hertford, NC	273	Gibson, IN	286	Ramsey, MN	300	Clinton, IN
244	Chester, SC	273	Posey, IN	286	Washington, MN	300	Tippecanoe, IN
244	York, SC	273	Spencer, IN	286	Polk, WI	300	White, IN
245	Hardin, TN	273	Vanderburgh, IN	287	Cook, IL	301	Columbia, WI
245	McNairy, TN	273	Warrick, IN	287	DuPage, IL	301	Dane, WI
246	Georgetown, SC	274	Livingston, MI	287	Lake, IL	301	Grant, WI
246	Horry, SC	274	Macomb, MI	287	McHenry, IL	301	Iowa, WI
247	Fayette, AL	274	Oakland, MI	288	Ashtabula, OH	301	Marquette, WI
247	Marion, AL	274	Washtenaw, MI	288	Cuyahoga, OH	301	Richland, WI
248	Dyer, TN	274	Wayne, MI	288	Geauga, OH	301	Sauk, WI
248	Lake, TN	275	Hendricks, IN	288	Lake, OH	302	Dubuque, IA
248	Lauderdale, TN	275	Johnson, IN	289	Carlton, MN	302	Jackson, IA
249	Kershaw, SC	275	Marion, IN	289	Cook, MN	302	Jo Daviess, IL
249	Lancaster, SC	275	Morgan, IN	289	Itasca, MN	302	Stephenson, IL
250	Jefferson, GA	275	Putnam, IN	289	Koochiching, MN	303	Grundy, IL
250	Washington, GA	275	Rush, IN	289	Lake, MN	303	Will, IL
251	Putnam, FL	275	Shelby, IN	289	Pine, MN	304	Allen, IN
251	St. Johns, FL	276	Monroe, MI	289	St. Louis, MN	304	DeKalb, IN
252	Cocke, TN	276	Fulton, OH	289	Douglas, WI	304	Lagrange, IN
252	Greene, TN	276	Lucas, OH	290	Allamakee, IA	304	Noble, IN
253	Elbert, GA	276	Ottawa, OH	290	Houston, MN	304	Steuben, IN
253	Wilkes, GA	276	Wood, OH	290	LaCrosse, WI	304	Whitley, IN
254	Colquitt, GA	277	Fulton, IL	290	Monroe, WI	305	Macon, IL
256	Wilkes, NC	277	Marshall, IL	290	Trempealeau, WI	305	Moultrie, IL
257	Osceola, FL	277	Mason, IL	290	Vernon, WI	305	Piatt, IL
258	Cherokee, NC	277	Peoria, IL	291	Boone, IL	305	Shelby, IL
258	Clay, NC	277	Tazewell, IL	291	Lee, IL	306	Dodge, WI
259	Butler, AL	278	Brown, WI	291	Ogle, IL	306	Fond Du Lac, WI
260	Bedford, TN	278	Door, WI	291	Winnebago, IL	306	Green Lake, WI
261	McDowell, NC	278	Kewaunee, WI	292	Allen, OH	306	Waushara, WI
262	Cumberland, NC	278	Oconto, WI	292	Auglaize, OH	306	Winnebago, WI
262	Sampson, NC	279	Champaign, IL	292	Hardin, OH	307	Henry, IL
263	Scott, TN	279	Coles, IL	292	Mercer, OH	307	Mercer, IL
264	Camden, NC	279	Cumberland, IL	292	Putnam, OH	307	Rock Island, IL
264	Dare, NC	279	Douglas, IL	292	Van Wert, OH	307	Stark, IL
264	Pasquotank, NC	279	Ford, IL	293	Alger, MI	308	Jasper, IN
264	Perquimans, NC	280	Milwaukee, WI	293	Delta, MI	308	Lake, IN
266	Manatee, FL	280	Ozaukee, WI	293	Luce, MI	308	Newton, IN
267	Alamance, NC	280	Washington, WI	293	Marquette, MI	308	Porter, IN
268	Rabun, GA	280	Waukesha, WI	293	Schoolcraft, MI	309	Gratiot, MI
269	Lamar, GA	281	Delaware, OH	294	Charlevoix, MI	309	Ionia, MI
269	Pike, GA	281	Fayette, OH	294	Cheboygan, MI	309	Kent, MI
269	Upson, GA	281	Franklin, OH	294	Chippewa, MI	309	Mecosta, MI
270	Franklin, IN	281	Madison, OH	294	Emmet, MI	309	Montcalm, MI
270	Adams, OH	281	Pickaway, OH	294	Mackinac, MI	310	Crawford, IL
270	Brown, OH	282	Clark, WI	295	Darke, OH	310	Lawrence, IL
270	Butler, OH	282	Lincoln, WI	295	Greene, OH	310	Daviess, IN
270	Clermont, OH	282	Marathon, WI	295	Montgomery, OH	310	Knox, IN
270	Hamilton, OH	282	Taylor, WI	295	Preble, OH	310	Martin, IN
270	Warren, OH	282	Wood, WI	296	Mason, MI	310	Pike, IN
271	Antrim, MI	283	Gallia, OH	296	Muskegon, MI	311	Clark, IL
271	Benzie, MI	283	Jackson, OH	296	Newaygo, MI	311	Clay, IN
271	Grand Traverse, MI	283	Meigs, OH	296	Oceana, MI	311	Parke, IN
271	Kalkaska, MI	283	Mason, WV	297	Sanilac, MI	311	Sullivan, IN
271	Leelanau, MI	284	Gogebic, MI	297	St. Clair, MI	311	Vermillion, IN
271	Manistee, MI	284	Ontonagon, MI	298	Buffalo, WI	311	Vigo, IN
272	Bullitt, KY	284	Forest, WI	298	Chippewa, WI	312	Fulton, IN
272	Henry, KY	284	Iron, WI	298	Dunn, WI	312	Marshall, IN
272	Jefferson, KY	284	Oneida, WI	298	Eau Claire, WI	312	Pulaski, IN
272	Marion, KY	284	Vilas, WI	298	Pepin, WI	312	St. Joseph, IN

Appendix B: Health Service Area Definitions

Table B-2: Numeric List of Health Service Areas

313 Bartholomew, IN	331 Franklin, IL	351 Jasper, IL	372 Clinton, OH
313 Decatur, IN	331 Jackson, IL	351 Richland, IL	372 Highland, OH
313 Jackson, IN	331 Perry, IL	352 Medina, OH	373 DeKalb, IL
313 Jennings, IN	331 Williamson, IL	352 Portage, OH	373 Kane, IL
314 Burnett, WI	332 Adams, IN	352 Summit, OH	373 Kendall, IL
314 Washburn, WI	332 Huntington, IN	353 Adams, IL	374 Barron, WI
315 Dickinson, MI	332 Jay, IN	353 Pike, IL	374 Rusk, WI
315 Iron, MI	332 Wells, IN	353 Lewis, MO	375 Branch, MI
315 Menominee, MI	333 Edgar, IL	353 Marion, MO	375 Hillsdale, MI
315 Florence, WI	333 Vermilion, IL	353 Pike, MO	375 Jackson, MI
315 Marinette, WI	333 Fountain, IN	353 Ralls, MO	375 Lenawee, MI
316 Perry, IN	333 Warren, IN	354 Crawford, OH	376 Miami, OH
316 Daviess, KY	334 Macoupin, IL	354 Marion, OH	376 Shelby, OH
316 Hancock, KY	334 Montgomery, IL	354 Morrow, OH	377 Coshocton, OH
316 McLean, KY	335 Jefferson, IL	354 Union, OH	377 Guernsey, OH
316 Ohio, KY	335 Wayne, IL	354 Wyandot, OH	377 Morgan, OH
317 Lake, MI	336 Bureau, IL	355 Calumet, WI	377 Muskingum, OH
317 Missaukee, MI	336 LaSalle, IL	355 Manitowoc, WI	377 Noble, OH
317 Osceola, MI	336 Livingston, IL	355 Sheboygan, WI	377 Perry, OH
317 Wexford, MI	336 Putnam, IL	356 Defiance, OH	378 LaPorte, IN
318 Brown, IL	337 Lewis, KY	356 Henry, OH	378 Starke, IN
318 Cass, IL	337 Pike, OH	356 Paulding, OH	379 Langlade, WI
318 Christian, IL	337 Ross, OH	356 Williams, OH	379 Menominee, WI
318 Logan, IL	337 Scioto, OH	357 Ashland, WI	379 Shawano, WI
318 McDonough, IL	338 DeWitt, IL	357 Bayfield, WI	380 Columbiana, OH
318 Menard, IL	338 McLean, IL	357 Price, WI	380 Brooke, WV
318 Sangamon, IL	338 Woodford, IL	357 Sawyer, WI	380 Hancock, WV
318 Schuyler, IL	339 Crawford, IN	358 Marion, IL	381 Barry, MI
319 Greene, IL	339 Floyd, IN	358 Washington, IL	381 Calhoun, MI
319 Morgan, IL	339 Harrison, IN	359 Baraga, MI	382 Kenosha, WI
319 Scott, IL	339 Washington, IN	359 Houghton, MI	382 Racine, WI
320 Allegan, MI	340 Des Moines, IA	359 Keweenaw, MI	383 Hamilton, IL
320 Ottawa, MI	340 Henry, IA	360 Harrison, OH	383 White, IL
321 Dearborn, IN	340 Henderson, IL	360 Jefferson, OH	384 Gallatin, IL
321 Jefferson, IN	341 Brown, IN	361 Clinton, IA	384 Hardin, IL
321 Ohio, IN	341 Greene, IN	361 Carroll, IL	384 Pope, IL
321 Ripley, IN	341 Monroe, IN	361 Whiteside, IL	384 Saline, IL
321 Switzerland, IN	341 Owen, IN	362 Hancock, IN	385 Fayette, IN
321 Carroll, KY	342 Arenac, MI	362 Henry, IN	385 Union, IN
321 Trimble, KY	342 Bay, MI	363 Effingham, IL	385 Wayne, IN
322 Huron, MI	342 Iosco, MI	363 Fayette, IL	386 Hancock, OH
322 Saginaw, MI	342 Ogemaw, MI	364 Cass, IN	386 Seneca, OH
322 Tuscola, MI	342 Oscoda, MI	364 Howard, IN	387 Jefferson, WI
323 Blackford, IN	343 Iroquois, IL	364 Tipton, IN	387 Walworth, WI
323 Delaware, IN	343 Kankakee, IL	365 Clark, IN	388 Knox, OH
323 Randolph, IN	344 Outagamie, WI	365 Scott, IN	388 Licking, OH
324 Knox, IL	344 Waupaca, WI	366 Erie, OH	389 Grant, IN
324 Warren, IL	345 Mahoning, OH	366 Huron, OH	389 Miami, IN
325 Clinton, IL	345 Trumbull, OH	366 Lorain, OH	389 Wabash, IN
325 Monroe, IL	345 Mercer, PA	366 Sandusky, OH	390 Hamilton, IN
325 Randolph, IL	346 Champaign, OH	367 Lee, IA	390 Madison, IN
325 St. Clair, IL	346 Clark, OH	367 Hancock, IL	391 Adams, WI
326 Green, WI	347 Carroll, OH	367 Clark, MO	391 Juneau, WI
326 Lafayette, WI	347 Holmes, OH	368 Athens, OH	392 Crawford, MI
326 Rock, WI	347 Stark, OH	368 Fairfield, OH	392 Otsego, MI
327 Berrien, MI	347 Tuscarawas, OH	368 Hocking, OH	392 Roscommon, MI
327 Cass, MI	347 Wayne, OH	368 Vinton, OH	394 Dubois, IN
327 Van Buren, MI	348 Kalamazoo, MI	369 Ashland, OH	395 Winneshiek, IA
328 Genesee, MI	348 St. Joseph, MI	369 Richland, OH	396 Rice, MN
328 Lapeer, MI	349 Elkhart, IN	370 Goodhue, MN	398 Logan, OH
329 Lawrence, IN	349 Kosciusko, IN	370 Pierce, WI	399 Jackson, WI
329 Orange, IN	350 Clayton, IA	370 St. Croix, WI	400 Portage, WI
330 Clare, MI	350 Delaware, IA	371 Alcona, MI	401 Boone, IN
330 Gladwin, MI	350 Crawford, WI	371 Alpena, MI	402 Montgomery, IN
330 Isabella, MI	351 Clay, IL	371 Montmorency, MI	403 Jefferson, LA
330 Midland, MI	351 Edwards, IL	371 Presque Isle, MI	403 Orleans, LA

Table B-2: Numeric List of Health Service Areas

403 Plaquemines, LA	410 Medina, TX	420 Young, TX	432 Perry, AR
403 St. Bernard, LA	410 Wilson, TX	421 Crawford, AR	432 Prairie, AR
403 St. Charles, LA	410 Zavala, TX	421 Franklin, AR	432 Pulaski, AR
403 St. James, LA	411 Attala, MS	421 Logan, AR	432 Saline, AR
403 St. John the Baptist, LA	411 Hinds, MS	421 Scott, AR	432 Van Buren, AR
404 Hempstead, AR	411 Holmes, MS	421 Sebastian, AR	433 Calhoun, TX
404 Howard, AR	411 Leake, MS	421 Haskell, OK	433 De Witt, TX
404 Lafayette, AR	411 Madison, MS	421 Le Flore, OK	433 Goliad, TX
404 Little River, AR	411 Rankin, MS	421 Sequoyah, OK	433 Jackson, TX
404 Miller, AR	411 Scott, MS	422 Coahoma, MS	433 Lavaca, TX
404 Nevada, AR	411 Simpson, MS	422 Quitman, MS	433 Refugio, TX
404 Sevier, AR	412 Choctaw, AL	422 Tallahatchie, MS	433 Victoria, TX
404 McCurtain, OK	412 Sumter, AL	423 St. Helena, LA	434 Hood, TX
404 Bowie, TX	412 Clarke, MS	423 Tangipahoa, LA	434 Johnson, TX
405 Armstrong, TX	412 Kemper, MS	424 Acadia, LA	434 Parker, TX
405 Briscoe, TX	412 Lauderdale, MS	424 Iberia, LA	434 Somervell, TX
405 Carson, TX	412 Neshoba, MS	424 Lafayette, LA	434 Tarrant, TX
405 Dallam, TX	412 Newton, MS	424 St. Martin, LA	435 Concordia, LA
405 Donley, TX	413 Hardin, TX	424 Vermilion, LA	435 Tensas, LA
405 Hansford, TX	413 Jasper, TX	425 Bastrop, TX	435 Adams, MS
405 Hartley, TX	413 Jefferson, TX	425 Burnet, TX	435 Franklin, MS
405 Hutchinson, TX	413 Newton, TX	425 Lee, TX	435 Jefferson, MS
405 Moore, TX	413 Orange, TX	425 Llano, TX	436 Atoka, OK
405 Ochiltree, TX	413 Tyler, TX	425 Travis, TX	436 Bryan, OK
405 Oldham, TX	414 Craig, OK	425 Williamson, TX	436 Fannin, TX
405 Potter, TX	414 Creek, OK	426 Coke, TX	436 Grayson, TX
405 Randall, TX	414 Mayes, OK	426 Concho, TX	437 Aransas, TX
405 Sherman, TX	414 Ottawa, OK	426 Crockett, TX	437 Brooks, TX
405 Swisher, TX	414 Rogers, OK	426 Irion, TX	437 Duval, TX
406 Bailey, TX	414 Tulsa, OK	426 McCulloch, TX	437 Jim Wells, TX
406 Borden, TX	415 Culberson, TX	426 Menard, TX	437 Kenedy, TX
406 Cochran, TX	415 El Paso, TX	426 Reagan, TX	437 Kleberg, TX
406 Crosby, TX	415 Hudspeth, TX	426 Runnels, TX	437 Live Oak, TX
406 Dawson, TX	415 Loving, TX	426 Schleicher, TX	437 Nueces, TX
406 Dickens, TX	416 Bossier, LA	426 Sterling, TX	437 San Patricio, TX
406 Garza, TX	416 Caddo, LA	426 Sutton, TX	438 Choctaw, OK
406 Hockley, TX	416 DeSoto, LA	426 Tom Green, TX	438 Delta, TX
406 King, TX	416 Natchitoches, LA	427 Hidalgo, TX	438 Lamar, TX
406 Lamb, TX	416 Red River, LA	427 Starr, TX	438 Red River, TX
406 Lubbock, TX	416 Sabine, LA	428 Callahan, TX	439 Bienville, LA
406 Lynn, TX	416 Webster, LA	428 Eastland, TX	439 Jackson, LA
406 Motley, TX	417 Canadian, OK	428 Haskell, TX	439 Lincoln, LA
407 Baxter, AR	417 Lincoln, OK	428 Jones, TX	439 Union, LA
407 Marion, AR	417 Logan, OK	428 Kent, TX	440 Beckham, OK
408 Austin, TX	417 Oklahoma, OK	428 Shackelford, TX	440 Roger Mills, OK
408 Chambers, TX	417 Pottawatomie, OK	428 Stephens, TX	441 Henderson, TX
408 Fort Bend, TX	418 Chickasaw, MS	428 Stonewall, TX	441 Smith, TX
408 Harris, TX	418 Itawamba, MS	428 Taylor, TX	441 Van Zandt, TX
408 Liberty, TX	418 Lee, MS	429 Alfalfa, OK	441 Wood, TX
408 Montgomery, TX	418 Monroe, MS	429 Blaine, OK	442 Pope, AR
408 San Jacinto, TX	418 Prentiss, MS	429 Garfield, OK	442 Yell, AR
408 Waller, TX	419 Ascension, LA	429 Grant, OK	443 Caldwell, LA
409 Covington, MS	419 East Baton Rouge, LA	429 Kingfisher, OK	443 East Carroll, LA
409 Forrest, MS	419 East Feliciana, LA	429 Major, OK	443 Franklin, LA
409 Greene, MS	419 Iberville, LA	429 Woods, OK	443 Morehouse, LA
409 Lamar, MS	419 Livingston, LA	430 Cleveland, OK	443 Ouachita, LA
409 Perry, MS	419 Pointe Coupee, LA	430 Garvin, OK	443 Richland, LA
410 Atascosa, TX	419 West Baton Rouge, LA	430 McClain, OK	443 West Carroll, LA
410 Bandera, TX	419 West Feliciana, LA	430 Murray, OK	444 Crane, TX
410 Bexar, TX	420 Archer, TX	431 Madison, LA	444 Ector, TX
410 Frio, TX	420 Baylor, TX	431 Claiborne, MS	444 Reeves, TX
410 Gonzales, TX	420 Clay, TX	431 Warren, MS	444 Ward, TX
410 Guadalupe, TX	420 Knox, TX	432 Conway, AR	444 Winkler, TX
410 Kendall, TX	420 Montague, TX	432 Faulkner, AR	445 Adair, OK
410 LaSalle, TX	420 Throckmorton, TX	432 Grant, AR	445 Cherokee, OK
410 McMullen, TX	420 Wichita, TX	432 Lonoke, AR	445 McIntosh, OK

Appendix B: Health Service Area Definitions

Table B-2: Numeric List of Health Service Areas

445 Muskogee, OK	461 Lamar, AL	478 Pontotoc, OK	500 Pearl River, MS
445 Wagoner, OK	461 Clay, MS	478 Seminole, OK	501 Leon, TX
446 Benton, AR	461 Lowndes, MS	479 Jack, TX	501 Madison, TX
446 Madison, AR	461 Noxubee, MS	479 Palo Pinto, TX	502 Carroll, MS
446 Washington, AR	462 Bosque, TX	480 Ashley, AR	502 Grenada, MS
446 Delaware, OK	462 Falls, TX	480 Chicot, AR	502 Montgomery, MS
447 Nacogdoches, TX	462 Hamilton, TX	481 Castro, TX	503 Fisher, TX
447 Sabine, TX	462 Hill, TX	481 Floyd, TX	503 Mitchell, TX
447 San Augustine, TX	462 Limestone, TX	481 Hale, TX	503 Nolan, TX
447 Shelby, TX	462 McLennan, TX	482 Pontotoc, MS	504 Jefferson Davis, MS
448 Clark, AR	463 Evangeline, LA	482 Tippah, MS	504 Lawrence, MS
448 Garland, AR	463 St. Landry, LA	482 Union, MS	505 Brazoria, TX
448 Hot Spring, AR	464 Brazos, TX	483 Greer, OK	505 Matagorda, TX
448 Montgomery, AR	464 Burleson, TX	483 Harmon, OK	505 Wharton, TX
448 Pike, AR	464 Grimes, TX	483 Jackson, OK	506 Blanco, TX
449 Angelina, TX	464 Robertson, TX	484 Choctaw, MS	506 Edwards, TX
449 Polk, TX	464 Washington, TX	484 Oktibbeha, MS	506 Gillespie, TX
449 Trinity, TX	465 Camp, TX	484 Webster, MS	506 Kerr, TX
449 Walker, TX	465 Franklin, TX	484 Winston, MS	506 Kimble, TX
450 Allen, LA	465 Morris, TX	485 Cass, TX	506 Mason, TX
450 Avoyelles, LA	465 Titus, TX	485 Harrison, TX	506 Real, TX
450 Catahoula, LA	466 Latimer, OK	485 Marion, TX	507 Comanche, TX
450 Grant, LA	466 Pittsburg, OK	486 Calhoun, AR	507 Erath, TX
450 LaSalle, LA	466 Pushmataha, OK	486 Columbia, AR	508 Lea, NM
450 Rapides, LA	467 Assumption, LA	486 Union, AR	508 Andrews, TX
451 Chautauqua, KS	467 Lafourche, LA	487 Bolivar, MS	508 Gaines, TX
451 Elk, KS	467 Terrebonne, LA	487 Humphreys, MS	509 Anderson, TX
451 Montgomery, KS	468 Brown, TX	487 Leflore, MS	509 Cherokee, TX
451 Nowata, OK	468 Coleman, TX	487 Sunflower, MS	509 Houston, TX
451 Washington, OK	468 Mills, TX	488 Issaquena, MS	510 Caldwell, TX
452 Bell, TX	468 San Saba, TX	488 Sharkey, MS	510 Hays, TX
452 Coryell, TX	469 Dewey, OK	488 Washington, MS	511 Copiah, MS
452 Lampasas, TX	469 Ellis, OK	489 Freestone, TX	511 Lincoln, MS
452 Milam, TX	469 Harper, OK	489 Navarro, TX	512 Childress, TX
453 Collin, TX	469 Woodward, OK	490 Colorado, TX	512 Cottle, TX
453 Dallas, TX	469 Lipscomb, TX	490 Fayette, TX	512 Hall, TX
453 Ellis, TX	470 Beauregard, LA	491 Deaf Smith, TX	513 Bee, TX
453 Hopkins, TX	470 Calcasieu, LA	491 Parmer, TX	513 Karnes, TX
453 Hunt, TX	470 Cameron, LA	492 Martin, TX	514 Terry, TX
453 Kaufman, TX	470 Jefferson Davis, LA	492 Midland, TX	514 Yoakum, TX
453 Rains, TX	470 Vernon, LA	492 Pecos, TX	515 Kay, OK
453 Rockwall, TX	471 George, MS	492 Terrell, TX	515 Osage, OK
454 Gregg, TX	471 Jackson, MS	492 Upton, TX	516 Kinney, TX
454 Panola, TX	472 Noble, OK	493 Comanche, OK	516 Maverick, TX
454 Rusk, TX	472 Pawnee, OK	493 Cotton, OK	516 Val Verde, TX
454 Upshur, TX	472 Payne, OK	493 Kiowa, OK	517 Comal, TX
455 Jasper, MS	473 Bradley, AR	493 Tillman, OK	518 Glasscock, TX
455 Jones, MS	473 Cleveland, AR	494 Boone, AR	518 Howard, TX
455 Smith, MS	473 Desha, AR	494 Carroll, AR	519 Scurry, TX
455 Wayne, MS	473 Drew, AR	494 Newton, AR	520 Cameron, TX
456 Hancock, MS	473 Jefferson, AR	494 Searcy, AR	520 Willacy, TX
456 Harrison, MS	473 Lincoln, AR	495 Cooke, TX	521 Jackson, AR
456 Stone, MS	474 Carter, OK	495 Denton, TX	522 Johnson, AR
457 Cleburne, AR	474 Johnston, OK	495 Wise, TX	523 Claiborne, LA
457 White, AR	474 Love, OK	496 Dallas, AR	524 Collingsworth, TX
457 Woodruff, AR	474 Marshall, OK	496 Ouachita, AR	525 Wilkinson, MS
458 Foard, TX	475 Custer, OK	497 Jefferson, OK	526 Brewster, TX
458 Hardeman, TX	475 Washita, OK	497 Stephens, OK	526 Jeff Davis, TX
458 Wilbarger, TX	476 Caddo, OK	498 Alcorn, MS	526 Presidio, TX
459 Calhoun, MS	476 Grady, OK	498 Tishomingo, MS	527 Arkansas, AR
459 Lafayette, MS	477 Amite, MS	499 Crittenden, AR	527 Monroe, AR
459 Yalobusha, MS	477 Marion, MS	499 Cross, AR	528 St. Mary, LA
460 Gray, TX	477 Pike, MS	499 Lee, AR	529 Okfuskee, OK
460 Hemphill, TX	477 Walthall, MS	499 St. Francis, AR	529 Okmulgee, OK
460 Roberts, TX	478 Coal, OK	500 St. Tammany, LA	530 Winn, LA
460 Wheeler, TX	478 Hughes, OK	500 Washington, LA	531 Dimmit, TX

Table B-2: Numeric List of Health Service Areas

532 Galveston, TX	545 Louisa, IA	552 Olmsted, MN	563 Pulaski, IL
533 Yazoo, MS	545 Washington, IA	552 Steele, MN	563 Union, IL
534 Polk, AR	546 Adair, IA	552 Wabasha, MN	563 Bollinger, MO
535 Beaver, OK	546 Clarke, IA	552 Winona, MN	563 Butler, MO
536 Uvalde, TX	546 Dallas, IA	553 Boone, MO	563 Cape Girardeau, MO
537 Phillips, AR	546 Decatur, IA	553 Chariton, MO	563 Carter, MO
538 Jim Hogg, TX	546 Jasper, IA	553 Cooper, MO	563 Mississippi, MO
538 Webb, TX	546 Madison, IA	553 Howard, MO	563 New Madrid, MO
538 Zapata, TX	546 Marion, IA	553 Macon, MO	563 Perry, MO
539 Cherokee, KS	546 Polk, IA	553 Randolph, MO	563 Ripley, MO
539 Barton, MO	546 Ringgold, IA	553 Shelby, MO	563 Scott, MO
539 Jasper, MO	546 Union, IA	554 Brown, KS	563 Stoddard, MO
539 McDonald, MO	546 Warren, IA	554 Jackson, KS	563 Wayne, MO
539 Newton, MO	547 Becker, MN	554 Jefferson, KS	564 Adams, NE
540 Anoka, MN	547 Clay, MN	554 Nemaha, KS	564 Clay, NE
540 Carver, MN	547 Mahnomen, MN	554 Osage, KS	564 Nuckolls, NE
540 Hennepin, MN	547 Norman, MN	554 Pottawatomie, KS	564 Webster, NE
540 Le Sueur, MN	547 Wilkin, MN	554 Riley, KS	565 Ellis, KS
540 McLeod, MN	547 Barnes, ND	554 Shawnee, KS	565 Gove, KS
540 Scott, MN	547 Cass, ND	554 Wabaunsee, KS	565 Graham, KS
540 Sherburne, MN	547 Griggs, ND	555 Greeley, NE	565 Logan, KS
540 Sibley, MN	547 Ransom, ND	555 Hall, NE	565 Rooks, KS
540 Wright, MN	547 Richland, ND	555 Hamilton, NE	565 Trego, KS
541 Franklin, MO	547 Sargent, ND	555 Howard, NE	566 Adair, MO
541 Iron, MO	547 Steele, ND	555 Merrick, NE	566 Knox, MO
541 Jefferson, MO	547 Traill, ND	556 Cerro Gordo, IA	566 Putnam, MO
541 St. Francois, MO	548 Caldwell, MO	556 Franklin, IA	566 Schuyler, MO
541 St. Genevieve, MO	548 Cass, MO	556 Hancock, IA	566 Scotland, MO
541 St. Louis, MO	548 Clay, MO	556 Kossuth, IA	566 Sullivan, MO
541 St. Louis City, MO	548 Clinton, MO	556 Winnebago, IA	567 Chase, KS
541 Washington, MO	548 Daviess, MO	556 Worth, IA	567 Coffey, KS
542 Burt, NE	548 Jackson, MO	557 Black Hawk, IA	567 Greenwood, KS
542 Cass, NE	548 Johnson, MO	557 Bremer, IA	567 Lyon, KS
542 Colfax, NE	548 Lafayette, MO	557 Buchanan, IA	568 Clark, SD
542 Cuming, NE	548 Platte, MO	557 Butler, IA	568 Codington, SD
542 Dodge, NE	548 Ray, MO	557 Fayette, IA	568 Deuel, SD
542 Douglas, NE	549 Barry, MO	557 Grundy, IA	568 Grant, SD
542 Sarpy, NE	549 Christian, MO	558 Butte, SD	568 Hamlin, SD
542 Saunders, NE	549 Dade, MO	558 Custer, SD	569 Ellsworth, KS
542 Washington, NE	549 Dallas, MO	558 Fall River, SD	569 Lincoln, KS
543 Burleigh, ND	549 Douglas, MO	558 Jackson, SD	569 Ottawa, KS
543 Emmons, ND	549 Greene, MO	558 Meade, SD	569 Saline, KS
543 Kidder, ND	549 Hickory, MO	558 Pennington, SD	570 Buffalo, NE
543 McLean, ND	549 Laclede, MO	559 Brown, NE	570 Dawson, NE
543 Mercer, ND	549 Lawrence, MO	559 Holt, NE	570 Franklin, NE
543 Morton, ND	549 Ozark, MO	559 Keya Paha, NE	570 Frontier, NE
543 Oliver, ND	549 Polk, MO	559 Rock, NE	570 Gosper, NE
543 Sheridan, ND	549 Stone, MO	560 Buena Vista, IA	570 Kearney, NE
543 Sioux, ND	549 Texas, MO	560 Cherokee, IA	570 Sherman, NE
544 Lyon, IA	549 Webster, MO	560 Ida, IA	571 Clay, AR
544 Pipestone, MN	549 Wright, MO	560 Monona, IA	571 Craighead, AR
544 Rock, MN	550 Bottineau, ND	560 Plymouth, IA	571 Greene, AR
544 Lake, SD	550 Burke, ND	560 Woodbury, IA	571 Lawrence, AR
544 Lincoln, SD	550 McHenry, ND	560 Dakota, NE	571 Poinsett, AR
544 McCook, SD	550 Mountrail, ND	560 Dixon, NE	571 Randolph, AR
544 Miner, SD	550 Renville, ND	560 Thurston, NE	571 Dunklin, MO
544 Minnehaha, SD	550 Ward, ND	561 Butler, NE	572 Brown, SD
544 Moody, SD	551 Clark, KS	561 Gage, NE	572 Day, SD
544 Turner, SD	551 Ford, KS	561 Jefferson, NE	572 Edmunds, SD
544 Union, SD	551 Gray, KS	561 Lancaster, NE	572 Faulk, SD
545 Benton, IA	551 Hodgeman, KS	561 Saline, NE	572 Marshall, SD
545 Cedar, IA	551 Meade, KS	561 Seward, NE	572 McPherson, SD
545 Iowa, IA	552 Howard, IA	562 Baca, CO	572 Spink, SD
545 Johnson, IA	552 Dodge, MN	562 Grant, KS	573 Blue Earth, MN
545 Jones, IA	552 Fillmore, MN	562 Stanton, KS	573 Nicollet, MN
545 Linn, IA	552 Mower, MN	563 Alexander, IL	573 Waseca, MN

TABLE B-2: NUMERIC LIST OF HEALTH SERVICE AREAS

573 Watonwan, MN	585 Pocahontas, IA	599 Warren, MO	618 Kiowa, KS
574 Fulton, AR	585 Webster, IA	600 Beadle, SD	618 Pratt, KS
574 Independence, AR	586 Lawrence, SD	600 Hand, SD	619 Cottonwood, MN
574 Izard, AR	586 Campbell, WY	600 Hyde, SD	619 Jackson, MN
574 Sharp, AR	586 Crook, WY	600 Jerauld, SD	619 Murray, MN
574 Stone, AR	587 Morton, KS	601 Allen, KS	619 Nobles, MN
574 Howell, MO	587 Seward, KS	601 Labette, KS	621 Leavenworth, KS
574 Oregon, MO	587 Cimarron, OK	601 Neosho, KS	621 Wyandotte, KS
574 Shannon, MO	587 Texas, OK	601 Woodson, KS	622 Jewell, KS
575 Finney, KS	588 Benton, MN	602 Brown, MN	622 Mitchell, KS
575 Hamilton, KS	588 Meeker, MN	602 Redwood, MN	622 Osborne, KS
575 Haskell, KS	588 Stearns, MN	602 Renville, MN	623 Dawes, NE
575 Kearny, KS	589 Jefferson, IA	603 Isanti, MN	623 Sheridan, NE
575 Lane, KS	589 Keokuk, IA	603 Kanabec, MN	623 Sioux, NE
575 Scott, KS	589 Mahaska, IA	603 Mille Lacs, MN	623 Bennett, SD
576 Butler, KS	589 Monroe, IA	604 Kittson, MN	623 Shannon, SD
576 Cowley, KS	589 Van Buren, IA	604 Marshall, MN	624 Anderson, KS
576 Harvey, KS	589 Wapello, IA	604 Pennington, MN	624 Douglas, KS
576 Marion, KS	590 Big Stone, MN	604 Red Lake, MN	624 Franklin, KS
576 Sedgwick, KS	590 Traverse, MN	605 Billings, ND	624 Johnson, KS
576 Sumner, KS	590 Roberts, SD	605 Dunn, ND	624 Miami, KS
577 Antelope, NE	591 Doniphan, KS	605 Golden Valley, ND	625 Clay, IA
577 Madison, NE	591 Andrew, MO	605 Stark, ND	625 Dickinson, IA
577 Pierce, NE	591 Buchanan, MO	606 Boone, IA	625 Palo Alto, IA
577 Stanton, NE	591 DeKalb, MO	606 Hamilton, IA	626 Emmet, IA
577 Wayne, NE	591 Gentry, MO	606 Hardin, IA	626 Martin, MN
578 Cedar, NE	591 Harrison, MO	606 Story, IA	627 Dent, MO
578 Knox, NE	591 Nodaway, MO	606 Wright, IA	627 Phelps, MO
578 Bon Homme, SD	591 Worth, MO	607 Bates, MO	627 Pulaski, MO
578 Clay, SD	592 Chippewa, MN	607 Henry, MO	627 Reynolds, MO
578 Hutchinson, SD	592 Kandiyohi, MN	607 St. Clair, MO	628 Pawnee, NE
578 Yankton, SD	592 Lac Qui Parle, MN	608 Douglas, MN	628 Richardson, NE
579 Divide, ND	592 Swift, MN	608 Pope, MN	629 Haakon, SD
579 McKenzie, ND	592 Yellow Medicine, MN	608 Stevens, MN	629 Hughes, SD
579 Williams, ND	593 Arthur, NE	609 Lincoln, MN	629 Jones, SD
580 Morrison, MN	593 Hooker, NE	609 Lyon, MN	629 Stanley, SD
580 Todd, MN	593 Keith, NE	610 Brookings, SD	629 Sully, SD
580 Banner, NE	593 Lincoln, NE	610 Kingsbury, SD	629 Ziebach, SD
580 Box Butte, NE	593 McPherson, NE	611 Polk, NE	630 Bourbon, KS
580 Garden, NE	593 Perkins, NE	611 York, NE	630 Crawford, KS
580 Grant, NE	594 Blaine, NE	612 Aitkin, MN	630 Linn, KS
580 Morrill, NE	594 Custer, NE	612 Cass, MN	631 Lake of the Woods, MN
580 Scotts Bluff, NE	594 Garfield, NE	612 Crow Wing, MN	631 Roseau, MN
580 Goshen, WY	594 Logan, NE	612 Hubbard, MN	632 Foster, ND
580 Niobrara, WY	594 Loup, NE	612 Wadena, MN	632 Stutsman, ND
581 Callaway, MO	594 Thomas, NE	613 Decatur, KS	632 Wells, ND
581 Cole, MO	594 Valley, NE	613 Sheridan, KS	633 Calhoun, IA
581 Crawford, MO	594 Wheeler, NE	613 Hitchcock, NE	633 Carroll, IA
581 Gasconade, MO	595 Boyd, NE	613 Red Willow, NE	633 Sac, IA
581 Maries, MO	595 Gregory, SD	614 Mississippi, AR	634 Chickasaw, IA
581 Miller, MO	595 Mellette, SD	614 Pemiscot, MO	634 Floyd, IA
581 Moniteau, MO	595 Todd, SD	615 Aurora, SD	635 Marshall, KS
581 Osage, MO	595 Tripp, SD	615 Brule, SD	635 Washington, KS
582 Grant, MN	596 Audubon, IA	615 Buffalo, SD	636 Cheyenne, KS
582 Otter Tail, MN	596 Cass, IA	615 Charles Mix, SD	636 Rawlins, KS
583 Barton, KS	596 Harrison, IA	615 Davison, SD	637 Norton, KS
583 Edwards, KS	596 Mills, IA	615 Douglas, SD	637 Phillips, KS
583 Pawnee, KS	596 Pottawattamie, IA	615 Hanson, SD	637 Smith, KS
583 Rush, KS	596 Shelby, IA	615 Lyman, SD	638 Pierce, ND
584 Polk, MN	597 Beltrami, MN	615 Sanborn, SD	638 Rolette, ND
584 Cavalier, ND	597 Clearwater, MN	616 Furnas, NE	638 Towner, ND
584 Grand Forks, ND	598 Reno, KS	616 Harlan, NE	639 Cedar, MO
584 Nelson, ND	598 Rice, KS	616 Phelps, NE	639 Vernon, MO
584 Pembina, ND	598 Stafford, KS	617 Greene, IA	640 Adams, ND
584 Walsh, ND	599 Lincoln, MO	617 Guthrie, IA	640 Bowman, ND
585 Humboldt, IA	599 St. Charles, MO	618 Comanche, KS	640 Hettinger, ND

Table B-2: Numeric List of Health Service Areas

640 Slope, ND	672 Sioux, IA	694 Nez Perce, ID	708 Salt Lake, UT
640 Harding, SD	673 Linn, MO	694 Asotin, WA	708 Summit, UT
640 Perkins, SD	674 Mcpherson, KS	694 Garfield, WA	708 Tooele, UT
641 Muscatine, IA	675 Wilson, KS	695 Gooding, ID	708 Uintah, UT
641 Scott, IA	676 Taney, MO	695 Jerome, ID	708 Wasatch, UT
642 Cloud, KS	678 Atchison, MO	695 Lincoln, ID	709 Eldorado, CA
642 Republic, KS	678 Holt, MO	695 Twin Falls, ID	709 Placer, CA
643 Greeley, KS	679 Marshall, IA	696 Bannock, ID	709 Sacramento, CA
643 Wichita, KS	679 Tama, IA	696 Bingham, ID	709 Yolo, CA
644 Fremont, IA	680 Dickey, ND	696 Caribou, ID	710 Modoc, CA
644 Page, IA	680 LaMoure, ND	696 Oneida, ID	710 Shasta, CA
644 Taylor, IA	681 Crawford, IA	696 Power, ID	710 Trinity, CA
645 Lucas, IA	682 Ness, KS	697 Butte, CA	711 Eagle, CO
645 Wayne, IA	683 Grundy, MO	697 Glenn, CA	711 Garfield, CO
646 Faribault, MN	683 Mercer, MO	697 Tehama, CA	711 Mesa, CO
646 Freeborn, MN	684 Logan, ND	698 Adams, WA	711 Pitkin, CO
647 Adams, IA	684 McIntosh, ND	698 Ferry, WA	711 Rio Blanco, CO
647 Montgomery, IA	685 Camden, MO	698 Lincoln, WA	711 Grand, UT
648 Campbell, SD	686 Poweshiek, IA	698 Pend Oreille, WA	712 Blaine, MT
648 Corson, SD	687 Nemaha, NE	698 Spokane, WA	712 Hill, MT
648 Dewey, SD	688 Adams, CO	698 Stevens, WA	712 Liberty, MT
648 Potter, SD	688 Arapahoe, CO	699 Coconino, AZ	712 Phillips, MT
648 Walworth, SD	688 Clear Creek, CO	699 Gila, AZ	713 Granite, MT
649 Appanoose, IA	688 Denver, CO	699 Maricopa, AZ	713 Lake, MT
649 Davis, IA	688 Douglas, CO	699 Pinal, AZ	713 Mineral, MT
650 Dickinson, KS	688 Elbert, CO	699 Yavapai, AZ	713 Missoula, MT
650 Geary, KS	688 Gilpin, CO	700 Cochise, AZ	713 Ravalli, MT
650 Morris, KS	688 Grand, CO	700 Graham, AZ	713 Sanders, MT
651 Boone, NE	688 Jefferson, CO	700 Greenlee, AZ	714 Carter, MT
651 Nance, NE	688 Park, CO	700 Pima, AZ	714 Custer, MT
651 Platte, NE	688 Summit, CO	700 Santa Cruz, AZ	714 Fallon, MT
652 Obrien, IA	689 Clackamas, OR	701 Alpine, CA	714 Garfield, MT
652 Osceola, IA	689 Clatsop, OR	701 Carson City, NV	714 Powder River, MT
654 Chase, NE	689 Columbia, OR	701 Churchill, NV	714 Prairie, MT
654 Dundy, NE	689 Multnomah, OR	701 Douglas, NV	715 Bear Lake, ID
654 Hayes, NE	689 Washington, OR	701 Humboldt, NV	715 Franklin, ID
655 Benson, ND	689 Clark, WA	701 Lyon, NV	715 Cache, UT
655 Eddy, ND	689 Cowlitz, WA	701 Mineral, NV	716 Ada, ID
655 Ramsey, ND	689 Wahkiakum, WA	701 Ormsby, NV	716 Boise, ID
656 Benton, MO	690 Colusa, CA	701 Pershing, NV	716 Canyon, ID
656 Morgan, MO	690 Sutter, CA	701 Storey, NV	716 Elmore, ID
656 Pettis, MO	690 Yuba, CA	701 Washoe, NV	716 Gem, ID
656 Saline, MO	691 Big Horn, MT	702 Benton, WA	716 Owyhee, ID
657 Carroll, MO	691 Carbon, MT	702 Franklin, WA	716 Valley, ID
657 Livingston, MO	691 Golden Valley, MT	703 Juab, UT	717 Morrow, OR
658 Fillmore, NE	691 Musselshell, MT	703 Millard, UT	717 Umatilla, OR
658 Thayer, NE	691 Rosebud, MT	703 Sanpete, UT	717 Columbia, WA
659 Sherman, KS	691 Stillwater, MT	703 Sevier, UT	717 Walla Walla, WA
659 Thomas, KS	691 Treasure, MT	703 Utah, UT	718 Fresno, CA
659 Wallace, KS	691 Yellowstone, MT	703 Wayne, UT	718 Kings, CA
660 Johnson, NE	691 Yellowstone Park, MT	704 Huerfano, CO	718 Madera, CA
660 Otoe, NE	692 Cascade, MT	704 Las Animas, CO	719 Crook, OR
661 Harper, KS	692 Chouteau, MT	704 Pueblo, CO	719 Deschutes, OR
661 Kingman, KS	692 Glacier, MT	704 Colfax, NM	719 Harney, OR
662 Clay, KS	692 Judith Basin, MT	705 Marion, OR	719 Jefferson, OR
663 Madison, MO	692 Pondera, MT	705 Polk, OR	719 Wheeler, OR
664 Stevens, KS	692 Teton, MT	705 Yamhill, OR	720 Elko, NV
665 Mitchell, IA	692 Toole, MT	707 Clark, NV	720 Eureka, NV
666 Audrain, MO	693 Bernalillo, NM	707 Esmeralda, NV	720 Lander, NV
666 Monroe, MO	693 Sandoval, NM	707 Lincoln, NV	721 Broadwater, MT
666 Montgomery, MO	693 Socorro, NM	707 Nye, NV	721 Jefferson, MT
667 Russell, KS	693 Torrance, NM	707 Garfield, UT	721 Lewis and Clark, MT
668 Cherry, NE	693 Valencia, NM	707 Kane, UT	722 Bonneville, ID
669 Barber, KS	694 Clearwater, ID	707 Piute, UT	722 Butte, ID
670 Grant, ND	694 Idaho, ID	707 Washington, UT	722 Clark, ID
671 Atchison, KS	694 Lewis, ID	708 Duchesne, UT	722 Custer, ID

Appendix B: Health Service Area Definitions **259**

Table B-2: Numeric List of Health Service Areas

722 Fremont, ID	740 San Juan, UT	760 Washington, CO	793 Catron, NM
722 Jefferson, ID	741 Cheyenne, NE	760 Weld, CO	793 Grant, NM
722 Madison, ID	741 Deuel, NE	760 Yuma, CO	793 Hidalgo, NM
722 Teton, ID	741 Kimball, NE	761 Delta, CO	794 Pierce, WA
723 Los Angeles, CA	741 Laramie, WY	761 Gunnison, CO	795 Boulder, CO
723 Orange, CA	742 Beaverhead, MT	761 Hinsdale, CO	796 Larimer, CO
724 Los Alamos, NM	742 Deer Lodge, MT	761 Montrose, CO	797 Platte, WY
724 Rio Arriba, NM	742 Silver Bow, MT	761 Ouray, CO	799 Daggett, UT
724 Santa Fe, NM	743 Klamath, OR	761 San Miguel, CO	799 Sweetwater, WY
724 Taos, NM	743 Lake, OR	763 Logan, CO	800 Humboldt, CA
725 Curry, NM	744 Box Elder, UT	763 Phillips, CO	801 Cibola, NM
725 De Baca, NM	744 Davis, UT	763 Sedgwick, CO	801 Guadalupe, NM
725 Quay, NM	744 Morgan, UT	764 Marin, CA	801 Harding, NM
725 Roosevelt, NM	744 Rich, UT	764 Sonoma, CA	801 Mora, NM
726 Converse, WY	744 Weber, UT	765 Apache, AZ	801 San Miguel, NM
726 Natrona, WY	745 Bent, CO	765 McKinley, NM	802 Santa Cruz, CA
727 Benton, OR	745 Crowley, CO	766 Alameda, CA	803 Mohave, AZ
727 Linn, OR	745 Kiowa, CO	766 Contra Costa, CA	804 Weston, WY
728 Flathead, MT	745 Otero, CO	767 Dawson, MT	805 White Pine, NV
728 Lincoln, MT	745 Prowers, CO	767 McCone, MT	806 Grant, OR
729 Adams, ID	746 Lake, CA	767 Richland, MT	807 Kern, CA
729 Payette, ID	746 Napa, CA	767 Wibaux, MT	808 Blaine, ID
729 Washington, ID	746 Solano, CA	768 Riverside, CA	808 Camas, ID
729 Malheur, OR	747 Chelan, WA	768 San Bernardino, CA	809 Carbon, UT
730 Cassia, ID	747 Douglas, WA	769 Lincoln, NM	809 Emery, UT
730 Minidoka, ID	747 Grant, WA	769 Otero, NM	810 Fergus, MT
731 Alamosa, CO	747 Okanogan, WA	770 Johnson, WY	810 Petroleum, MT
731 Conejos, CO	748 Gilliam, OR	770 Sheridan, WY	811 Mendocino, CA
731 Costilla, CO	748 Hood River, OR	771 Jackson, CO	812 Custer, CO
731 Mineral, CO	748 Sherman, OR	771 Albany, WY	812 Fremont, CO
731 Rio Grande, CO	748 Wasco, OR	771 Carbon, WY	813 Lemhi, ID
731 Saguache, CO	748 Klickitat, WA	772 Chaves, NM	814 Union, NM
732 Dona Ana, NM	748 Skamania, WA	772 Eddy, NM	815 Whatcom, WA
732 Luna, NM	749 Big Horn, WY	773 Gallatin, MT	816 Inyo, CA
732 Sierra, NM	749 Park, WY	773 Madison, MT	816 Mono, CA
733 Daniels, MT	750 Amador, CA	774 Imperial, CA	817 Ketchikan Gateway, AK
733 Sheridan, MT	750 Calaveras, CA	774 San Diego, CA	817 Outer Ketchikan, AK
734 Benewah, ID	750 San Joaquin, CA	775 Lincoln, WY	817 Prince of Wales, AK
734 Bonner, ID	751 Monterey, CA	775 Sublette, WY	817 Wrangell-Petersburg, AK
734 Boundary, ID	751 San Benito, CA	775 Teton, WY	818 Angoon, AK
734 Kootenai, ID	751 Santa Clara, CA	777 Fremont, WY	818 Haines, AK
734 Shoshone, ID	752 Siskiyou, CA	777 Hot Springs, WY	818 Juneau, AK
735 Moffat, CO	752 Jackson, OR	777 Washakie, WY	818 Sitka, AK
735 Routt, CO	752 Josephine, OR	778 Meagher, MT	818 Skagway-Yakutat, AK
736 Island, WA	753 Nevada, CA	778 Wheatland, MT	819 Fairbanks North Star, AK
736 King, WA	753 Sierra, CA	779 Roosevelt, MT	819 Southeast Fairbanks, AK
736 Kitsap, WA	754 Cheyenne, CO	779 Valley, MT	819 Upper Yukon, AK
736 San Juan, WA	754 El Paso, CO	780 Lassen, CA	819 Yukon-Koyukuk, AK
736 Skagit, WA	754 Kit Carson, CO	780 Plumas, CA	820 Aleutian Islands, AK
736 Snohomish, WA	754 Lincoln, CO	781 San Luis Obispo, CA	820 Anchorage, AK
737 Mariposa, CA	754 Teller, CO	781 Santa Barbara, CA	820 Barrow-North Slope, AK
737 Merced, CA	755 Beaver, UT	782 Douglas, OR	820 Bethel, AK
737 Stanislaus, CA	755 Iron, UT	782 Lane, OR	820 Bristol Bay, AK
737 Tuolumne, CA	756 Park, MT	783 Lincoln, OR	820 Bristol Bay Borough, AK
738 Del Norte, CA	756 Sweet Grass, MT	783 Tillamook, OR	820 Kenai-Cook Inlet, AK
738 Coos, OR	757 San Francisco, CA	784 Latah, ID	820 Kodiak Island, AK
738 Curry, OR	757 San Mateo, CA	784 Whitman, WA	820 Matanuska-Susitna, AK
739 Kittitas, WA	758 Grays Harbor, WA	785 Clallam, WA	820 Nome, AK
739 Yakima, WA	758 Lewis, WA	785 Jefferson, WA	820 Valdez-Chitina-Whittier, AK
740 Navajo, AZ	758 Mason, WA	786 Chaffee, CO	820 Wade Hampton, AK
740 Archuleta, CO	758 Pacific, WA	786 Lake, CO	821 Honolulu, HI
740 Dolores, CO	758 Thurston, WA	787 Yuma, AZ	821 Kalawao, HI
740 La Plata, CO	759 Baker, OR	788 Powell, MT	821 Maui, HI
740 Montezuma, CO	759 Union, OR	789 Tulare, CA	822 Kauai, HI
740 San Juan, CO	759 Wallowa, OR	790 Ventura, CA	823 Hawaii, HI
740 San Juan, NM	760 Morgan, CO	792 Uinta, WY	